# SOCIAL DETERMINANTS
## OF HEALTH

# SOCIAL DETERMINANTS
# OF HEALTH

## CANADIAN PERSPECTIVES

Editor:
Dennis Raphael

Canadian Scholars' Press Inc.
Toronto

**Social Determinants of Health: Canadian Perspectives**
Edited by Dennis Raphael

First published in 2004 by
**Canadian Scholars' Press Inc.**
180 Bloor Street West, Suite 801
Toronto, Ontario
M5S 2V6

**www.cspi.org**

Canadian Scholars' Press gratefully acknowledges financial support for our publishing activities from the Government of Canada through the Book Publishing Industry Development Program (BPIDP).

**Library and Archives Canada Cataloguing in Publication**

Social determinants of health : Canadian perspectives / editor: Dennis Raphael.

This volume contains extended and refined contributions from the conference Social Determinants of Health Across the Life Span, held at York University in Toronto November 2002.

Includes bibliographical references and index.
ISBN 1-55130-237-3

1. Public health—Social aspects—Canada—Congresses. I. Raphael, Dennis II. Social Determinants of Health Across the Life Span
(2002 : York University, Toronto, Ont.)

RA418.S63 2004          362.1          C2004-902880-4

Cover photo: *Children, Toronto, Canada*. Copyright Patrick Corrigan.
Cover design by Zack Taylor, www.zacktaylor.com
Page design and layout by Brad Horning

04 05 06 07 08 5 4 3 2

Printed and bound in Canada by AGMV Marquis Imprimeur Inc.

Canada

# TABLE OF CONTENTS

# FOREWORD

O NE OF THE KEY POINTS that I made in *Building on values: The future of health care in Canada* is that we have to set a national goal of making Canadians the healthiest people possible. One of the keys to achieving this goal is a greater emphasis on preventative health measures and improving population health outcomes.

Although I referenced this in my report, I will be the first to admit that even if all of my 47 recommendations are adopted, and even if they are implemented the way I would want them to be, it will only take us part way toward this goal.

A health care system—even the best health care system in the world—will be only one of the ingredients that determine whether your life will be long or short, healthy or sick, full of fulfillment, or empty with despair.

If we want Canadians to be the healthiest people in the world, we have to connect all of the dots that will take us there. To connect the dots, we have to know where they are. Those who have contributed to this volume have added valuable perspectives in this regard as they connect research and ideas on the social determinants of health to the health outcomes we seek as a nation.

Healthy lifestyle choices may be important and vital—and they are. A comprehensive, responsive and accountable national health care system may be important and vital—and it is.

But the main factors—the main "determinants" as the experts call them—that will likely shape our health and life span are the ones that affect society as a whole. And if we want Canadians to be the healthiest people in the world, we have to deal with them at that level.

The editor of this text, Dr. Raphael, has gathered together some of Canada's important thinkers on the key determinants. This volume provides the latest research and ideas regarding income distribution; the importance of a healthy workplace; the critical role that early childhood education, and public education generally, plays in the lifecycle process; the importance of food and shelter; and the importance of belonging reinforced by various views of social inclusion.

I noted recently that our policy-making and program-developing mechanisms in Canada are suffering from what I call "hardening of the categories." Something useful is proffered by one government department with the intended gains stifled by something counterproductive in another department.

Our policy-making processes need to be integrated and integrating. We need to move from an "illness model" to a "wellness" paradigm that connects the dots of all of the factors that contribute to health for individuals and society at large.

Even if we make great strides to improve our systems of health care in Canada, our genuine gains in health will be hindered unless we pay serious attention to the other determinants of health. At present, there are too many children going to school and to bed hungry, too many people living on our urban streets, an increasing number of working poor, and too many people feeling like they are on the outside looking in when it comes to decision-making in our communities.

How important is it that we think in new ways?

Historians and health experts tell us that we have had two great revolutions in the course of public health. The first was the control of infectious diseases, notwithstanding our current challenges. The second was the battle against non-communicable diseases.

The third great revolution is about moving from an illness model to all of those things that both prevent illness and promote a holistic sense of well-being.

In my view, the wellness model needs to be informed:

- by inspired leaders who genuinely share power with those less fortunate
- by a commitment to social inclusion and Civil Society that provide opportunities for all Canadians to participate in the things that count in our neighborhoods across this great country
- by an understanding that hopelessness kills and hopefulness with opportunity is a prescription for good health

That's my kind of revolution. It's the kind that will ensure that Canadians are the healthiest people we can be. It's also the kind of revolution that understands that the exceptional health we seek, and how we achieve it, can provide a Canadian model for the world to emulate.

*Social Determinants of Health* provides a rich companion to our work on health care and a useful springboard for integrated healthy public policy.

**The Hon. Roy J. Romanow, P.C., O.C., Q.C.**
**Saskatoon**
**February 2004**

# PREFACE

T HIS VOLUME PROVIDES an extensive portrait of the state of various social (societal) determinants of health in Canada. It represents a unique undertaking in the study of health and its social determinants. It has long been known that the roots of health can be found in the organization of society and how resources are distributed among it members; however, scholarship into these determinants of health has generally been limited to those in the health sciences. Those who study social determinants of health such as early childhood education and care, education and literacy, employment and working conditions, food security, health services, housing, income and its distribution, social exclusion, the social safety net, and unemployment and job insecurity have generally not considered these issues as health issues. For them, scholarship into the state and quality of these issues is an all-encompassing activity. They cannot be expected to be responsible for analyses of the health-related effects related to their areas of expertise.

There is a need then, to foster communication between those concerned with the current state of various social determinants of health and those knowledgeable about their health effects. This need is especially great in Canada as a consensus is emerging that the quality of many social determinants of health is deteriorating as a result of policy decisions being driven by various political, economic, and social forces. This recognition led me to apply for funding to the Health Policy Program of Health Canada for a conference entitled *Social determinants of health across the life-span* to take place at York University in Toronto in late November of 2002. The vision of this conference was simple: Invite an authority who would comment on the current state of an important social determinant of health followed by one who would present the health implications of the situation.

Organization of the conference was a collaboration between the School of Health Policy and Management of York University and the Centre for Social Justice in Toronto. Primary funding was provided by Health Canada with supplemental support from the Institute of Population and Public Health of the Canadian Institutes for Health Research (CIHR). Speakers addressed three objectives: (1) consider the state of key social determinants of health across Canada; (2) explore the implications of these conditions for the health of Canadians; and (3) outline policy directions to improve the health of Canadians by influencing the quality of these determinants of health. The immediate outcome of the project was the drafting by conference participants of *The Toronto charter for a healthy Canada* that is contained in this volume as an appendix. Health Canada has provided summary proceedings of the Conference. This volume contains extended and refined contributions by many of the presenters at the conference.

We very much appreciate the financial support provided by Health Canada and CIHR and the institutional support provided by York University and the Centre for Social Justice. The commitment to this project by the conference presenters and the 400 attendees of the York University conference, including the 90 who presented posters detailing their work on the social determinants of health, convinced me of the worthiness of this effort. The enthusiastic support of senior editor Megan Mueller of Canadian Scholars' Press Inc. was essential to completion of this volume. I hope the material contained in this volume will spur debate on the future of Canadian public policy with the aim of promoting the health and well-being of all Canadians.

**Dennis Raphael**
**March 2004**

# Chapter One

---

# INTRODUCTION TO THE
# SOCIAL DETERMINANTS OF HEALTH

## Dennis Raphael

## Introduction

Social determinants of health are the economic and social conditions that influence the health of individuals, communities, and jurisdictions as a whole. Social determinants of health determine whether individuals stay healthy or become ill (a narrow definition of health). Social determinants of health also determine the extent to which a person possesses the physical, social, and personal resources to identify and achieve personal aspirations, satisfy needs, and cope with the environment (a broader definition of health). Social determinants of health are about the quantity and quality of a variety of resources that a society makes available to its members.

These resources include—but are not limited to—conditions of childhood, income, availability of food, housing, employment and working conditions, and health and social services. An emphasis upon societal conditions as determinants of health contrasts with the traditional focus upon biomedical and behavioural risk factors such as cholesterol, body weight, physical activity, diet, and tobacco use. Since a social determinants of health approach sees the mainsprings of health as being how a society organises and distributes economic and social resources, it directs attention to economic and social policies as means of improving it.

A social determinants of health approach is not a wholly new development, but has its roots in critical examination of the causes of illness and disease that date from the mid-nineteenth century. More recently, British researchers have studied the sources of health inequalities among populations, thereby contributing much to our understanding of the importance of social determinants of health. Canadians have also developed health promotion and population health concepts that direct attention to various social determinants of health. But it appears that Canada is well behind other jurisdictions in applying this knowledge to developing economic and social policies that support health.

Canada's shortcomings in addressing the social determinants of health are surprising, as tremendous increases have occurred in our theoretical and empirical knowledge of how economic and social conditions determine health. Numerous studies indicate that various social determinants of health have far greater influence upon health and the incidence of illness than traditional biomedical and behavioural risk factors. There is also new scholarship on the state and quality of various social determinants of health in Canada and how these conditions affect the health of Canadians. Yet, for the most part policy-makers, the media, and the general public remain badly informed concerning these issues. Indeed, it has been suggested that much of the public policy agenda seems designed to threaten—rather than support—the health of Canadians by weakening the quality of many social determinants of health.

These concerns about the neglect of the importance of social determinants of health led to York University's School of Health Policy and Management applying to Health Canada's Policy Research Program for funding to organise a national conference entitled *Social determinants of health across the life-span: A current accounting and policy implications*. The purpose of the conference was to: (a) consider the state of several key social determinants of health across Canada; (b) explore the implications of these conditions for the health of Canadians; and (c) outline policy directions to strengthen these social determinants of health. This volume presents the findings from this conference.

In this introduction, I review the concept of social determinants of health and present recent theoretical developments and empirical findings. I provide the rationale for selecting the social determinants of health included in the volume and explore four key themes in the field. Throughout this presentation the social determinants of health approach is contrasted with the traditional approach to disease prevention focused on biomedical and behavioural risk factors. I conclude by asking the reader to consider how current Canadian policy environments affect both the quality of these social determinants of Canadians' health and Canadian policymakers' receptivity to the ideas contained within this volume.

## An historical perspective on the social determinants of health

During the mid 1800s political economist Friedrich Engels studied the health conditions of working people in England and identified the factors responsible for social class differences in health. His 1845 work, *The condition of the working class in England*, describes the horrendous living and working conditions which workers were forced to endure (Engels, 1845/1987). Engels showed, as one of many examples, how profoundly different death rates within a suburb of Manchester were directly correlated with quality of housing and quality of streets. He was remarkably perceptive in identifying the mechanisms by which disease and early death came to the working classes. He described how material conditions of life—poverty, poor housing, clothing, and diet, and lack of sanitation—directly led to the infections and diseases common among the poor. Engels also explored how the day-to-day stress of living under such conditions contributed to illness and injury. The adoption of health-threatening behaviours such as drink was seen as means of coping with such disastrous conditions of life. Engels concluded:

> All conceivable evils are heaped
> upon the poor … They are given
> damp dwellings, cellar dens that are

not waterproof from below or garrets that leak from above ... They are supplied bad, tattered, or rotten clothing, adulterated and indigestible food. They are exposed to the most exciting changes of mental condition, the most violent vibrations between hope and fear ... They are deprived of all enjoyments except sexual indulgence and drunkenness and are worked every day to the point of complete exhaustion of their mental and physical energies ... (Engels, 1845/1987, p. 129).

## British contributions

More recently, re-interest in the social determinants of health was sparked by the publication of the *Black report* and the *Health divide* (Townsend et al., 1992). These UK reports described how lowest employment-level groups showed a greater likelihood of suffering from a wide range of diseases and dying prematurely from illness or injury at every stage of the life cycle. Additionally, health differences occurred in a step-wise progression across the socio-economic range with professionals having the best health and manual labourers the worst. Skilled workers' health was midway between the extremes. These two reports—and the many that have followed up on these themes—stimulated the study of health inequalities and the factors that determine these inequalities and directed attention to the role public policy plays in either increasing or reducing health inequalities.

Health inequalities and the social determinants of these inequalities are active areas of inquiry among British researchers. Their studies frequently focus on inequalities in health among members of different employment strata with recognition that

---

### Box 1.1: Rudolf Virchow and the social determinants of health

German physician Rudolf Virchow's (1821–1902) medical discoveries were so extensive that he is known as the "Father of Modern Pathology." But he was also a trailblazer in identifying how societal policies determine health. In 1848, Virchow was sent by the Berlin authorities to investigate the epidemic of typhus in Upper Silesia. His *Report on the Typhus epidemic prevailing in Upper Silesia* argued that lack of democracy, feudalism, and unfair tax policies in the province were the primary determinants of the inhabitants' poor living conditions, inadequate diet, and poor hygiene that fuelled the epidemic.

Virchow stated that *Disease is not something personal and special, but only a manifestation of life under modified (pathological) conditions.* Arguing *Medicine is a social science and politics is nothing else but medicine on a large scale,* Virchow drew the direct links between social conditions and health. He argued that improved health required recognition that: *If medicine is to fulfil her great task, then she must enter the political and social life. Do we not always find the diseases of the populace traceable to defects in society?* (Virchow, 1848/1985).

The authorities were not happy with the report and Virchow was relieved of his government position. But he continued his pathology research within university settings and went on to a parallel career as a member of Berlin City Council and the Prussian Diet where he focused on public health issues consistent with his Upper Silesia report. Virchow also bitterly opposed Otto Von Bismarck's plans for national rearmament and was challenged to a duel by the said gentleman. Virchow declined participation.

---

membership in such groups is strongly correlated with income and education levels. British researchers also study the health effects of poverty and how indicators of disadvantage usually cluster together. Much of the available data on social determinants of health is British, as are some of the best theorisations of how these factors influence health across the life span. The United Kingdom is also the source of many ideas on how to apply these findings to promote health.

## Canadian contributions

Canadians have actively theorised the relationship between economic and social conditions and health. In 1974 the federal government's *A new perspective on the health of Canadians* identified human biology, environment, lifestyle, and health care organization as determinants of health (Lalonde, 1974). The document was important in that it identified determinants of health other than the health care system.

Another Canadian government document, *Achieving health for all: A framework for health promotion*, outlined reducing inequities between income groups as an important goal of government policy (Epp, 1986). This would be accomplished by influencing policies that have a direct bearing on health. The list of policy areas is long and includes, among others, income security, employment, education, housing, business, agriculture, transportation, justice and technology. Health Canada's *Taking action on population health: A position paper for health promotion and programs branch staff* states:

There is strong evidence indicating that factors outside the health care system significantly affect health. These "determinants of health"

include income and social status, social support networks, education, employment and working conditions, physical environments, social environments, biology and genetic endowment, personal health practices and coping skills, healthy child development, health services, gender and culture (Health Canada, 1998, p. 1).

Canadian Public Health Association (CPHA) documents tell a similar story. In 1986, its *Action statement for health promotion in Canada* identified advocating for healthy public policies as the single best strategy to affect the determinants of health. Priority actions included reducing inequalities in income and wealth, and strengthening communities through local alliances to change unhealthy living conditions. In 2000, the CPHA endorsed an action plan that recognised how poverty profoundly influenced health and identified means by which poverty would be reduced. Other CPHA reports document the health effects of unemployment, income insecurity, homelessness, and general economic conditions (Canadian Public Health Association, 2003).

Canadian studies usually focus on income—and the incidence of poverty—and how these are related to inequalities in health. There is also increasing emphasis in Canada, the United Kingdom, and other European nations on viewing health inequalities as a result of citizens experiencing systematic material, social, cultural, and political exclusion from mainstream society. Understanding and reducing these processes of "social exclusion" requires consideration of broader societal forces and how these influence the health of Canadians.

The study of the social determinants of health therefore deals with two key problems: *What are the societal factors (e.g., income, education, employment conditions, etc.) that lead to health inequalities?* and *What are the societal forces (e.g., economic, social, and political policies, etc.) that shape the quality of these societal factors?* In the next section various frameworks for considering the social determinants of health are presented.

## What are social determinants of health?

The term *social determinants of health* appears to have grown out of the search by researchers to identify the specific exposures by which members of different socio-economic groups come to experience varying degrees of health and illness. While it was well documented that individuals in various socio-economic groups experienced differing health outcomes, the specific factors and means by which these factors led to illness remained to be identified.

One of the first modern efforts to identify these factors was seen in the 1996 volume *Health and social organization: Towards a health policy for the 21ˢᵗ century* (Blane, Brunner, and Wilkinson, 1996). In the chapter *Social determinants of health: The sociobiological translation*, Tarlov (1996) took the environment health field from the Lalonde report—the others being biology and genes, health care, and lifestyle—and fleshed out these environmental determinants of health. In his model, inequalities in the quality of social determinants of housing, education, social acceptance, employment, and income become translated into disease-related processes.

Another stimulus to developing the concept of the social determinants of health was findings of national differences in overall population health. As one illustration, the health of Americans compares unfavourably to the health of citizens in most other industrialised nations (Raphael, 2003). This is the case for life expectancy, infant mortality, and death by childhood injury despite the U.S.'s overall greater wealth. In contrast, the population health of the Scandinavian nations is generally superior to most other nations. Could the same factors that explain health differences among groups within nations explain the differences seen between national populations?

## Current concepts of the social determinants of health

There are a variety of contemporary approaches to social determinants of health. The commonalities among these are particularly illuminative.

The *Ottawa charter for health promotion* identifies the *prerequisites for health* as peace, shelter, education, food, income, a stable ecosystem, sustainable resources, social justice, and equity (World Health Organization, 1986). These prerequisites of health are concerned with structural aspects of society and the organisation and distribution of economic and social resources.

Health Canada outlines various *determinants of health*—some of which are social determinants—of income and social status, social support networks, education, employment and working conditions, physical and social environments, biology and genetic endowment, personal health practices and coping skills, healthy child development, health services, gender, and culture (Health Canada, 1998). Within this framework, the specific concepts of physical and social environments can be criticised for lacking grounding in concrete experiences of peoples' lives and lacking policy relevance—i.e. there usually is no *Ministry of Physical Environments* or *Ministry of Social Environments.*

A British working group charged with the specific task of identifying *social determinants of health* named the social [class health] gradient, stress, early life, social exclusion, work, unemployment, social support, addiction, food, and transport (Wilkinson and Marmot, 2003). This listing is more grounded in the everyday experience of people's lives and policy-making structures and avoids the potential problem of policy irrelevance. Indeed, the stimulus for this work was the European Office of the World Health Organization wanting to raise these issues among policy-makers and the public.

The organisers of the 2002 York University *Social determinants of health across the life span* conference synthesised these formulations to identify eleven key social determinants of health especially relevant to Canadians (see Box 1.2). Four criteria were used to identify these social determinants of health.

The first criterion was that the social determinant be consistent with most existing formulations of the social determinants of health and associated with an existing empirical literature as to its relevance to health. *All these social determinants of health are important to the health of Canadians.*

The second criterion was that the social determinant of health be consistent with lay/public understandings of the factors that influence health and well-being. This was ascertained through assessment of available empirical work on Canadians' under-standings of what aspects of Canadian life contribute to health and well-being. *All these social determinants of health are understandable to Canadians.*

The third criterion was that the social determinant of health be clearly aligned with existing governmental structures and policy frameworks (e.g., Ministries of Housing, Native Affairs, Labour, Education, etc.). *All these social determinants of health have clear policy relevance to Canadian decision-makers and citizens.*

The fourth criterion was that the social determinant of health be an area of either active governmental policy activity (e.g.,

---

**Box 1.2: York University's social determinants of health**

The 11 social determinants of health identified by the organizers of the York University conference form the basis for the content of this volume. These are:
- Aboriginal status
- early life
- education
- employment and working conditions
- food security
- health care services
- housing
- income and its distribution
- social safety net
- social exclusion
- unemployment and employment security.

health care services, education) or policy inactivity that have provoked sustained criticism (e.g. food security, housing, social safety net). *All these social determinants of health are especially timely and relevant.*

The inclusion of health services, housing, and the social safety net as social determinants of health is unusual. Health services are included in the belief that a well-organised and rationalised health care system could be an important social determinant of health—if this is not currently the case. Housing is normally included within another determinant (e.g., physical environments or social exclusion) which is surprising considering its centrality to human health and well-being. The social safety net is increasingly recognised as an important determinant of the health of populations but to date is not explicitly included in available formulations. Aboriginal status is another social determinant of health that is not explicitly explored in most conceptual-isations of social determinants of health. It represents the interaction of culture, public policy, and the mechanisms by which systematic exclusion from participation in Canadian life profoundly affects health.

Gender and how its meaning is constructed within Canadian society is another important social determinant of health. It interacts with all other social determinants of health to influence the health and well-being of Canadians. Rather than limit its examination to a single section of this volume, all authors systematically consider how its impact upon and interaction with their specific social determinant of health influences health.

## Current themes in the social determinants of health

Four important themes are apparent within the study of social determinants of health that can guide understanding of the material in this volume. These are: (a) empirical evidence concerning the social determinants of health; (b) mechanisms and pathways by which social determinants of health influence health; (c) the importance of a life course perspective; and (d) the role of policy environments in determining the quality of the social determinants of health within jurisdictions. Each is considered in turn.

### Theme 1: Empirical evidence of the importance of the social determinants of health

Evidence is converging that the quality of various social determinants of health provide explanations for: (a) improvement in health among Canadians over the past 100 years; (b) persistent differences in health among Canadians; and (c) differences in overall health among Canada and other developed nations.

*The social determinants of improved health among Canadian since 1900*

Profound improvements in health have occurred in industrialised nations such as Canada since 1900. It has been hypothesised that access to improved medical care is responsible for such differences, but best estimates are that only 10–15 percent of increased longevity since 1900 is due to improved care (McKinlay and McKinlay, 1987). As one illustration, the advent of vaccines and medical treatments are usually said to be responsible for the profound declines in mortality from infectious diseases in Canada since 1900. But by the time vaccines for diseases such as measles, influenza, and polio and treatments for scarlet fever, typhoid, and diphtheria appeared, dramatic declines in mortality had already occurred. Improvements in behaviour (e.g., reductions in tobacco use, changes in diet, etc.) have also been hypothesised as responsible for improved longevity, but most analysts conclude that improvements in health are due to the improving material conditions of everyday life experienced by Canadians since 1900.

These improvements occurred in the areas of early childhood, education, food processing and availability, health and social services, housing, and every other social determinant of health. Much of the current volume is concerned with the present state of these social determinants of health and their influence upon the health of Canadians. Particularly important is the question of how recent policy decisions are either improving or weakening the quality of these social determinants of health.

*The social determinants of health inequalities among Canadians*

Despite dramatic improvements in health in general, significant inequalities in health among Canadians persist (Wilkins et al., 2002). Medicare in Canada weakens the argument that this is due to lack of access for some to quality health care. As for differences in health behaviours (e.g., tobacco use, diet, and physical activity), studies from as early as the mid 1970s— reinforced by many more studies since then—find their impact upon health is minor as compared to social determinants of health such as income and others examined in this volume (Raphael, 2002).

Health differences among Canadians result primarily from experiences of qualitatively different environments associated with the social determinants of health. In this section, an overview of the magnitude of differences in health that are related to the social determinant of health of income is provided. Income is especially important as it serves as a marker of different experiences with many social determinants of health. Income is a determinant of health in itself, but it is also a determinant of the quality of early life, education, employment and working conditions, and food security. Income also is a determinant of the quality of housing, need for a social safety net, the experience of social exclusion, and the experience of unemployment and employment insecurity across the life span. Also, a key aspect of Aboriginal life and the experience of women in Canada is their greater likelihood of living under conditions of low income.

Income is a prime determinant of Canadians' premature years of life lost and premature mortality from a range of diseases (see Box 1.3). Numerous studies indicate that income levels during early childhood, adolescence, and adulthood are all independent predictors of who will develop and eventually succumb to disease (Davey Smith, 2003).

The figure of 23% in figure 1.1 is calculated by using the mortality rates in the wealthiest quintile of neighbourhoods as a baseline and considering all deaths above that rate to be excess related to income differences. Therefore, 23% of all of the premature years of life lost to Canadians can be accounted for by differences existing among wealthy, middle-and low-income Canadians.

What are the diseases that differentially afflict people of varying income levels? If the total number of premature years of life lost attributed to income differences are related to specific diseases, the data presented in Figure 1.2 is obtained. The specific diseases that are most related to income differences in mortality are heart disease and stroke. Importantly, premature death by injuries, cancers, infectious disease, and others are all strongly related to income differences among Canadians.

## Box 1.3: Statistics Canada study of income-related premature mortality

In Canada, data on individuals' income and social status are not routinely collected at death, so national examination of the relationship between income and mortality from various diseases uses census tract of residence to estimate individuals' income. There is potential for error in these analyses that relate income to death based on residential area, since some low income people live in well-off neighbourhoods and vice versa. Essentially, these analyses are conservative estimates of the relationship between income level and death rates. The most recent available data shows that in 1996, Canadians living within the poorest 20% of urban neighbourhoods were more likely to die from cardiovascular disease, cancer, diabetes, and respiratory diseases—among other diseases—than other Canadians (Wilkins et al., 2002).

Figure 1.1 shows the percentage of premature years of life lost in urban Canada than can be attributed to various diseases and to income differences. Cancers are the leading cause of premature years of life lost accounting for 31% of these. Injuries and circulatory diseases (heart disease and stroke) are also leading causes of premature years of life lost. However, the percentage of premature years of life lost that can be attributed to income differences among Canadians is also very high at 23%, a magnitude that is greater than all years lost to either injuries or circulatory disease and approaching the level of cancers.

---

### Figure 1.1: Percentage of premature years of life lost (0–74 years) to Canadians in urban Canada due to various causes, 1996

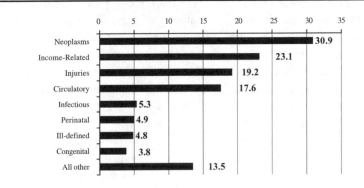

Source: "Percentage of premature years of life lost (0–74 yrs) to Canadians in urban Canada due to various causes, 1996," adapted from the Statistics Canada publication "Health reports—supplement," Catalogue 82-003, Volume 13, *2002 Annual Report*, Chart 9, p. 54.

---

In 2002, Statistics Canada examined the predictors of life expectancy, disability-free life expectancy, and the presence of fair or poor health among residents of 136 regions across Canada (Shields and Tremblay, 2002). The predictors employed included socio-demographic factors (proportion of Aboriginal population, proportion of visible

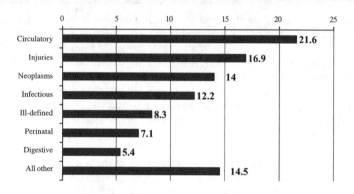

**Figure 1.2: Percentage of income-related premature years of life lost (0–74 yrs) caused by specific diseases in urban Canada, 1996**

Circulatory: 21.6
Injuries: 16.9
Neoplasms: 14
Infectious: 12.2
Ill-defined: 8.3
Perinatal: 7.1
Digestive: 5.4
All other: 14.5

Source: "Percentage of income-related premature years of life lost (0–74 yrs) caused by specific diseases in urban Canada, 1996," adapted from the Statistics Canada publication "Health reports—supplement," Catalogue 82-003, Volume 13, *2002 Annual Report*, Chart 10, p. 54.

minority population, unemployment rate, population size, percentage of population aged 65 or over, average income, and average number of years of schooling). Also placed into the analysis were daily smoking rate, obesity rate, infrequent exercise rate, heavy drinking rate, high stress rate, and depression rate. Table 1.1 shows the proportion of variation (the total is 100%) in health outcomes explained by each of these predictors. Consistent with most other research, behavioural risk factors are rather weak predictors of health status as compared to socio-economic and demographic measures of which income is a major component.

These differences in premature mortality are mirrored in greater incidence of just about every affliction that Canadians experience. This is especially the case for chronic diseases such as heart disease and stroke, diabetes, cancers, as well as injuries and infectious disease.

Incidence of, and mortality from, heart disease and stroke, and adult-onset or type 2 diabetes are especially good examples of the importance of the social determinants of health (Raphael and Farrell, 2002; Raphael et al., 2003). While governments, medical researchers, and public health workers continue to emphasise the importance of traditional adult risk factors (e.g., cholesterol, diet, physical activity, and tobacco use), it is well established that these are relatively poor predictors of heart disease, stroke, and type 2 diabetes rates among populations. The factors that do make a difference are living under conditions of material deprivation as children and adults, stress associated with such conditions, and the adoption of health threatening behaviours as means of coping with these difficult circumstances. In fact, difficult living circumstances during childhood are especially good predictors of these diseases.

In addition to predicting adult incidence and death from disease, income differences—and the other social determinants of health related to income—are also related to the health of Canadian

**Table 1.1: Proportion of variation in life expectancy, disability-free life expectancy, and proportion of citizens reporting fair or poor health explained by different factors at the health region level in Canada (total variation for each outcome measure = 100%)**

| Predictors | Life expectancy | Disability-free life expectancy | Fair or poor health |
|---|---|---|---|
| Socio-demographic factors only | 56% | 32% | 25% |
| *Additional variation predicted by:* | | | |
| Daily smoking rate | 8% | 6% | 4% |
| Obesity rate | 1% | 5% | 10% |
| Infrequent exercise rate | 0% | 3% | 0% |
| Heavy drinking rate | 1% | 3% | 1% |
| High stress rate | 0% | 0% | 1% |
| Depression rate | 0% | 8% | 9% |

Source: Shields, M. and Tremblay, S. (2002), "The health of Canada's communities," *Health reports—supplement* 13 (July), p. 13.

children and youth. Canadian children living in low-income families are more likely to experience greater incidence of a variety of illnesses, hospital stays, accidental injuries, mental health problems, lower school achievement and early drop-out, family violence and child abuse, among others (Canadian Institute for Children's Health, 2000). In fact, low-income children show higher incidences of just about any health-, social-, or education-related problem, however defined. These differences in problem incidence occur across the income range but are most concentrated among low-income children.

*The social determinants of health differences between nations*

National differences in health indicators such as life expectancy, infant mortality, incidence of disease, and death from injuries exist (Raphael, 2003). Concerning the sources of these differences between Canadians and citizens elsewhere, these same social determinants of health are implicated.

Differences in social determinants of health such as income and its distribution, quality of early childhood, and employment and working conditions explain much of the differences in health among citizens of Canada, the USA and various European nations. Table 1.2 shows how the USA, Canada, and Sweden fare on a number of social determinants of health and indicators of population health. The concluding chapter of this volume explores the meaning of these international differences in social determinants of health and policy implications.

**Theme 2: Mechanisms and pathways by which social determinants of health influence health**

It is important to understand how social determinants of health come to influence health and cause disease. Recent theoretical thinking considers how social determinants of health "get under the skin" to influence health. The *Black* and the *Health divide* reports considered two primary mechanisms

**Table 1.2: USA, Canada, and Sweden rankings on selected social determinants of health and indicators of population health in comparison to other industrialized nations (2000–2002)**

| Measure | (Ranking, 1 is best) | | |
| --- | --- | --- | --- |
| | USA | Canada | Sweden |
| % in Child poverty | 22 of 23 | 17 | 1 |
| Income inequality | 18 of 21 | 13 | 3 |
| % in Low paid employment | 24 of 24 | 20 | 1 |
| Public social expenditure | 24 of 28 | 23 | 1 |
| Public share health spending | 28 of 29 | 23 | 1 |
| Life expectancy | 20 of 26 | 5 | 4 |
| Infant mortality | 24 of 30 | 16 | 1 |
| Child injury mortality | 23 of 26 | 18 | 1 |

Source: Raphael, D. (2003). "A society in decline: the social, economic, and political determinants of health inequalities in the USA," in Hofrichter, R. (Ed.), *Health and social justice: A reader on politics, ideology, and inequity in the distribution of disease.* San Francisco: Jossey Bass/Wiley, 59–88.

for understanding health inequalities: *cultural/ behavioural* and *materialist/structuralist* (Townsend et al., 1992).

The *cultural/behavioural explanation* was that individuals' behavioural choices (e.g., tobacco and alcohol use, diet, physical activity, etc.) were responsible for their developing and dying from a variety of diseases. Both the *Black* and *Health divide* reports however, showed that behavioural choices are heavily structured by one's material conditions of life. And—consistent with mounting evidence—these behavioural risk factors account for a relatively small proportion of variation in the incidence and death from various diseases. The *materialist/ structuralist* explanation emphasises the material conditions under which people live their lives. These conditions include availability of resources to access the amenities of life, working conditions, and quality of available food and housing among others.

The author of the *Health divide* concluded: *The weight of evidence continues to point to explanations which suggest that socio-economic circumstances play the major part in subsequent health differences.* Despite this conclusion and increasing evidence in favour of this view, much of the Canadian public discourse on health and disease remains focused on "life-style" approaches to disease prevention. The *Traditional ten tips for better health* reflect this life-style orientation while the *Social determinants of health ten tips for better health* are consistent with more advanced thinking (see Box 1.4).

These conceptualisations have been refined such that analysis is now focused upon three frameworks by which social determinants of health come to influence health. These frameworks are: (a) materialist; (b) neo-materialist; and (c) psychosocial comparison.

*Materialist approach: Conditions of living as determinants of health*

The materialist explanation of how social determinants influence health is based on the observation that individuals are exposed to varying degrees of positive and negative exposures over the course of their lives. These exposures accumulate to produce health outcomes in adulthood. Socio-

## Box 1.4: Which tips for better health are consistent with research evidence?

The messages given to the public by governments, health associations, and health workers are heavily influenced by the ways in which health issues are understood. Contrast the two sets of messages provided below. The first set is individually-oriented and assumes individuals can control the factors that determine their health. The second set is societally-oriented and assumes the most important determinants of health are beyond the control of most individuals. Which set of tips is most consistent with the available evidence on the determinants of health?

### The traditional ten tips for better health

1. Don't smoke. If you can, stop. If you can't, cut down.
2. Follow a balanced diet with plenty of fruit and vegetables.
3. Keep physically active.
4. Manage stress by, for example, talking things through and making time to relax.
5. If you drink alcohol, do so in moderation.
6. Cover up in the sun, and protect children from sunburn.
7. Practice safer sex.
8. Take up cancer screening opportunities.
9. Be safe on the roads: follow the Highway Code.
10. Learn the First Aid ABCs: airways, breathing, circulation. (Donaldson, 1999)

### The social determinants ten tips for better health

1. Don't be poor. If you can, stop. If you can't, try not to be poor for long.
2. Don't have poor parents.
3. Own a car.
4. Don't work in a stressful, low paid manual job.
5. Don't live in damp, low quality housing.
6. Be able to afford to go on a foreign holiday and sunbathe.
7. Practice not losing your job and don't become unemployed.
8. Take up all benefits you are entitled to, if you are unemployed, retired or sick or disabled.
9. Don't live next to a busy major road or near a polluting factory.
10. Learn how to fill in the complex housing benefit/ asylum application forms before you become homeless and destitute. (Gordon, 1999; personal communication)

economic and income status are powerful predictors of health as they serve as indicators of material advantage or disadvantage that accumulate over the life-span. "The social structure is characterized by a finely graded scale of advantage and disadvantage, with individuals differing in terms of the length and level of their exposure to a particular factor and in terms of the number of factors to which they are exposed" (Shaw et al., 1999, p.102).

Material conditions of life influence health by determining the quality of individual development, family life and interaction, and community environments. Material conditions of life result in differing likelihood of physical (infections, malnutrition, chronic disease and injuries), developmental (delayed or impaired cognitive, personality, and social development), educational (learning disabilities, poor learning, early school leaving), and social (socialization, preparation for work and family life) problems.

Second, differences in material conditions of life lead to differences in the experience of psychosocial stress (Brunner and Marmot, 1999). The fight and flight reaction—chronically elicited in response to continuing threats such as income, housing and food insecurity, among others—threatens health. Such threats lead to weakening of the immune system, increased insulin resistance, and greater incidence of lipid and clotting disorders and other biomedical injuries that serve as precursors of disease in adulthood.

Third, adoption of health-threatening behaviours is a response to material deprivation and stress (Jarvis and Wardle, 1999). Social and economic environments determine whether individuals take up tobacco, use alcohol, have poor diets, and engage in physical activity. Tobacco use, excessive alcohol use and carbohydrate-dense diets result from lack of material resources and are also means of coping with such circumstances.

Materialist arguments are useful for understanding the sources of health inequalities among Canadians. Health inequalities result from differences in material conditions of life that are mediated through the social determinants of health. Materialist arguments also help explain health differences among developed nations. For example, the U.S. has higher rates of infant mortality, lower life expectancy, and greater mortality from heart disease and diabetes than Canada. As explanation, the U.S. has higher rates of family and child poverty, and lower-end workers earn far less than do lower-end workers in Canada.

*Neo-materialist approach: Conditions of living and social infrastructure as determinants of health*

Differences in health among nations, regions, and cities are related to how income and other resources are distributed among the population (Lynch et al., 2000). American states and cities with more unequal distribution of income have greater proportions of low-income people and greater income gaps between rich and poor. They also invest less in public infrastructure such as education, health and social services, health insurance, supports for the unemployed and those with disabilities, and spending on education and libraries. Such unequal jurisdictions have much poorer health profiles.

Similarly, Canada has a smaller proportion of lower-income people, a smaller gap between rich and poor, and spends relatively more on public infrastructure than the U.S. (Ross et al., 2000). Canada also enjoys better overall health than the U.S. in terms of infant mortality, life expectancy, and childhood injuries. Neither nation does as well as Sweden where distribution of resources is much more equalitarian, low-income rates are very low, and health indicators are among the best in the world.

The neo-materialist view directs attention to both the effects of living conditions on individuals' health but also the societal factors that determine the quality of these social determinants of health. Jurisdictions with large rich-poor gaps are poor for health since *"the effect of income inequality on health reflects a combination of negative exposures and lack of resources held by individuals, along with systematic underinvestment across a wide range of human, physical, health, and social infrastructure"* (Lynch et al., 2000, p. 1202). The neo-materialist view directs attention to how a society's decisions on how to distribute resources affects the quality of various social determinants of health, thereby influencing the health of Canadians.

*Social comparison approach: Hierarchy and social distance as determinants of health*

The social comparison explanation argues that health inequalities in developed nations such as Canada are not primarily due to material deprivation, but rather to citizens' interpretations of their standings in the social hierarchy (Kawachi and Kennedy, 2002). There are two mechanisms by which this occurs.

At the individual level, the perception and experience of hierarchy in unequal societies lead to stress and poor health. Comparing themselves—their status, possessions, and other life circumstances—to others, individuals experience ongoing feelings of shame, worthlessness, and envy. These perceptions have psycho-biological effects that lead to poor health. These comparisons also lead to attempts to alleviate such feelings through overspending, taking on additional employment responsibilities that threaten health, and adopting health-threatening coping behaviours such as overeating and use of alcohol and tobacco.

At the communal level, the widening and strengthening of hierarchy weakens social cohesion—a determinant of health. Individuals become more distrusting and suspicious of others thereby weakening support for communal structures such as public education, health, and social programs. An exaggerated desire for tax reductions on the part of the public that result in weakened public infrastructure can be one result of these processes.

While these processes are clearly provoked by aspects of the material world, the focus in this model is upon increased hierarchy, unfavourable self-social comparison, and weakening of social cohesion as pathways to poor health. This model directs attention to the psychosocial effects that public policies that weaken the social determinants of health may have upon Canadians. An important issue is the extent to which material aspects of society—such as those described in the materialist and neo-materialist approaches—are the prime determinants of these processes.

**Theme 3: The importance of a life-course perspective**

Traditional approaches to health and disease prevention have a distinctly non-historical emphasis. Usually adults, and increasingly adolescents and youth are urged to adopt "healthy lifestyles" as a means of preventing the development of chronic diseases such as heart disease and diabetes, among others. In contrast to these approaches, life-course approaches emphasise the accumulated effects of experience across the life span in understanding the maintenance of health and the onset of disease. It has been argued:

> The prevailing aetiological model for adult disease which emphasizes adult risk factors, particularly aspects of adult life style, has been

challenged in recent years by research that has shown that poor growth and development and adverse early environmental conditions are associated with an increased risk of adult chronic disease. (Kuh and Ben-Shlomo, 1997, p. 3)

More specifically, it is apparent that the economic and social conditions—the social determinants of health—under which individuals live their lives have a cumulative effect upon the probability of developing any number of diseases. This has been repeatedly demonstrated in longitudinal studies—the U.S. National Longitudinal Survey, the West of Scotland Collaborative Study, Norwegian and Finnish linked data—which follow individuals across their lives (Blane, 1999). This has been most clearly demonstrated in the case of heart disease and stroke. And most recently, studies into the childhood and adulthood antecedents of adult-onset diabetes show how adverse economic and social conditions across the life span predispose individuals to this disorder (Raphael and Farrell, 2002; Raphael et al., 2003).

A recent volume brings together some of the most important work concerning the importance of a life-course perspective for understanding the importance of social determinants (Davey Smith, 2003). Adopting a life-course perspective directs attention to how social determinants of health operate at every level of development—early childhood, childhood, adolescence, and adulthood—to both immediately influence health as well as provide the basis for health or illness during following stages of the life course.

## Theme 4: The role of policy environments

An important purpose of this volume is to outline policy options for strengthening these social determinants of health. Strengthening social determinants of health would reduce health inequalities, thereby improving the population health of Canadians. This being the case, it would be expected that governments would be responsive to these ideas. This may not be the case. *In fact, Canada has fallen behind countries such as the United Kingdom and Sweden and even some jurisdictions in the United States in applying the population health knowledge base that has been largely developed in Canada* (Canadian Population Health Initiative, 2002, p. 1).

This policy vacuum on social determinants of health exists within a broader context. Canadian political economist Gary Teeple argues that strong national identities and the need to mitigate class conflict at the end of World War II led to the development of the Canadian welfare state (Teeple, 2000). This process strengthened the social determinants of health. The Canadian welfare state was associated with more equitable distribution of income and wealth through social, economic, and political reforms. These reforms included progressive tax structures, social programs, and governmental structures that mitigated conflicts between business and labour, among others.

These reforms are being weakened through economic globalization. Since the early 1970s, a fundamental change has occurred in national and global economies. In Canada, governments have adopted neo-liberal approaches that by emphasizing the role of markets in organizing and allocating resources, have weakened the structures associated with the welfare state. Federal program spending as a percentage of GDP is now at 1950s levels, and government policies have increased income and wealth inequalities, created crises in housing and food security, and increased the precariousness of employment (Raphael, 2001). Can social determinants of health be strengthened in such an environment?

## Conclusion

The pages to follow contain assessments of the current state of 11 key social determinants of health in Canada and analyses of how these conditions affect the health of Canadians. Consider how each theoretical framework presented—the materialist, neo-materialist, and psycho-social comparison—helps to explain how these social determinants come to influence health. Consider how the quality of these social determinants of health are influenced by decisions made by Canadian policy-makers in Ottawa, your province, and your local municipality.

As you read the policy options that are provided for improving both the state of these determinants and the health of Canadians, keep in mind the importance of the broader political, economic, and social environments in which Canadians are now living. To what extent do these environments influence the receptivity of policymakers to these ideas and what can be done to see these ideas put into practice? What are the means by which these ideas can be implemented to reduce health inequalities and improve the overall health of Canadians?

## Recommended readings

Bartley, M. (2003). *Health inequality: An introduction to concepts, theories and methods.* Cambridge: Polity Press.

Large differences in life expectancy exist between the most privileged and the most disadvantaged social groups in industrial societies. This book assists in understanding the four most widely accepted theories of what lies behind inequalities in health: behavioural, psycho-social, material, and life-course approaches.

Hofrichter, R. (Ed.). (2003). *Health and social justice: Politics, ideology, and inequity in the distribution of disease.* San Francisco: Jossey-Bass.

This volume offers a comprehensive collection of articles written by expert contributors representing the fields of sociology, epidemiology, public health, ecology, politics, organizing, and advocacy. Each article explores a particular aspect of health inequalities and demonstrates how these are rooted in injustices associated with racism, sex discrimination, and social class.

Davey Smith, G. (2003). *Health inequalities: Life-course approaches.* Bristol: Policy Press.

The life-course perspective on adult health and health inequalities is an important development in epidemiology and public health. This volume presents innovative, empirical research that shows how social disadvantage throughout the life-course leads to inequalities in life expectancy, death rates, and health status in adulthood.

Raphael, D. (2002). *Social justice is good for our hearts: Why societal factors—not lifestyles—are major causes of heart disease in Canada and elsewhere.* Toronto: Centre for Social Justice. Online at www.socialjustice.org.

This work details how income inequality and the social exclusion that results from it, are directly related to illness and death from heart disease in Canada and other developed nations. It shows how the Canadian tradition of maintaining equity and social and health services is weakening, thereby creating direct threats to the health of Canadians.

# Related websites

Canadian Centre for Policy Alternatives (CCPA)—www.policyalternatives.ca
The Centre monitors developments and promotes research on economic and social issues facing Canada. It provides alternatives to the views of business research institutes and many government agencies by publishing research reports, sponsoring conferences, organizing briefings and providing informed comment on the issues of the day from a non-partisan perspective.

Canadian Council on Social Development (CCSD)—www.ccsd.ca
The CCSD is a social policy and research organization focusing on social welfare and development issues of poverty, social inclusion, disability, cultural diversity, child well-being, employment, and housing. It provides statistics and reports on the state of poverty and income inequality in Canada and policy options for improving the health and well-being of Canadians.

Centre for Social Justice (CSJ)—www.socialjustice.org
The CSJ's work is focused on narrowing the gap between rich and poor, challenging corporate domination of Canadian politics, and pressing for policy changes that promote economic and social justice. It provides information, statistics and reports on the gap between rich and poor, housing, and other issues related to social determinants of health.

National Council of Welfare (NCW)—www.ncwcnbes.net
The NCW advises the Canadian government on matters related to social welfare and the needs of low-income Canadians. NCW publishes several reports each year on poverty and social policy issues, presents submissions to Parliamentary Committees and Royal Commissions, and provides information on poverty and social policy.

Population Health Forum (PHF)—depts.washington.edu/eqhlth/
The PHF's mission is to raise awareness and initiate dialogue about the ways in which political, economic, and social inequalities interact to affect the overall health status of US society. It achieves its goals of promoting knowledge and advocating for action in service of a healthier society by providing information, statistics, and relevant reports and articles.

# Part One

————●————

# INCOME SECURITY
## AND EMPLOYMENT IN CANADA

INCOME AND ITS DISTRIBUTION, the availability and security of employment, and conditions of employment, are prime social determinants of health. The availability of income, much of this a result of employment, serves as a determinant of other social determinants of health. Without adequate income, access to food, housing, and other basic prerequisites of health, is increasingly difficult. Without adequate income, the likelihood of social exclusion increases as more and more Canadians are unable to participate in commonly assumed economic, social, cultural, and political activities. And even when employment is available, deteriorating working conditions, wages, and benefits, and increasing employment insecurity threaten health. Employment insecurity is a result of increasing economic globalization and the power of corporations and other employers. The contributions in this section document how Canadians are experiencing clear threats to health through the weakening of these social determinants of health. The sources of the deterioration of these social determinants of health are identified as being political, economic, and social policy decisions being made by governments. The contributors probe the origins of these decisions and present alternative policy futures to address these concerns.

**Ann Curry-Stevens** provides an overview of the meaning and importance of income and wealth inequality as well as the latest Canadian statistics. Despite long standing beliefs about the equalitarian nature of Canadian society, not only is inequality increasing, but it is Canadians at the very bottom who are losing ground while those at the very top benefit. And non-white and new Canadians are especially likely to be losing ground. This skewing of Canadian society results from having governments leaving issues of income distribution to the marketplace and abrogating their responsibilities to meet the basic needs of many Canadians.

**Nathalie Auger, Marie-France Raynault, Richard Lessard, and Robert Choinière** provide an overview of what is known about the relationship between income and health. They provide different ways of measuring income and how these measures can be related to health. Their review provides conclusive evidence that income is a key social determinant of health. Detailed findings from recent studies on the relationship between income and health in Montreal drive home these points. The authors conclude that little will be accomplished in terms of improving Canadians' health without focus on issues of income distribution, poverty reduction, and providing Canadians with the basic prerequisites of health.

**Dianne-Gabrielle Tremblay** discusses how recent economic and demographic transformations are influencing the current Canadian employment market. Various definitions of employment insecurity are presented. Increases in "boundaryless careers," in contrast to those jobs where some degree of security and upward progression could be expected, leads to increasing precariousness of employment. This is especially the case among Canadian women. The sources of these changes are a combination of economic and social forces, but their effects are strongly mediated by policy responses within nations. U.S. and Canadian approaches are contrasted with those seen among Scandinavian nations where full employment and job retraining efforts are more valued.

**Michael Polanyi, Emile Tompa, and Janice Foley** focus on the productivity and health effects of increased labour market flexibility. While it is believed that such approaches increase productivity and efficiency, the evidence concerning this is mixed. What is clearer is that such approaches increase worker insecurity and threaten health and well-being. These negative effects are more likely to accrue to women, Canadians of colour, and those at the lower end of the economic ladder. The authors provide a range of ways by which economic competitiveness and employee health needs can be balanced. These include policy changes to balance power between employers and employees, research and education, and cultural and institutional changes to support health and well-being.

**Andrew Jackson** explains how a good job involves security, adequate conditions including pace and stress, opportunities for self-expression and individual development at work, participation, and work-life balance. Evidence is systematically provided that indicates that there is significant deterioration in many of these workplace characteristics in Canada. One factor strongly related to working conditions is degree of unionization whereby unionization is associated with improved conditions, security, and benefits. The Canadian scene is contrasted to that of European nations that direct resources to improving employment and employment training. Improvement will occur when governments help equalize bargaining power between workers and employers.

**Michael Polanyi** provides recent findings concerning major work dimensions and their influence upon health. He focuses on availability, adequacy of income, appropriateness of work arrangements with respect to non-work responsibilities and needs, and appreciation or involvement of workers as active workplace participants and contributors to society. Concepts such as "flexisecurity" and provision of a basic income are potential means of improving workplace conditions and improving health. He also suggests means by which available evidence can be translated into action involving democratizing policy-making processes and providing citizens with opportunities for meaningful engagement in democratic deliberation.

# Chapter Two

## INCOME AND INCOME DISTRIBUTION

### Ann Curry-Stevens

## Introduction

Income inequality (also generically titled the "growing gap") has generated significant attention over the last 5 years, with a substantial body of research profiling various elements of the gap. This chapter will walk the reader through an array of measures of inequality and unearth the learnings from such research. It is hoped that, simultaneously, the readers will become critical consumers of such statistical information, building skills to evaluate the adequacy of future data to which they are exposed. New research has also been done for this chapter—research that exposes the changing class structure of Canada, molding us increasingly towards the poignant image of a rotten apple, eroding the middle class and growing the rich and the poor.

We then place this research in the broader social and political context of the turn of the century, with two decades under our belts of the erosion of the social safety net and greater reliance on the market for meeting our economic needs. In conclusion, we profile the various forms of solutions that exist including policy solutions, campaign solutions and vision-based solutions.[1]

## Misleading "average" income reports

When incomes are said to be growing, the data typically refers to a single measure of incomes, the mean (or average) for the entire population. One accentuated example reveals the inadequacy of this measure:

If there are five people making $20,000/year and one person making $200,000/year, then the mean income level for those six people is $50,000/year. But to what degree does this measure reflect the real experience of those six people? Very little, for any of those involved.

In real life, Canadian families had an average market income, which in 2001 was $63,700, up from $63,200 in 2000. This is an increase, in one year, of 0.79%; not bad considering that economic growth had been borderline—almost a recession (as measured by GDP figures). From first glance, it would appear as though the economy is serving us well, in that our incomes were still rising, despite stagnant economic growth. But remembering the illustration used above, the average income might be misleading, as it might be unduly high if the incomes at the top are skewing the average to higher values. This is exactly what is happening.

## Measures of income distribution: Market incomes

Market incomes are the topic of discussion for the next few sections of this chapter, as we focus on how well the market serves our income needs, across the income spectrum. In later sections, we will examine other measures of income, including income measures that include the effects of transfers (such as unemployment insurance, child tax benefits, pensions, and social assistance) and taxes (provincial and federal income tax). Wealth measures (the total value of assets minus debts) are covered at the close of the review of income measures.

### a. Median incomes

The median income indicates the actual income of the middle-income earner in the population. In the scenario above, the median income would be that of the midpoint between the 3rd and 4th income earner. The middle-income earner is making $20,000/year, a picture that illustrates the actual environment for the majority, but does not provide any evidence of the incomes for anyone else. In reality, the difference between the average and median incomes of all Canadians is substantial. The average income in 2000 was $29,769 while the median income was $7500 less, at $22,120

(Statistics Canada, 2001a). It is interesting to note the difference between the mean and the median—when the mean is higher, it has been swayed by the preponderance of very high incomes.

The problem with both the average and the median income measures is that they tell us very little about the incomes of those outside of the middle range—and the average actually tells us nothing about income earners at all, as our hypothetical example shows us. For those of us wanting to uncover the lived reality for Canadians, we have to turn to other income measures that explore various income groups, how they change in relationship over time and reveal the trends that occur during various time periods, such as the last generation, the last decade and different cycles of booms and busts.

### b. Quintiles

A recent study by the Canadian Labour Congress (2003) reveals how the most recent changes in income are spread across different slices of the population, namely quintiles (or 20% segments) of the population.

From this analysis, we can establish that, in fact, the reported gains in income for Canadian families over the past year were misleading. It is unequally borne by different sections of the population; the poorer one is, the more likely one is to have actually lost income during this last year.

One might claim that this loss is not much of a difference. In reality, the loss at the bottom was quite minimal (just over $400). So maybe we are just making a fuss over relatively inconsequential issues. The value of these dollars for low income earners is, however, significant as $400 can represent the purchase of winter clothing for your children or being able to sustain telephone service.

## Table 2.1: Distribution of market income by quintile, 2000 and 2001

| Market income | 2000 | 2001 | % Change 2000–2001 |
|---|---|---|---|
| Bottom Quintile | $8,781 | $8,362 | -4.77% |
| Second Quintile | $32,688 | $32,362 | -1.00% |
| Middle Quintile | $54,115 | $54,127 | +0.02% |
| Fourth Quintile | $78,039 | $78,389 | +0.45% |
| Top Quintile | $142,451 | $145,580 | +2.20% |

Data Source: Statistics Canada, Survey of Labour and Income Dynamics

Market income is income earned through employment (waged and self-employment) plus the value of gains on investments cashed in during the year.

Source: Canadian Labour Congress. (2003). *Economy: Economic review and outlook* 14(2). Fall. Ottawa: Canadian Labour Congress.

To establish if these findings are typical or atypical, we need to turn to both longer term analysis and more detailed analysis, for the quintile investigation likely smooths over variations within these groups.

### c. Deciles and ratios

In 1998, the Centre for Social Justice published an explosive report on the growing gap in Canada—an attempt to understand the nature of inequality in Canada and how it had changed over time. This study turned away from the traditional evaluation of quintiles in favor of deciles and allowed for exploration of greater nuances of life at both margins—the top 10% of income earners and the bottom 10% of income earners. The preferred statistic in this situation was the ratio of the top and bottom 10%, and an assessment of how they had varied over time. The study in 1998 was repeated in 1999, with the cumulative findings replicated below.

These findings revealed burgeoning inequality (as the ratio exploded from double to triple digits) yet showed some good news in its narrowing from 1993 to 1997. This good news appeared to stem from an eventual improvement of low income four years into an unprecedented economic boom.

## Table 2.2: Distribution of market income by decile

| Market income earnings | 1981 | 1984 | 1989 | 1993 | 1997 |
|---|---|---|---|---|---|
| Poorest 10% | 4,866 | 1,938 | 3,741 | 511 | 1,255 |
| Richest 10% | 122,964 | 125,056 | 144,699 | 131,412 | 136,394 |
| Ratio | 25.27 | 64.53 | 36.68 | 257.17 | 108.68 |

Data Source: Statistics Canada, Survey of Consumer Finances

Source: Yalnizyan, A. (1998). *The growing gap: A report on growing inequality between the rich and poor in Canada.* Toronto: Centre for Social Justice; Yalnizyan, A. (2000). *Canada's great divide: The politics of the growing gap between rich and poor in the 1990s.* Toronto: Centre for Social Justice.

**d. Horizontal measures: Boom and bust cycles**

The next report from the Centre for Social Justice (Curry-Stevens, 2001) used a different measure of inequality. The measure used in the earlier reports was unduly influenced by relatively small increases in income, resulting in a shrinking of the gap during the economic boom cycle of the last ten years. The calculations work as follows:

Let's say that the poorest Canadian families earned $1,000 in 1995 and the richest earned $100,000. Using the ratio measure, the gap ratio is 100, that is the richest 10% earn 100 times more than the poorest 10%. Let's then say that in the next year, the poorest Canadians earn $2,000 and the richest earn $110,000. According to the ratio calculation, the measure of inequality drops to 55—and it appears that there is a drastic shrinking of inequality in the country. Yet the distance between the two income earning groups has increased since the poor got richer by only $1,000 while the richest earned an additional $10,000. It is the significance of the changes in incomes of the poorest that unduly influence this measure—and we know that their incomes are highly volatile.

Seeking to remedy this situation, the third report on the status of inequality in Canada from the Centre for Social Justice turned to a horizontal measure of inequality (as used in the report of the Canadian Labour Congress), that of measuring the performance of each decile over time and comparing the performance of different income groups. Additionally, the CSJ report analyzed the trends within economic cycles to see how incomes were affected by upturns and downturns in the economy. Those seeking to silence complaints about the market had increasingly voiced an argument akin to, "Well, we are likely entering a recession, so it is more important that we do x, y or z than to put more money into income supports for poor people" (feel free to put whatever policy alternative you want in this sentence, such as cut program spending, reduce corporate taxes, weaken labour legislation that in reality makes life more difficult for many Canadians).

The CSJ report, entitled "When markets fail people" was prepared with the intention of exploring the income performance of the deciles over the last two recessions (1981–1984 and 1989–1993) and the last three recovery periods (1973–1981, 1984–1989, and 1993–1998). The patterns of economic performance were dramatic. For the bottom income earners, the last two recessions saw a drop in income of 60% and 86%, yet their income recovery performance during the boom years were actually negative in the first boom, significant during the next (up by $1,803) and marginal in the third (up by $584). The companion data for the wealthiest Canadian families were that in the first recession they actually gained ground and had their incomes increase by 2%; the second saw their incomes drop by 9%. Yet during the recovery years, their incomes surged by $11,964, $19,643, and $17,158.

Turning our analysis to recovery periods, we find that all income groups eventually gain ground (with the sole exception of the poorest decile in the boom of the 1970s), but inequality widens dramatically as top incomes surge over the meager improvements made at lower levels. A supplemental calculation of "fair shares"

**Table 2.3: Market incomes during recessions (1981–1984 and 1989–1993)**

| | 1981 | 1984 | 1989 | 1993 | 1981 to 1984 | % Change | 1989 to 1993 | % Change |
|---|---|---|---|---|---|---|---|---|
| Decile 1 | 4,866 | 1,938 | 3,741 | 511 | -2,928 | 60% drop | -3,230 | 86% drop |
| Decile 2 | 21,296 | 14,853 | 19,000 | 10,392 | -6,443 | 30% drop | -8,608 | 45% drop |
| Decile 3 | 31,747 | 26,250 | 30,614 | 22,306 | -5,497 | 17% drop | -8,308 | 21% drop |
| Decile 4 | 39,395 | 35,117 | 39,879 | 32,314 | -4,278 | 11% drop | -7,565 | 16% drop |
| Decile 5 | 46,498 | 42,911 | 47,813 | 40,946 | -3,587 | 8% drop | -6,867 | 14% drop |
| Decile 6 | 53,187 | 50,073 | 55,508 | 49,611 | -3,114 | 6% drop | -5,897 | 11% drop |
| Decile 7 | 60,886 | 57,708 | 63,945 | 59,216 | -3,178 | 5% drop | -4,729 | 7% drop |
| Decile 8 | 69,739 | 66,739 | 74,681 | 70,012 | -3,000 | 4% drop | -4,669 | 6% drop |
| Decile 9 | 83,169 | 80,433 | 89,707 | 84,782 | -2,736 | 3% drop | -4,925 | 5% drop |
| Decile 10 | 122,964 | 125,056 | 144,699 | 131,412 | +2,092 | 2% increase | -13,287 | 9% drop |

Date source: Unpublished data from Statistics Canada, Survey of Consumer Finances. All figures are in constant 1997 dollars.

Source: Curry-Stevens, A. (2001). When markets fail people: Exploring the widening gap between rich and poor in Canada. Toronto: CSJ Foundation for Research and Education.

was done on the data—if the data distribution was to stay constant, each decile would receive 10% of the income gains. Our analysis revealed that every decile below 7— for every economic boom over the last 30 years—got less than their fair share. It is only the top three deciles that got more than their fair share. As consistent with our growing pessimism about the market, we find that the top decile takes the lion's share of all income improvements and that this share accelerates across the decades.

Noted is the failure to achieve fairness. This "fair share" approach would have sustained existing levels of inequality. We did not even consider whether remedial

**Table 2.4: Market incomes during recoveries (1973–1981, 1984–1989, and 1994–1998)**

| | 1973 | 1981 | 1884 | 1989 | 1994 | 1998 | 1973 –81 | 1984 –89 | 1994 –98 |
|---|---|---|---|---|---|---|---|---|---|
| Decile 1 | 5,386 | 4,866 | 1,938 | 3,741 | 733 | 1,317 | ($520) | $1,803 | $584 |
| Decile 2 | 20,245 | 21,296 | 14,853 | 19,000 | 11,874 | 13,809 | $1,051 | $4,147 | $1,935 |
| Decile 3 | 29,189 | 31,747 | 26,250 | 30,614 | 24,715 | 26,093 | $2,558 | $4,364 | $1,378 |
| Decile 4 | 35,824 | 39,395 | 35,117 | 39,879 | 34,761 | 36,456 | $3,571 | $4,762 | $1,695 |
| Decile 5 | 41,752 | 46,498 | 42,911 | 47,813 | 43,510 | 46,073 | $4,746 | $4,902 | $2,563 |
| Decile 6 | 47,747 | 53,187 | 50,073 | 55,508 | 52,117 | 55,679 | $5,440 | $5,435 | $3,562 |
| Decile 7 | 54,239 | 60,886 | 57,708 | 63,945 | 61,091 | 65,562 | $6,647 | $6,237 | $4,471 |
| Decile 8 | 62,495 | 69,739 | 66,739 | 74,681 | 71,615 | 76,851 | $7,244 | $7,942 | $5,236 |
| Decile 9 | 74,113 | 83,169 | 80,433 | 89,707 | 87,225 | 94,122 | $9,056 | $9,274 | $6,897 |
| Decile 10 | 111,000 | 122,964 | 125,056 | 144,699 | 135,509 | 152,667 | $11,964 | $19,643 | $17,158 |

Data source: Unpublished data from Statistics Canada, Survey of Labour and Income Dynamics, and Survey of Consumer Finances. All figures are in constant 1997 dollars.

Source: Curry-Stevens, A. (2001) When markets fail people: Exploring the widening gap between rich and poor in Canada. Toronto: CSJ Foundation for Research and Education.

allocations of income could occur whereby the poor would receive more income gains than the rich, reducing the gap.

The comparison of these two performances is dramatic. Recessions cause the poor to lose far more earning power than any other group; yet after shouldering these huge losses, they fail to catch up during recoveries—putting to rest the possibility that when full economic cycles are considered, these trends have a negligible effect on inequality. For decades, we have asked the working class to tighten their belts during recessions and have made promises that when the economy improves, more benefits will be allocated. Recovery times allow the rich to accelerate their earnings with minor gains resulting for the poor. This performance is pervasive over each economic cycle, and throughout the last generation (approximately 25 years); the trends have worsened with inequality being experienced more deeply across the population.

The data reveals a deeply troubling finding—that the market incomes of the bottom 30% of Canadian families were less in 1998 than they were in 1973. Troubling trends also exist for the middle class, who are basically treading water, gaining little ground, and have to cope with the rapid distancing of those richer than they.

## Population measures of inequality

We now turn our attention to the shifting profile of the population and explore the numbers of people living at these different income levels. Such investigation provides insights as to the changing nature of our class structure. First let us explore this theoretically. Prior to the rapid expansion of waged labour and the industrial revolution

in the 19th century, the distribution of the population was pyramid-shaped, with the vast majority living in poverty. Through the 19th century and much of the 20th century, there was a massive expansion of the middle class as many moved up the income ladder and, to a lesser degree, an expansion of the wealthy. These trends resulted in the class structure becoming "apple-shaped," and it was seen as a healthy sign of a flourishing democracy. A strong and stable middle class, with potentiality for upward mobility, seemed to mark the golden age of capitalism (1940s to 1970s). We now investigate, statistically, the form that our population now takes.

Yalnizyan (1998) profiled the proportion of Canadian families in 1973 and in 1996 who were living at different income levels. Taking the decile distribution of 1973 and then measuring how much of the population was now based at those levels, she uncovered a grave hollowing out of the middle class. Where middle-income earners formerly composed 60% of the population, this value slipped to just 44% by 1996. While the middle class shrank, the ranks of the very poor and the very rich rose significantly. This was the generational picture of the inequality from 1973 to 1996— but without the fuller picture of distribution for 1973, we do not know what form our class structure had, although we know it was more divided and polarized from that time on.

Subsequently, Curry-Stevens (2003) examined the shifting concentration along various ranges of income, and provides a clearer picture of how the population is shaped at the start and the end of the last two decades.

From this study, we can see that the income distribution of Canadian families is changing quite dramatically, especially if we examine how the recovery and recession

Social Determinants of Health

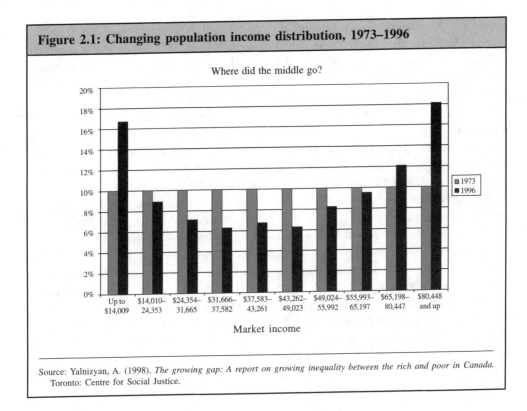

Figure 2.1: Changing population income distribution, 1973–1996

Where did the middle go?

Market income

Source: Yalnizyan, A. (1998). *The growing gap: A report on growing inequality between the rich and poor in Canada.* Toronto: Centre for Social Justice.

times impact the population. The size of the middle class, relative to other income groups, decreased by 17% over the last 20 years.

Surprisingly, losses are experienced in both the recovery (-5.6%) and recession (-5.0%) periods. This is counterintuitive. We would

Table 2.5: Distribution of market incomes of Canadian families 1980 to 2000, highlighting most recent recession and recovery data, as well as data for last 2 decades.

|  | Poor | Working poor | Struggling | Middle class | Well off | Rich | Very rich | TOTAL |
|---|---|---|---|---|---|---|---|---|
|  | < $5,000 | $5,000 - $19,999 | $20,000 - $29,999 | $30,000 - $59,999 | $60,000 - $99,999 | $100,000 - $149,999 | >$150,000 | rounded to nearest 1% |
| 1980 | 7.3% | 10.1% | 8.1% | 34.7% | 29.7% | 8.0% | 2.2% | 100% |
| 1989 | 7.7% | 10.6% | 8.5% | 32.1% | 28.1% | 9.6% | 2.9% | 100% |
| 1993 | 10.9% | 12.9% | 9.9% | 30.5% | 25.0% | 8.4% | 2.3% | 100% |
| 2000 | 7.3% | 12.0% | 8.7% | 28.8% | 27.9% | 11.1% | 4.3% | 100% |
| Calculations |  |  |  |  |  |  |  |  |
| Recovery | -33.0% | -7.0% | -12.1% | -5.6% | 11.6% | 32.1% | 87.0% |  |
| Recession | 41.6% | 21.7% | 16.5% | -5.0% | -11.0% | -12.5% | -20.7% |  |
| 2 Decades | 0.0% | 23.0% | 6.9% | -17.0% | -6.1% | 38.8% | 95.5% |  |

Source: Curry-Stevens, A. (2003). "Arrogant capitalism: Changing futures, changing lives," *Canadian review of social policy* 51(June), 137–142.

expect that the economy would generate an increasing middle class as the ranks of the poor and struggling move up the ladder. We were led to believe that a thriving middle class is the foundation of a healthy democracy. However the economy is not generating such an outcome.

The chart also reveals another troubling dynamic. Note the pattern of those earning between $60,000 and $99,999 a year. This well off group has shrunk by 6.1% over the last two decades. The erosion of the size of this group creates a structural barrier to a more affluent Canada, whereby decreasing odds of moving up thwarts the middle class. The ranks of the economic elite are growing in strength, drawing in numbers from those well off, but not being replaced by mobility upwards from the middle class.

New research more fully examines the profile of our changing class structure over the last 21 years. For this study, we profile the population distribution according to income levels and compare the 1980 and 2001 patterns. Such investigation allows us to address the shifting structures and companion problems.

We can see that population measures of economic inequality reveal profound changes in our class structure, with the predominant features of the 1973 to 1996 being an erosion of the middle class and rising ranks of the wealthy and the poor. This hollowing out brings to mind an image of the "apple" going rotten. The data taking us to 2001 shows that not only are Canadians marginally more likely to be destitute (making less than $10,000) but are also more likely to be working poor (earning less than $30,000). They are also much less likely to earn incomes up to $80,000, and join the ranks of the well off. Yet they are more likely to be rich and very rich—meager consolation given the scenario facing the majority of Canadians.

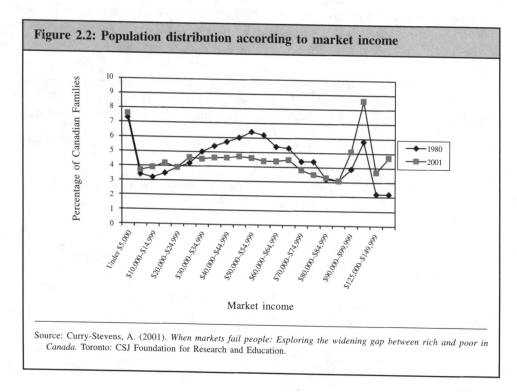

**Figure 2.2: Population distribution according to market income**

Percentage of Canadian Families

Market income

Source: Curry-Stevens, A. (2001). *When markets fail people: Exploring the widening gap between rich and poor in Canada.* Toronto: CSJ Foundation for Research and Education.

Social Determinants of Health

## Taxes and transfers: Establishing our lived experiences

We have been reviewing market incomes in Canada because of their prime generative role in creating inequality. Turning to the role of transfers and taxes (the redistributive factors), we simultaneously focus on the incomes that people actually live on. Government transfers provide them with additional income through pensions, welfare and unemployment benefits (the principal transfers), but taxes reduce income in order to pay for essential services and such transfers. Overall, these interventions have an equalizing effect, as they serve to raise the incomes of those at the bottom (through transfers) and lower the incomes at the top (through income taxes). Our key areas of concern are the trends in these taxes and transfers—issues that rest with the government and various politicians in power. It is government policy that determines levels of taxes and transfers, and thus patterns of redistribution.

Overall, this redistributive effect serves to dramatically reduce inequality. Before taxes and transfers, the inequality between rich and poor is in the triple digits—with the richest 10% earning 109 times the income of the poorest 10%. When taxes and transfers are added, the ratio drops (in 1997) to 7.15 (Yalnizyan, 2000). The cumulative effect is obviously significant and progressive. But the study of Yalnizyan was not a good news story. For while this ratio shows the moderating effect of government policy, it also showed that this effect has become less significant over the last generation. Her data revealed that the ratio has been growing for the last 4 years, from a low of 6.22 to levels not seen since the early 1980s.

Put another way, our governments have become increasingly tolerant of income inequality and are cutting the mechanisms that promote income equality. Specifically,

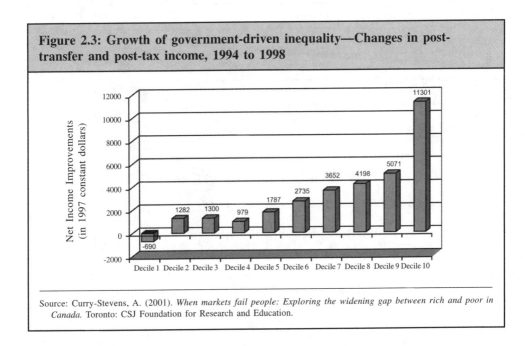

**Figure 2.3: Growth of government-driven inequality—Changes in post-transfer and post-tax income, 1994 to 1998**

Source: Curry-Stevens, A. (2001). *When markets fail people: Exploring the widening gap between rich and poor in Canada.* Toronto: CSJ Foundation for Research and Education.

drops in income transfers (with employment insurance coverage being dramatically reduced at the federal level and social assistance reduced in many provinces) and decreased progressivity in our income tax system serve to increase inequality. The significance of these mechanisms must be appreciated—for as the attack on government spending occurred at the start of the 1980s, so too did the attack on the progressive tax system.

From the perspective of those concerned with equality, such moves by the federal and provincial governments are indefensible, leading as they have to a net loss of income at the bottom decile during this most recent era of economic growth. Again, we witness the pulling away of the top income group—in whose ranks we find our political and economic leaders. This trend generates concerns about the growing social isolation of the rich from the majority population below them.

## Wealth measures

A final method to measure inequality is the measure of wealth. This is the total sum of the value of all assets minus all debts owed, and allows us to review the cumulative impact of years of differential incomes on the net assets of various groups within the population. The years of available statistics are limited to 1984 and 1999, a problem moderated somewhat by the more stable nature of wealth—as opposed to income measures (Statistics Canada, 2001b). The exception to this stability is the value of assets held in the stock market, volatile in recent years, and substantially more

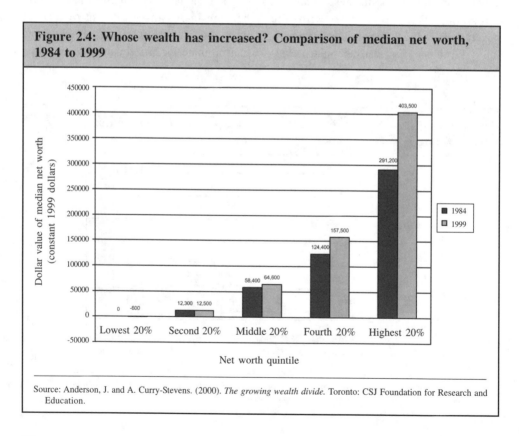

**Figure 2.4: Whose wealth has increased? Comparison of median net worth, 1984 to 1999**

Source: Anderson, J. and A. Curry-Stevens. (2000). *The growing wealth divide*. Toronto: CSJ Foundation for Research and Education.

Social Determinants of Health

significant for upper income groups and of rapidly shrinking significance as one moves down the prosperity ladder.

Again, the average wealth measure paints a rosy picture, with an 11% increase measured in median wealth of Canadian families. The decile picture reveals an answer to the question: "For whom is this true?" by showing the distribution of these effects. The poorest 10% of Canadian families actually lost ground and now owe more than they own, with their median net worth set at -$2100. The richest 10% of families saw their wealth increase by a dramatic 53% to a value of $703,500, while the richest 20% of families had their wealth rise by 39%. Figure 2.4 shows the uneven distribution of improvements (by quintile) in wealth over the last 15 years.

## Hardest hit populations

Within patterns of income are features that put a face to inequality today. Increasingly, that face is racialized, destitute, and young. These features are not exclusive to such groups, but market and government trends have been most damaging to them. As we consider the growth in income inequality, severe social consequences in different communities emerge. Two such communities are covered in this chapter: the poorest Canadians and people of colour.

### a. The poorest Canadians

Those at the bottom of the income ladder, in the poorest decile and quintile, have already been shown to be exhibiting the worst form of market failure—for their incomes are completely insufficient to sustain their families or themselves. They lose by far the most in recessions (up to 86% of their incomes were lost in the last recession) and fail to gain much ground in recoveries (earning only another $584 in the last recovery). In fact, when surveying the total income for the bottom decile, Curry-Stevens (2001) showed that 91% of the total income derives from government transfers. In an era of cuts to transfers (most notably employment insurance and welfare), it is the poorest income groups that suffer by far the most. It is perhaps noteworthy that more than 40% of families derive at least 10% of their incomes from government transfers—and that this level drops below 5% for the top four deciles.

The poverty rates themselves have fluctuated according to the point within the economic cycle in which they are measured. While the incidence of poverty has gone down in this last economic boom (and this is truly good news), it remains higher than the level reached in 1989. Scott (2002) has compiled the rates shown in Table 2.6.

Further calculations by Scott reveal that the news is not as good as originally assessed.

---

**Box 2.1**

"It is common, among the non-poor, to think of poverty as a sustainable condition—austere, perhaps, but they get by somehow, don't they? They are always 'with us.' What is harder for the non-poor to see is poverty as acute distress: The lunch that consists of Doritos or hot dog rolls, leading to faintness before the end of the shift. The 'home' is also a car or a van. The illness or injury that must be 'worked through' with gritted teeth because there's no sick pay and the loss of one day's pay will mean no groceries for the next." (Ehrenreich, 2001, p. 214)

---

## Table 2.6: Selected poverty rates

| Rate of Poverty | 1989 | 1993 | 1996 | 2000 |
|---|---|---|---|---|
| All Canadians | 13.9% | 17.7% | 18.5% | 14.7% |
| Children | 14.7% | 21.0% | 21.1% | 16.5% |
| Working age | 12.1% | 15.7% | 17.3% | 13.7% |
| Seniors | 22.5% | 22.7% | 19.7% | 16.4% |

Based on before-tax "Low Income Cut-Offs"

Source: Scott, K. (2002). *A lost decade: Income inequality and the health of Canadians.* Presentation to the *Social determinants of health across the lifespan* conference. Toronto: November 2002.

While the levels of poverty have gone down, the depths of poverty have increased. The poverty gap measures the distance below the poverty line that the poor live. All groups except lone-parent families are worse off than they were in 1989, living typically $1,000 deeper in poverty.

### b. People of colour

Racialized groups in Canada face a strong earnings disadvantage compared to whites. In 1998, the racialized population earned 30% less than whites, and they were 2.3 times more likely to live in poverty (Galabuzi, 2001). Furthermore, the economic performance of recent immigrants is deteriorating, with real incomes falling, on average, 7% from 1980 to 2000—this despite general income growth of 7% for Canadian-born men (Frenette and Morisette, 2003).

Several hypotheses have surfaced to explain these differences. Each one is refuted in turn:

1. It is because they are immigrants. No. White immigrants earn an average of 22% more than immigrants of colour—thus showing that most of the difference is a function of skin colour and much less due to immigrant status (Galabuzi, 2001).

2. It is because they are not as well educated. No. When we compare recent immigrants to the Canadian-born population, 44% of recent male immigrants have a university degree while only 19% of those Canadian-born are similarly accomplished. The pattern for women is similar but less pronounced. Even in the 1980s, the educational attainment of new immigrants was double that of the Canadian-born (Frenette and Morisette, 2001).

3. It is because of their language skills. No. The Canadian government demands competency in one of the two official languages to be eligible for immigration. They may be strongly accented but will have English language proficiency.

There is one other possible causative factor—that the length of time in Canada affects the type of jobs available, and thus it would be unreasonable to expect that new entries to the job market would have earnings parity with more seasoned workers. In considering this issue, we turn to Frenette and Morisette (2003). Seeking to understand how earnings between immigrants and non-immigrants could achieve parity, they

Social Determinants of Health

reviewed the economic performance of immigrants who arrived during different time periods with those Canadian-born. For immigrants who arrived within the last 5 years, incomes have been dramatically lower than the Canadian-born workers. In 2000, recent immigrant men earned 28% less than Canadian men. This is double the rate of 1980, indicating a deepening of the employment crisis for new immigrants. For women, the difference is even greater; they earn 31% less than their Canadian-born counterparts.

Frenette and Morisette's investigation of the longer-term impact of immigration status is also profoundly unsettling. Fifteen years after arrival, immigrants who arrived between 1985 and 1989 earned between 15% and 24% less than non-immigrants. Earlier immigrants fared better—those arriving from 1975–1979 earned only 13% less. One troubling consequence is the "potential drop in immigrants' permanent income, and, in the absence of offsetting changes in their savings rates, a potential decline in immigrants' wealth and precautionary savings .... Recent immigrants will be more likely to have difficulty making ends meet and will also be more vulnerable to shocks such as job loss or unexpected expenditures" (Frenette and Morisette, 2003, p. 15).

Immigrant workers can be expected to sustain this pattern over time, unless there is "abnormally high earnings growth in the future" (Frenette and Morisette, 2003, p. 1). Such "abnormal" growth could be induced by an array of policy initiatives such as employment equity or acceptance at par of foreign credentials or foreign work experience, interventions that have been largely voluntary as opposed to mandatory (with the notable exception of the federal government's commitment to employment equity within the public service).

It seems we are ignoring the obvious— that instead of immigration status, education or language skills, the problem is one of skin colour, and that racism in our institutions and individual behaviors is the strongest component of the differential earnings level.

Is this a fair accusation to level at Canadian society—a country that prides itself in its racial diversity and its embrace of immigrants from all countries around the world? Digging a little below this superficial image, one finds a strong legacy of racism, land theft, colonization, occupational segregation, and even slavery. Few know it, but 200 years of slavery existed from the early 1600s to 1833, followed shortly thereafter by ongoing segregation in schools and other institutions. Racism was deemed legal by Canada's highest court (until 1939) and Ontario segregated Black students up until 1964.

The marginalization of Native people that began in the 1600s continues today, with Aboriginal rights limited to reserves— severely curtailing the political and social rights of Aboriginals who live off-reserve. The continued failure of the federal government to introduce Aboriginal self-government and to resolve outstanding land claims serves to maintain the marginalization and exploitation of Aboriginals. The residential school system of 1879 to the mid-1980s served to forcibly remove children from their homes, deny them access to their families and culture and force British culture into their mouths and bodies. Aboriginal communities throughout the country continue to struggle with recovery.

What do we imagine the impact of this history to be? Pronounced labour issues that exist today carry over from more clearly apparent exploitation. Modern-day servants exist in the form of those who clean our toilets, wash our dishes, package our foods, mow our lawns, care for our children, sew our clothes, drive us around, and harvest our foods. Such occupations are typically low-wage and rely heavily on the labour of racialized groups. We must ask ourselves how much our legacy of slavery creates the employment conditions of these occupations. Is our ongoing failure to adequately pay those who service the needs of whites a carry over of slavery and how we view those who perform such tasks?

We must face this history, and the companion evidence of reports that illustrate racism is embedded in various Canadian systems: criminal justice (Commission on Systemic Racism in the Ontario Criminal Justice System, 1994), education (Canadian Race Relations Foundation, 1999; Lewis, 1992), immigration (Canadian Council for Refugees, 2000), public service (Task Force on the Participation of Visible Minorities in the Federal Public Service, 2000), housing (Ornstein, 1994 and 1999), and employment (Abella, 1984; Canada Employment and Immigration Advisory Council, 1992).

## Summary of findings

Reviewing the data in this chapter, we uncover the following problems with the distribution of market income, total income, and wealth:

1.  Inequality is growing, with the performance of the market serving to deepen the economic (and consequently social) gap between rich and poor.
2.  The severity of these problems is accelerating through the last generation, as incomes at the top surge and those at the bottom falter.
3.  There is much greater income volatility at the bottom of the income ladder, and less as the ladder

is climbed. This form of insecurity (the unpredictability of poverty in any given time-span) necessitates assured incomes through social transfers.

4.  The lowest incomes are completely inadequate to live on, with the bottom decile being destitute and the next decile earners living well below the poverty line. Even the third decile is below the poverty line. Despite recent improvements in the poverty levels, they still are higher than 1989—leading us to conclude that the market is unable to provide sufficient work or income for the most marginal Canadians.

5.  The ratio of top earners to bottom earners moves from double digits in the 1970s and 1980s and enters triple digit inequality in the 1990s. Different measures of this gap generate different theories as to whether the gap is widening or narrowing. Earlier ratio measures have been discarded in favor of absolute measures.

5.  Upward income mobility is harder to achieve today than 20 years ago. There has been an erosion of upper (but not top) income groups in society; it is harder today to break out of middle incomes and into upper incomes.

7.  Governments today are tolerating more inequality; the post-tax, post-transfer income measures reveal a trend towards greater inequality. The erosion of the progressive nature of income taxes and transfers is responsible for this change.

8.  Greater reliance on markets for the overall financial well-being of its

citizens can be proclaimed a dismal failure—for both absolute and relative inequality, but most poignantly for relative inequality. Today we are a much more socially and economically divided nation, with lives increasingly prescribed by the fortunes and misfortunes of our birth.

9. The particularly vulnerable position for people of colour reflects deep racial divisions within our society, divisions that are exacerbated by income inequality and occupational segregation.

## Solutions

Let us distinguish the various forms of solution that exist—policy solutions, campaign solutions and vision-based solutions—all of which provide insights as to how to reduce income inequality. While more questions may surface as one becomes familiar with the existing research, this author gives little priority to further research. The trends are established, are durable, and are largely resistant to minor tinkering. We have proven our case—it is time to move to solutions.

There are several sources for quite comprehensive "shopping lists" of policy solutions. We direct the reader to those covered in each of the three Centre for Social Justice reports on the growing gap. Items covered include strategies to address jobs, wages, services, and supports and specifically include items such as a living wage, increased access to unionized jobs, employment equity, and reversing the trends towards free trade and corporate globalization.

Specific attractive policies include improved unionization access—for the median income for non unionized workers in 2002 is $13.80/hour while those who are union covered earn $19.60/hour—a union wage advantage of $5.80/hour (Canadian Labour Congress, 2003). Such too is the benefit for racialized workers, as the union advantage for racialized workers serves to dramatically lower the earnings gap from approximately 30% to 8%, meaning that racialized workers earn incomes that much more closely reach those of whites when they are union members (Galabuzi, 2001).

These lists are a combination of returning to what worked in the past (more reliance on progressive taxation, higher overall tax revenues and increased social spending on both services and income supports) and innovative solutions that have worked in other countries (guaranteed annual incomes, living wages that take income earners above the poverty line, reduced work weeks that increase overall employment levels and creation of disincentives for excessive corporate incomes). While there is reticence on the part of the progressive community to return to the days of old (especially given the successful campaigns of the right that have undermined support for a healthy tax base), it was a system that worked to provide base minimums of support to those who needed it. Ask anyone denied employment insurance or who suffered cuts to welfare cheques, to whom the days of old look pretty good.

The problem with such shopping lists is that they are just that—a list of possible interventions. When proposed, they offer no sense of strategic priorities or sense of agreement on which interventions would yield better results than others. That is the job of social movement organizations and coalitions that would actually select one or two specific initiatives that then form the base for a campaign. In order to shift from the shopping list to the campaign priorities, we need an assessment of the viability of various policy initiatives, which in turn requires assessments of the resources within social movements and which issues stand a chance of winning—entailing full consideration of the decision makers on the issues, whether broad public support can be activated, and whether political will can be generated for the initiative.

Vision-based solutions attempt to present a different vision for Canada, serving to galvanize citizens around particular objectives and directions. While most typically articulated by political parties (especially during political campaigns), the lack of such political visioning has given rise to non-governmental groups doing such work. One example is the process conducted by the Canadian Policy Research Network, as they engaged 408 citizens in a dialogue on Canada's future.

Occasionally, governments themselves pass motions that are visionary in orientation. The all-party motion passed in 1989 to end child poverty by the year 2000 was one such initiative that served to generate considerable public interest, yet failed dismally in ending or even reducing child poverty.

We close with a vision for the future of economic inequality that stems from the analysis conducted in this paper:

We must proclaim that the market fails more and more of us at an accelerated pace, resulting in a growth of both absolute and relative inequality. The most significant of these trends is the growing social exclusion of the economic and political elite who exhibit their arrogance by an array of both social and economic policies that serve narrow self-interests. Their isolation by gender, race and class serves to deepen the emerging crisis of mistrust in our political leadership. It is time for a redirection of our collective resources that ensures that the social identity of our birth does not dictate our life's achievements. It is time to educate ourselves as to this reality and build a nation that ensures decency of jobs and wages for all working people and extends compassionate support to those who slip through our existing systems.

## Conclusion

As we enter 2004, cracks are appearing in the armor of conservative pundits—who have, through their faulty economic performance, induced their own political losses in several areas of Canada, most notably Ontario and Toronto. The Tory agenda of downsizing, privatization, and deregulation has destabilized quality of life and moved political sensibilities further to the left. Concurrently, movements for democratic reforms are moving to the forefront—for the problems of income inequality have strong ties to the activities of our political leadership (including both elected officials and top bureaucrats).

It is imperative for us to loudly proclaim the failures of the market to deliver enough decent jobs, especially for those at and close to the bottom of the income ladder. The incomes are insufficient, and the burdens placed on the tax and transfer system (i.e., the

"Now that the overwhelming majority of the poor are out there toiling in Wal-Mart or Wendy's—well, what are we to think of them? Disapproval or condescension no longer apply, so what outlook makes sense? Guilt, you may be thinking warily. Isn't that what we're supposed to feel? But guilt doesn't go anywhere near far enough; the appropriate emotion is shame—shame at our own dependency, in this case, on the underpaid labour of others. When someone works for less pay than she can live on—when, for example, she goes hungry so that you can eat more cheaply and conveniently—then she has made a great sacrifice for you, she has made you a gift of some part of her abilities, her health and her life ... the working poor neglect their own children so that the children of others will be cared for; they live in substandard housing so that other homes will be shiny and perfect; they endure privation so that inflation will be low and stock prices high ... Some day, of course ... they are bound to tire of getting so little in return and demand to be paid what they're worth. There'll be lots of anger when that day comes, and strikes and disruption. But the sky will not fall and we will all be better off for it in the end."
(Ehrenreich, 2001, p. 221)

government) to remedy this situation poise us for a deepening of the tax revolt movement, as Canadians seem inclined to focus their blame at the taxes they must pay as opposed to their low and stagnating incomes levels. Blame squarely rests with the market, and its inability to offer a decent living to enough of us.

So, what are we to do? The task is simultaneously pragmatic, tactical, and visionary. At its root, we must ensure that our politicians work in the best interests of us all. They must be separated from the moneyed interests that undermine their capacity to work for the common good, and be held to standards that illustrate deep understanding of their own privilege. It is time to engender boldness and courage in all of us to build a society with justice for all.

## Note

1. Most data in this chapter uses income measures on families—in which 85% of us reside. The reported data from the Centre for Social Justice refers to families (with one or two parents) raising dependent children.

## Recommended readings

Canadian Centre for Policy Alternatives. (2004). *The alternative federal budget 2004: Rebuilding the foundations.* Ottawa: Canadian Centre for Policy Alternatives.
    This document provides an excellent assessment of government spending and income collection—and yields a balanced budget that favors the interests of middle and lower income Canadians. Anyone seriously interested in the alternatives to corporate domination and the levers that exist for governments to generate better incomes and services for the majority of Canadians should become familiar with the alternative budget process, conducted yearly by the CCPA.

Ehrenreich, B. (2001). *Nickel and dimes: On (not) getting by in America.* New York: Owl Books.
    This book is a profound narrative of the experiences of a journalist who goes undercover and works in several different low wage jobs, attempting to make ends meet. She works as a waitress, hotel maid, house

cleaner, nursing home aide, and Wal-Mart salesperson. This book is an easy and evocative read, leading the reader to contemplate issues of privilege and build considerable empathy with and outrage on behalf of the low wage workers of North America.

Ross, D., Scott, K., and Smith, P. (2000). *The Canadian fact book on poverty 2000*. Ottawa: Canadian Council on Social Development.

The CCSD makes a significant contribution to researchers by compiling and releasing data on that status of poverty in Canada. This text is supplemented by other reports on the progress of Canada's children and various policy discussions on issues related to social development. Its website (www.ccsd.ca) provides an excellent set of online resources.

Robinson, D. (2002). *The state of the economy.* Ottawa: Canadian Centre for Policy Alternatives.

This set of papers regularly published and available online at www.policyalternatives.ca is a current reading of the state of the economy, citing issues such as employment rates, economic growth, levels of debt and deficits and balance of payments with our trading partners. It goes further to document federal policy decisions and the impact they have on both revenues and expenditures.

Yalnizyan, A. (1998). *The growing gap: A report on growing inequality between the rich and poor in Canada.* Toronto: Centre for Social Justice.

This is the most comprehensive profile of the growing gap in Canada. Covering the broad measures as well as population-specific issues (gender, youth and seniors), this report provokes alarm and documents alternate policy options to narrow the gap. A must-read for beginning researchers on economic inequality in Canada.

## Related websites

Centre for Social Justice—www.socialjustice.org
  a.   Three annual reports on the status of inequality in Canada, published in 1998, 2000, and 2001.
  b.   Fact sheets on tax cuts and various other issues related to economic inequality and the growing gap. These fact sheets are very useful for education on inequality.

Canadian Centre for Policy Alternatives—www.policyalternatives.ca
  a.   The real bottom line. Issue #1—Taxes.
  b.   Ten tax myths, by Murray Dobbin (1999).
  c.   Tall tales about taxes, by Marc Lee (2000).
There is a significant but untold story about taxes, progressivity, and hidden bias towards the wealthy, as embedded in both federal and provincial taxes. These resources provide a great introduction to the current and pressing tax issues that have dramatic effects on inequality.

Campaign 2000 and the Child Poverty Working Groups—www.campaign2000.ca
  This website is an excellent source of child-centred information on federal and provincial budgets, political debates, and demographic reports. The campaign began shortly after the all-party motion to end child poverty by the year 2000. When it appeared that little progress was underway, a group of NGOs and associated researchers came together to influence public policy and to strengthen family life in Canada, with the goal of making sure that no Canadian child is raised in poverty. The deadline has come and gone, with 1/6 of Canadian children living in poverty.

# Chapter Three

## INCOME AND HEALTH IN CANADA

Nathalie Auger, Marie-France Raynault,
Richard Lessard, and Robert Choinière

## Introduction

Canadian social policies have for some time included poverty reduction as a goal. There has been a particular focus in eliminating poverty in groups at risk. Some policies have been successful, such as those focusing on poverty reduction among the elderly, and others unsuccessful, such as policies for reduction of childhood poverty (Barrett et al., 2003). Canada has also been a leader in generating income-related health research. In fact, many Canadian studies have shown there is a positive association between income and health (Wilkins et al., 2002).

At the provincial level, there is also a great interest in income issues by public health. For example, Quebec has for some time had provincial objectives for population health. These began with the 1992 Politique de la Santé et du Bien-Être which outlined six strategies for reaching nineteen population health objectives (MSSS, 1992). The strategies focused on developing personal skills, creating supportive environments, building healthy public policy, working with high risk groups, and improving life conditions. In the latter strategy, one specific objective was poverty reduction in families with young children. The 1992 objectives evolved over time into the current National Public Health Program which includes a multitude of health objectives in the domains of chronic disease, unintentional injury, infectious disease, environmental health, work-place health, and social health (Massé and Gilbert, 2003).

Even before Quebec's orientation towards poverty became explicit, public health officials in Montreal have been preoccupied with the effects of poverty on health. This concern led up to a 1998 study in the city of Montreal which showed that socio-economic differences had a large impact on the health of Montrealers at all stages of the life cycle (Lessard et al., 1998). This study, and other Quebec studies, have had a significant impact on public health policy in the province. They have also generated further research on income-related health inequality in Montreal.

In this chapter, we will focus on Canadian studies assessing the relationship between income and health. There are two general types of studies looking at income and health:

(1) those assessing the relationship between income and health, and (2) those assessing the relationship between income inequality and health. In Canada, most studies have been done using income per se. Consequently, this chapter focuses mainly on studies of income and health. Nevertheless, the relationship between income inequality and health remains important. Before turning to a discussion of these studies, a brief mention of their inherent characteristics and weaknesses is warranted.

## Characteristics of income–health studies

The problems found in studies assessing the relationship between income and health have been reviewed in detail elsewhere (Kawachi, 2000; Phipps, 2003). In this section, we will only provide a general overview in order to better understand the underlying concepts. Many of the critiques pertain to defining poverty. Others pertain to finding a suitable measure of poverty, which usually involves a measure of income. Unfortunately, income measures do not necessarily encompass factors such as social deprivation and social capital: the social aspects of poverty.

To further complicate matters, studies may use data in which the unit of measurement is at the macro (population) level, rather than at the micro (individual) level. The former have been called ecologic studies. Macro level analyses may also be subject to a bias called the ecologic fallacy, which occurs when macro level data are used to make inferences at the individual level. There are also criticisms of individual-level study designs. For example, cross-sectional studies which assess the poverty-health relationship at one point in time do not allow one to determine whether poverty preceded poor health. In fact, it is feasible that poor health precedes poverty. This bias has been called reverse causation (Phipps, 2003).

We will first discuss the definition of poverty. There is no clear consensus on what is meant by poverty. Although all measures of poverty are essentially relative, one option is to conceptualise poverty along the following aspects: absolute, relative, and subjective poverty (Phipps, 2003). (1) Absolute poverty usually refers to having less than an absolute minimum income level based on the cost of basic needs. One of the disadvantages of this definition is that it is difficult to objectively select a minimum set of necessities. Another disadvantage is that the cut-off changes over time. Although there is no official poverty line in Canada, the Statistics Canada low income cut-off has traditionally been used as such (Phipps, 2003). Recently, the market basket measure has been introduced as another tool to measure poverty (Human Resources Development Canada, 2003). (2) Relative poverty usually refers to having less than the average standard in society. This form of poverty is often measured as the proportion of individuals below a certain percentage of the median income (Phipps, 2003). (3) Subjective poverty refers to individuals feeling they do not have enough to meet their needs. Information on subjective poverty can be obtained from surveys. In industrialised countries, there is a general consensus that relative measures of poverty are more appropriate for studies on income and health (Phipps, 2003). In practice, however, studies tend to vary greatly on the type of indicator used to measure poverty.

Some of the indicators used to measure poverty in ecologic studies of income inequality include: (1) Proportion of aggregate income earned by the poorest proportion of households, (2) Ratio of income shares earned by the upper 90th percentile to the 10th percentile of households, and (3) a multitude of other indices. These studies have been critiqued for arbitrarily choosing indicators or for using data driven indicators (Kawachi, 2000). This critique has, however, been countered and it has been shown that income inequality studies usually reach the same conclusion irrespective of the indicator used (Kawachi, 1997).

The indicators selected for study may have other drawbacks, some of which may have implications for identifying the income-health relationship (Phipps, 2003): (1) The indicator may not reflect annual disposable income. Ideally, income should be calculated after taxes and governmental transfers. Likewise, income should take into account the costs of public services. If services such as health care are not publicly financed, disposable income will be reduced since individuals who rely more heavily on these services will have to pay out of pocket. (2) In households composed of more than one person, the indicator may not take into account the advantage of shared resources. Researchers have proposed equivalence scales to calculate income per person; however, the choice of equivalence scale may not be objective. Also, equivalence scales may not adjust for unequal sharing of resources within families. (3) The indicator may not take into account volatility of income. Long-term measures of income may be more appropriate. Alternatively, it may be that acute changes in income are more important determinants of health. (4) Indicators do not take into account accumulated assets or debts. (5) Indicators do not account for time required to acquire income. (6) It may be that depth of poverty,

or just how far income falls short of the poverty line, is more important. (7) Similarly, duration of poverty may be important. (8) The timing of poverty during the life cycle may play a role. Exposure to poverty during the early years of a child's life may have a greater effect on health (Phipps, 2003). (9) The study may not adequately adjust for other factors, known as confounders, that could account for the income-health relationship (Kawachi, 2000). Some studies use other measures of socio-economic status as a proxy for income (e.g., place of residence). This is because socio-economic data on ill or deceased individuals is not routinely collected in Canada.

These methodological constraints would lead one to question the validity of the income–health relationship. However, many researchers have countered these criticisms with credible arguments (Kawachi, 2000). Also, given that the number of studies finding positive associations between income and health continues to increase, the importance of income as a determinant of health becomes clear. We now turn to a discussion of some of the most recent studies.

## Canadian studies on income and health

In this section, we will focus only on a few of the studies that have been done in Canada, with a particular emphasis on a recent study done in an urban area of Quebec (Lessard et al., 2002). The Canadian evidence has been reviewed elsewhere and it is not the purpose of this chapter to repeat the findings (Wilkins et al., 2002; Phipps, 2003). Suffice to say that at least 17 Canadian studies of individual-level income data and 11 studies of small geographic area-based socio-economic data have found a link of income with health (Wilkins et al., 2002).

We will first mention an ecologic study done by Ross et al. (2000), which assessed the relation between income inequality and mortality in Canada and the United States using census data and vital statistics. Income inequality was defined as percentage of total household income received by the poorest 50% of households. The authors found that income inequality was lower in Canada than in the United States. They also found no statistical relation between income inequality and mortality at either the provincial or municipal level in Canada, while a strong relation existed in the United States. The authors speculate that the social policies widely present in Canada, but less so in the United States, could partly account for the differences in mortality (Ross et al., 2000). One of the implications of this study is that policies which reduce income inequality may be favourable for public health. However, this is questionable since recent evidence indicates that income inequality *is in itself* probably not responsible for poor population health (Mackenbach, 2002).

There is a large body of evidence linking income and health status in Canadian children (Phipps, 2003). The evidence has been summarised by the Canadian Institute of Child Health (Kidder et al., 2000). Briefly, this organisation has found income to be associated with low birth weight, injury-related mortality including fire and homicide deaths, developmental problems such as hyperactivity, psychosocial problems, delinquent behaviour, and delayed vocabulary development, amongst others. For many of these analyses, data was taken from the *National longitudinal survey of children and youth* and the *National population health survey* (Ross and Roberts, 1999). In a separate study by the Institut de la statistique du Québec, the investigators examined data from the 1998 *Longitudinal study of child development in Québec* (Séguin et al., 2001). They found that both overall and perceived health varied with income in 5-month olds, even after taking into account health at birth and other socio-demographics. However, some recent Canadian studies have found the relationship between income and children's health to be small in magnitude or statistically insignificant, especially when level of education of the mother is taken into account (Phipps, 2003). This relationship remains an ongoing debate.

Few Canadian studies have looked at trends over time. This issue was addressed in a recent ecologic study by Wilkins et al. (2002). The investigators examined changes in mortality rates by income in small geographic areas of urban Canada from 1971 to 1996. They divided their population into quintiles based on proportion of people in the neighbourhood below the low income cut-off. They measured life expectancy at birth, infant mortality, potential years of life lost (PYLL), income-related excess PYLL before age 75, cause-specific mortality rates, and various other indicators of health. They found that for most causes of death, differences in mortality between rich and poor neighbourhoods had diminished over the study period. However, some causes of death changed little and some, such as suicide mortality among females, had increased. They also estimated that, in 1996, 24% of total PYLL were related to income differences.

A recent study by the Institut de la statistique du Québec looked at the association between income and health over time using individual level data (Ferland, 2003). All data was taken from the 1987 Santé Québec survey and the 1998 *Enquête sociale et de santé*. In this study, individuals were classified into five groups based on gross income before taxes adjusted for household size. Health status for several outcomes (perceived health, mental health, long-term activity limitation, psychological stress, and functional gastrointestinal problems) was found to be negatively associated with gross annual income. Furthermore, the study concluded that there had been no weakening of the income-health relationship over time. In fact, for one health outcome, psychological stress, there appeared to be an increase in inequality of health outcomes between the richest and poorest individuals (Ferland, 2003).

The association between income and health has also been documented for risk factors of cardiovascular diseases in Canadian adults. In a cross-sectional study of data taken from the 1986 to 1992 provincial Canadian heart health surveys, increases in annual income were found to be associated with a progressive decrease in the prevalence of smoking, overweight, and physical inactivity (Choinière et al., 2000). Furthermore, the inverse relationship could also be seen when the analysis was repeated for each of the three regions of Canada (Atlantic, Central, and Western). The authors also found that level of education was highly associated with cardiovascular risk factors, even more so than income.

We will now turn to a study that was done on the urban health of Montrealers in 2002 (Lessard et al., 2002). But first, we will provide some background in order to better understand the origins of the Montreal study.

## The history of research on income and health in Montreal

The history of public health in Montreal dates back to the late nineteenth century when knowledge of infectious disease epidemiology was just beginning to develop. The first population health report, written in 1875, showed that mortality rates were not equal in the different neighbourhoods of Montreal. During epidemics of smallpox and scarlet fever in Montreal in the 1880s, poorer populations were found to be more susceptible to these diseases (Gaumer et al., 2002).

Since the 1970s, Canada has recognised that environmental factors have an important impact on the health of populations (Lalonde, 1974; Epp, 1986). In Quebec, public health departments began implementing programs to diminish the impact of poverty on the population. Despite these programs, little was known about the role of income on health in Montreal. This led up to a 1998 study in Montreal which looked closely at social inequality and its impact on health (Lessard et al., 1998). The study showed that poverty in Montreal was associated with health at all stages of the life cycle, including infant mortality, lung cancer, fertility rates, psychological distress, and suicide. The study, which was widely circulated in Quebec, spurred greater interest in social inequality as a determinant of health in Montrealers.

In a follow-up to the 1998 report, a more widespread study was conducted in 2002 on the urban health of Montrealers (Lessard et al., 2002). This second study included an analysis of the association between various indicators of socio-economic status and health. It confirmed the findings of the 1998 study and demonstrated that the health gap between rich and poor continued to exist in Montreal.

## The methods used in the 2002 Montreal study

Although the study looked at different factors affecting health, this discussion will focus mainly on the relationship between income and health. All health data were taken from provincial vital statistics, registries, and surveys (Lessard et al., 2002). Unfortunately, information on individual income is not available from most of these sources. The investigators therefore used proxy measures of income. The ecologic analysis was done in two ways (Choinière et al., 2003):

1. First, the investigators obtained income information by linking health data sets to the population census via the census tract. Like Wilkins et al. (2002), the analysis was based on the classification of census tracts according to proportion of individuals living below the low income cut-off before taxes. The low income cut-off is considered by Statistics Canada to be the income level where a family tends to spend a significantly higher proportion of its income on food, shelter, and clothing compared to the average family (Webber, 1998). It is based on family and community size. The investigators next stratified census tracts into five income groups (low, low average, average, high average, high) and examined a variety of health indicators by income quintile. For infant mortality, there was sufficient data to assess trends over time.

2. Second, the investigators examined health outcomes in different geographic areas of Montreal by linking health data sets to the population census via the CLSC district. The CLSC is a local community health centre that services a delineated district. There are 29 CLSC districts in Montreal.

These districts are relatively heterogeneous in terms of socio-demographic characteristics when compared to one another. The 29 CLSCs can be further grouped into six administrative sub-regions. These sub-regions were originally created by the Régie régionale de la santé et des services sociaux de Montréal-Centre for health planning purposes. They are referred to as West, West-central, North, South-west, East-central, and East. Morbidity and mortality was calculated for both CLSC districts and geographic sub-regions.

Lastly, the investigators made comparisons to other major Canadian cities. The investigators chose five Canadian cities with similar demographics, these being Ottawa, Toronto, Winnipeg, Calgary, and Vancouver. This part of the analysis was based on data from Statistics Canada and the Canadian Institute for Health Information (Choinière et al., 2003). Adjusted rates for a variety of health outcomes were compared between cities.

## What were the findings of the study?

Montreal is a city of 1.8 million residents living on an area about 500 km$^2$. About a quarter of the inhabitants are immigrants from outside Canada. Compared to the other Canadian cities in the study, Montreal fared relatively poorly for many of the socioeconomic indicators (Lessard et al., 2002). In 2000, Montreal had the lowest median income per household at $35,910, with Vancouver second at $42,026. In that same year, 29% of households lived below the Statistics Canada low income cut-off, while this figure was 14.1% in Calgary. In

1995, Montreal had the highest proportion of income derived from government transfers (16.5%). The proportion of income earned by the poorest half of households in that year was the lowest in the country at 18%; much lower than Ottawa and Calgary which were over 22%. Montreal had the highest unemployment rate at 10% in 2001, followed by Toronto's at 7.3%. In fact, Montreal has been called Canada's poverty capital (Lessard et al., 2002). Recently, however, analyses done using the market basket measure which takes into account the lower housing costs in Montreal have found Montrealers to be less poor than once thought (Human Resources Development Canada, 2003).

In terms of health status, Montreal varied markedly. The life expectancy of Montrealers is amongst the lowest of Canadian urban cities. Montreal has some of the highest rates for the leading causes of mortality. The adjusted cancer mortality in 1996 was 199.1 (per 100 000 inhabi-

tants), the highest of all cities. Vancouver's rate was only 156.9. The adjusted circulatory system mortality was 242.1, ranking second only to Winnipeg with a rate of 261. There were, however, health outcomes for which Montreal fared well, such as mortality from accidental wounds (Lessard et al., 2002). The reasons for these differences are unclear. Although socio-economic discrepancies clearly exist between the major urban centres of Canada, the restricted analysis that was done in this study may partly account for the differences. We therefore turn to the intra-municipal analysis, which was more detailed.

Within Montreal, a relationship across the income quintiles was found for several health indicators. The lowest income quintile consistently had poorer measures of health, including infant mortality. Infant mortality is widely regarded as a general indicator of population health and adequacy of social services. Figure 3.1 shows infant mortality over time by income quintile in Montreal.

**Figure 3.1: Infant mortality rate, by income status, Montreal, 1989–1993 to 1994–1998**

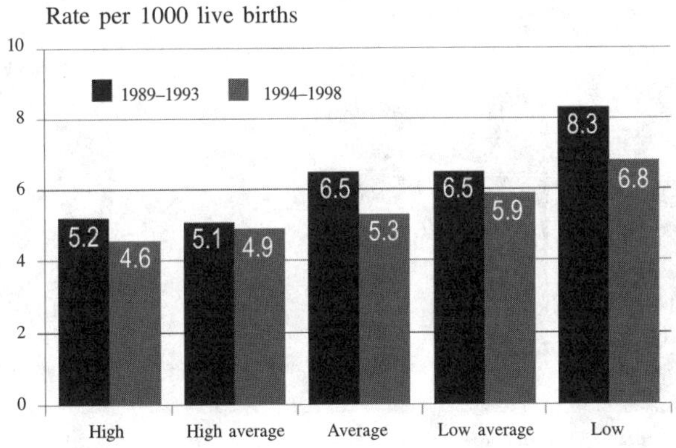

Source: Lessard, R., Roy, D., Choinière, R., Lévesque, J.F., Perron, S., *Urban health: A vital factor in Montreal's development*. Montreal: Direction de santé publique, 2002. Online at www.santepub-mtl.qc.ca/Publication/autres/annualreport2002.html.

This figure illustrates following three points:

1. Infant mortality fell in all income quintiles over the decade.
2. Despite the above finding, infant mortality is highest in low income quintiles.
3. The increase in infant mortality is relatively constant as we move from high to low income quintiles.

A similar trend was seen in gender and life expectancy. Figure 3.2 shows life expectancy at birth by sex and income quintile at one point in time. This figure illustrates the following:

1. Life expectancy is highest in high income quintiles.
2. Life expectancy decreases steadily as we move from higher to lower income quintiles.
3. This decrease is more pronounced in men than in women. In fact, men in the low income quintile can expect to live 6.6 years less than high income men, whereas this is only 3.6 years for women.

Figure 3.3 indicates that mortality rates for the leading causes of death differ depending on income quintile. Strikingly, the trend can be seen for all four leading causes of death (cancer, circulatory system, respiratory tract, and accidental injury). Note that this trend could be seen for even those diseases on which Montreal performed well compared to other major urban centres.

For the sake of completeness, behavioural risk factors such as physical inactivity, eating habits, and smoking followed a similar pattern as mortality indicators. These risk factors were found at a higher rate in low income groups.

Another interesting finding in the 2002 report was the association between geographic sub-regions and health. The six sub-regions were found to vary on a wide range of socio-demographic and socio-

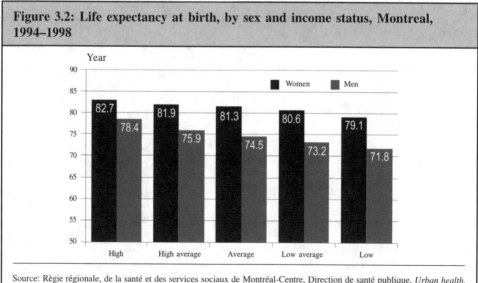

Figure 3.2: Life expectancy at birth, by sex and income status, Montreal, 1994–1998

Source: Règie régionale, de la santé et des services sociaux de Montréal-Centre, Direction de santé publique, *Urban health, A vital factor in Montréal's development.* 2002 Annual Report on the Health of the Population, Montréal, 2002. Online at www.santepub-mtl.qc.ca/Publication/rapportannue/2002/annualreport2002.html.

Social Determinants of Health

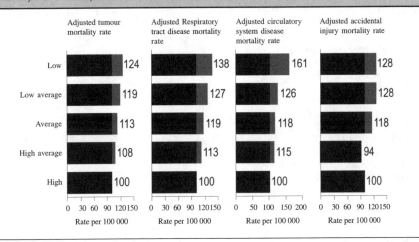

**Figure 3.3: Mortality rate for the four leading causes of death, by income status, Montreal, 1994–1998**

| | Adjusted tumour mortality rate | Adjusted Respiratory tract disease mortality rate | Adjusted circulatory system disease mortality rate | Adjusted accidental injury mortality rate |
|---|---|---|---|---|
| Low | 124 | 138 | 161 | 128 |
| Low average | 119 | 127 | 126 | 128 |
| Average | 113 | 119 | 118 | 118 |
| High average | 108 | 113 | 115 | 94 |
| High | 100 | 100 | 100 | 100 |

Rate per 100 000

Source: Régie régionale, de la santé et des services sociaux de Montréal-Centre, Direction de santé publique, *Urban health, A vital factor in Montréal's development*. 2002 Annual Report on the Health of the Population, Montréal, 2002. Online at www.santepub-mtl.qc.ca/Publication/rapportannue/2002/annualreport2002.html.

economic indicators, some of which are shown in Table 3.1. This table shows that the South-west and East-central sub-regions are relatively poor compared to other sub-regions. In contrast, the West and West-central sub-regions are the most well off. The table shows a striking geographic variation in childhood poverty in Montreal. In the poorest sub-regions, more than half of children under five years old lived under the low-income cut-off in 1995. Meanwhile, the richest region had less than a quarter of children living under the cut-off. It is also interesting to note that the two poorest sub-regions were also those that reported the lowest perceived neighbourhood quality of life and perceived neighbourhood safety. These two measures have been identified as components of social capital, which may be important since social capital may be an upstream determinant of health (Kawachi et al., 1997).

Table 3.2 demonstrates the inequalities in health between the richer west side and the poorer east side of Montreal. A man living in East-central could expect to live 6.5 years less than a male living in the west sub-region. Although not shown in the table, the difference in life expectancy between CLSC districts is as high as 13.5 years among men and 8 years among women. In addition, Table 3.2 shows that the divide between the east and west side of Montreal also applies to cancer, circulatory system, and respiratory tract deaths.

Although not shown in the table, lung and colon cancer incidence and mortality also followed a similar geographic trend. Breast cancer, however, followed a different pattern. The incidence of breast cancer was highest in socio-economically advantaged sub-regions. This finding is not surprising given that there is a greater risk of breast cancer in high socio-economic status women. What is surprising, however, is that breast cancer mortality was paradoxically higher in poorer sub-regions. The reasons for this association are unclear. It may be

## Table 3.1: Comparison of Montreal's sub-regions

| Indicator | West | West central | North | South-west | Centre-east | East |
|---|---|---|---|---|---|---|
| Proportion of employment-assistance beneficiaries, 2002 | 4.5% | 9.6% | 15.7% | 17.4% | 18.1% | 14.5% |
| Proportion of single-parent families with children under 18 years of age, 1996 | 16% | 24% | 30% | 35% | 36% | 32% |
| Proportion of the population under 5 years of age living under the low-income cutoff, 1995 | 22% | 42% | 53% | 50% | 58% | 46% |
| Proportion of residents who believe that their neighbourhood does not enjoy good quality of life, 2000 | 8.2% | 8.9% | 13.2% | 18.3% | 23.0% | 14.1% |
| Proportion of residents who do not consider their neighbourhood to be safe, 2000 | 5.6% | 7.3% | 7.7% | 10.8% | 17.1% | 9.8% |

Source: Lessard, R., Roy, D., Choinière, R., Lévesque, J.F., Perron, S., *Urban health: A vital factor in Montreal's development*. Montreal: Direction de santé publique, 2002. Online at www.santepub-mtl.qc.ca/Publication/autres/annualreport2002.html.


## Table 3.2: Comparison of Montreal's sub-regions

| Indicator | West | West central | North | South-west | East-central | East |
|---|---|---|---|---|---|---|
| Life expectancy at birth, men, 1994–1998 (years) | 77.2 | 75.9 | 77.4 | 73.1 | 70.7 | 73.8 |
| Life expectancy at birth, women, 1994–1998 (years) | 82.1 | 82.0 | 82.6 | 79.5 | 79.4 | 80.4 |
| Adjusted mortality rate, cancer, 1994–1998 (rate per 100,000) | 230 | 237 | 216 | 295 | 296 | 266 |
| Adjusted mortality rate, circulatory system disease, 1994–1998 (rate per 100,000) | 290 | 307 | 267 | 369 | 371 | 349 |
| Adjusted mortality rate, respiratory tract disease, 1994–1998 (rate per 100,000) | 71 | 67 | 65 | 100 | 93 | 89 |
| Adjusted mortality rate, accidental injuries, 1994–1998 (rate per 100,000) | 22 | 21 | 2 | 22 | 30 | 23 |

Source: Lessard, R., Roy, D., Choinière, R., Lévesque, J.F., Perron, S., *Urban health: A vital factor in Montreal's development*. Montreal: Direction de santé publique, 2002. Online at /www.santepub-mtl.qc.ca/Publication/autres/annualreport2002.html.

that individuals living in poor neighbourhoods have more limited access to health systems than their rich counterparts.

Furthermore, the rate of suicide was significantly higher in the East-central sub-region compared to the West (adjusted

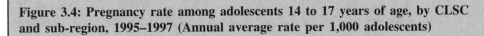

**Figure 3.4: Pregnancy rate among adolescents 14 to 17 years of age, by CLSC and sub-region, 1995–1997 (Annual average rate per 1,000 adolescents)**

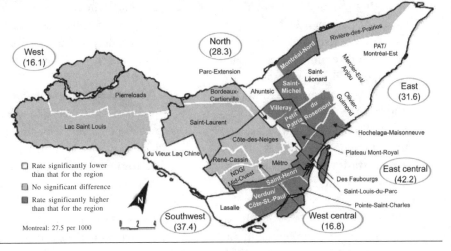

West (16.1)

North (28.3)

Parc-Extension

Pierreloads

Bordeaux-Cartierville

Ahuntsic

Saint-Michel

Saint-Léonard

Montréal-Nord

Rivière-des-Prairies

PAT/ Montréal-Est

Mercier-Est/ Anjou

Olivier-Guimond

East (31.6)

Lac Saint Louis

Saint-Laurent

Villeray

Petit Patrie

du Rosemont

Hochelaga-Maisonneuve

Côte-des-Neiges

du Vieux Laq Chine

René-Cassin

Métro

Plateau Mont-Royal

☐ Rate significantly lower than that for the region

◼ No significant difference

◼ Rate significantly higher than that for the region

Montreal: 27.5 per 1000

NDG/ Mid-Ouest

Saint-Henri

Verdun/ Côte-St-Paul

Lasalle

Des Faubourgs

Saint-Louis-du-Parc

Pointe-Saint-Charles

East central (42.2)

N

Southwest (37.4)

West central (16.8)

Source: Lessard, R., Roy, D., Choinière, R., Lévesque, J.F., Perron, S., *Urban health: A vital factor in Montreal's development*. Montreal: Direction de santé publique, 2002. Online at www.santepub-mtl.qc.ca/Publication/autres/annualreport2002.html.

suicide mortality rate per 100,000 inhabitants was 23 versus 9). The pregnancy rate amongst adolescents was also much higher in poorer neighbourhoods (42.2 versus 16.1 per 1,000 fourteen to seventeen year olds), as shown in Figure 3.4. Likewise, a multitude of other health outcomes were systematically more frequent in the poorer neighbourhoods.

In summary, this study shows that socio-economic conditions in Montreal are strongly associated with a variety of health outcomes.

## Theories explaining income and health

Having demonstrated the relationship between income and health indicators, it is pertinent to wonder why such a link exists. In fact, several theories have been proposed in the literature (Phipps, 2003). In general,

these can be divided into two types, those pertaining to absolute income per se and those pertaining to relative inequality of income.

Briefly, the absolute income hypothesis proposes there is a positive association between personal income and health, but that the association is non-linear. That is, even though the health of both rich and poor increases with income, the poor are much more responsive to income changes. The implication is that redistribution of income from rich to poor should cause average health to improve (Phipps, 2003). The absolute deprivation hypothesis goes even further to say that income below a certain deprivation threshold is adverse for health, but once past this threshold, there are minimal gains in health to be made (Phipps, 2003).

There are at least three theories explaining how income inequality affects health (Kawachi, 2000):

1. Income inequality may result in underinvestment in human capital, manifested through lower social spending in sectors such as education. This may be because, in societies with rising inequalities, the rich have diverging interests from the poor and exert pressure to decrease public spending (Kawachi, 2000). A variant is the neo-materialist hypothesis which states that income inequality is a manifestation of underlying historical, political, cultural, and economic processes (Lynch et al., 2000). These processes result in systematic underinvestment in public infrastructure including education, health services, transportation, housing, occupational regulations, etc. The result is that not only do individuals have a lack of private resources, but there is also reduced access to material infrastructure necessary for health.

2. Income inequality leads to underinvestment in social capital by diminishing community solidarity and social cohesion (Kawachi, 2000).

3. The third pathway occurs through psychosocially mediated effects, in which perceived widening of the income gap leads to frustration and biological processes that are harmful to health (Kawachi, 2000).

Some authors have argued that the link between income inequality and population health could be a statistical artefact. However, several authors have demonstrated that statistical issues cannot entirely account for the link between income and health (Phipps, 2003).

## Conclusion

The studies in Montreal and the rest of Canada contribute to the growing evidence confirming the link between poverty and health. Economic policies in Canada have not been entirely successful in reducing poverty, as evidenced by the increase in childhood poverty over time and the growing income inequality between the richest and poorest members of society (see chapter 2). The finding by the United Nations Development Programme (UNDP, 2003) that Canada's performance on human development has recently fallen compared to other developed countries, in part due to poverty in Canada, illustrates the growing importance of this problem.

Poverty has a significant impact on health, as stated by the Director of the Montreal Public Health Department (Lessard et al., 1998, p. 60):

Having scanned the health and well-being of Montrealers from one end of the life cycle to the other, we note the important role played by poverty. Inequalities in health and well-being can be traced back to socioeconomic inequalities, that is to the harsh living conditions which marginalize so many of our fellow citizens, not only limiting their access to essential goods, but depriving them as well of any meaningful role in social life.

Poverty weighs heavily on health in both its material and social dimensions: poor education, dependence, precarious jobs, inactivity. And the consequences of this are reflected in most of our social and health indicators: globally, in reduced life expectancy and, more particularly, in the higher proportion of diseases or psychosocial problems, in low-birth-weight babies, in developmental problems, in school dropout rates, in adolescent pregnancies, in psychosocial distress, etc.

If, as a society, we want to make significant gains on the health front, we must energetically pursue our efforts to improve living conditions. It is no exaggeration to say that poverty in Montreal constitutes a major health problem— a problem all the more worrisome seeing that it persists in a global context of unprecedented wealth and technological progress.

The original 1998 report by the Montreal Public Health Director led to the development of the Observatoire montréalais des inegalitées sociales et de la santé (OMISS), an organisation whose mission is to reduce social and health inequalities by encouraging knowledge development and linking research to decision-making. The work of OMISS and the continuing efforts in Montreal and other regions could have a significant impact on policies for poverty reduction. In 2002, the government of Quebec adopted Bill 112, a law to combat poverty and social exclusion (Bill 112, 2002). Bill 112 describes a provincial strategy to combat poverty and includes five key action areas: (1) prevention of poverty, with a focus on developing the potential of individuals, (2) strengthening social and economic safety nets, (3) promoting access to employment, (4) promoting the involvement of society as a whole, and (5) ensuring intervention at all levels. This law is unique in North America and is a significant step in recognising poverty as a priority for policy-making (Nöel, 2002).

Without fighting poverty, we have little hope of improving public health. The importance of this task is even more evident when we see that, in many of Montreal's neighbourhoods, more than 50 percent of children live under the low income cut-off. Public health policies in Canada necessarily must address the upstream determinants of health, particularly that of poverty.

## Recommended readings

Lessard R., Roy D., Choinière R., Bujold R., et al. (1998). *Social inequalities in health: Annual report of the health of the population.* Direction de santé publique, Montreal. Online at www.santepub-mtl.qc.ca/Publication/autres/rapport1998.html#english.

This report is the first time an annual report was published by the Montreal Public Health Unit. Social inequalities was selected as a focus because of the importance to health of poverty in Montreal.

Lessard R., Roy D., Choinière R., Lévesque J.F., and Perron S. (2002). *Urban health: A vital factor in Montreal's development.* Direction de santé publique Montreal. Online at www.santepub-mtl.qc.ca/Publication/autres/annualreport2002.html

This report is the fifth annual report of the Montreal Public Health Unit. It touches upon social inequality as one risk factor amongst others in the urban environment.

Nöel, A. (2002). *A law against poverty: Quebec's new approach to combating poverty and social exclusion.* Background Paper-Family Network, Canadian Policy Research Networks, December 2002. Online at www.cpds.umontreal.ca/fichier/cahiercpds03-01.pdf.

This paper was written as a backgrounder to the new Quebec anti-poverty law. Its purpose was to make the law better known and to open a discussion on the law.

Phipps, Shelley. (2003). *The impact of poverty on health: A scan of research literature.* Canadian Institute for Health Information, June 2003. Online at http://secure.cihi.ca/cihiweb/dispPage.jsp?cw_page=GR_323_E

This paper, prepared by the Canadian Population Health Initiative, serves as a summary of the state of knowledge between poverty and health.

## Related websites

The four websites that follow contain extensive information on poverty and health at the local, national, and international levels. They also provide links to additional relevant web sites.
- The Montreal Public Health Unit—www.santepub-mtl.qc.ca/
- Canadian Institute for Health Information—secure.cihi.ca/cihiweb/splash.html
- Observatoire montréalais des inegalitées sociales et de la santé (OMISS)—www.omiss.ca/english/index.html
- The University of Montreal (in French)—politiquessociales.net/

# Chapter Four

———⬤———

# UNEMPLOYMENT AND
# THE LABOUR MARKET

## Diane-Gabrielle Tremblay

## Introduction

This chapter deals with unemployment and transformations within the labour market. We are interested in those issues arising from the perspective of economic security and insecurity of individuals. We will first locate our position in the general context of economic transformation, the evolution toward a knowledge economy, and the effects this evolution may have for individuals, particularly from the perspective of the transformation of careers. The current context also translates into new modes of learning which are more informal and less focussed on internal labour markets, and which also have an effect on job security or insecurity. This raises issues about individuals' employment possibilities. The chapter will deal generally with seven questions and is therefore divided into the following seven sections:

1. What are the main labour market transformations and their effects?
2. What does job security mean today?
3. What is the definition of "insecurity"? What are its causes?
4. What are the connections between jobs and security/insecurity?
5. What effects do employment and social policies have on job security?
6. Is job security still important? If so—
7. How can job security be ensured?

## Transformation of the labour market

For a number of decades, certain regions of Canada have known relatively high levels of unemployment. While the situation has improved, especially in the central regions, a number of regions still experience problems, particularly those that depend on natural resources.

In the context of the knowledge economy, careers are increasingly fragmented, with individuals being involved in a growing number of jobs, projects, and businesses over the course of their working lives. This reinforces both the problems faced by some unskilled people and certain regions where the percentage of people without high education is lower.

The knowledge economy also translates into the development of "projects." In this context, the intelligence of a business is a function of the quality of the "skill network" it contains, rather than the skills of its individual employees (Tremblay, 2003a, 2003d, 2002b). Thus, both young people entering the labour market and those undergoing a career change must face new labour market realities, broadly determined by the development of the new knowledge economy (Tremblay, 2003c, 2003f).

Knowledge economy businesses, with their focus on projects, bring into question a number of the dominant principles and theories of labour economics, particularly with regard to the advantages of internal markets that allow individuals to develop skills and careers within an organization (Tremblay, 1997).

The new boundaryless careers follow a different pattern than careers on a vertical promotion ladder as are found in internal labour market models, and particularly in the internal markets model (Tremblay, 1997). In the latter model, careers were lived out within a single company, and often within a single union. These new nomadic careers present new challenges for both individuals and organizations.

## Boundaryless careers

Careers have most often been analyzed in the context of an internal labour market, or within the context of large hierarchical companies, frequently unionized ones, where one "moves up" the hierarchy in one's career. Horizontal and other forms of mobility have received less attention, partly because these forms are traditionally seen as non-promotion and therefore, non-career moves. This may also be due to the fact that unions have strongly adopted the ladder, or closed internal market model as the archetypal career (Tremblay and Rolland, 1998). However, in recent years, the concept of career has evolved (Cadin et al., 2000). Some career theorists have begun to show evidence of a different vision of careers. Some have even spoken of a new paradigm which is counter-posed to the dominant hierarchical ascending career model. I refer here to the concept of "boundaryless careers" (Arthur and Rousseau, 1996; Tremblay, 2003a).

In a number of sectors, new forms of organization of work and collaboration are being developed, such as team work, network, and virtual communities of practice (Tremblay, 2004). However, while such developments may be positive for certain sectors, they entail precariousness, lack of stability, and the lack of a career for others. New types of employment often arise. As examples we have the case of self-employment, and "false" self-employment, that is those who are dependent on one or more order-givers (Tremblay and Chevrier, 2002b).

In general, the context of new organizations entails more flexibility, often through development of multi-skilling and enriched jobs, but just as frequently through the development of a greater range of tasks at one level. This includes rotation through a number of equivalent tasks, as well as the development of precarious conditions of work.

The following question thus arises: Where have all the permanent industrial workers, the ones who had job security and a guaranteed salary, gone? In the past, the standard-bearer for job security was the male industrial worker, with a full-time, unionized job. He had protection, a stable, "permanent" job, and any interruptions in continuity of his employment were covered by unemployment insurance, which protected the family income. Today, this worker hardly exists.

We have entered the age of flexibility. This has meant a range of new employment statuses and periods of unemployment (Tremblay, 2003a, 2003b, 1990). But it has also entailed variable intensity of employment, including part-time, casual, and contract work. The types of work and levels of income are variable, and according to labour market experts, are leading to a review of the traditional definitions of the various groups within the labour force (Standing, 2000; Tremblay, 1997).

While the foregoing poses definite challenges for economic theory, it challenges income security as well! In fact, it leads us to wonder how unemployment and insecurity should be redefined in this new context, given that the unemployment rate no longer offers a correct measurement of the true supply of labour or insecurity. This situation is clearly seen in the case of self-employed workers (Tremblay and Chevrier, 2002b). The traditional categories within

labour economics are no longer sufficient. The categories of employees, unemployed people and inactive members of the labour force are too simplistic for an analysis of the reality of self-employment or the new diversity of employment status (casual, temporary, reduced-time, part-time, etc.).

Therefore, the concept of "active labour force" itself becomes questionable, given the diversity of forms of employment explained above. The various forms of work (third sector, social economy, non-governmental organizations, volunteers, and informal) are multiplying; some are more recognized than others. Homework, parenting, and care-giving is increasingly recognized as legitimate, which raises the issue of distinctions between work and non-work, and, accordingly, between the active and inactive labour force, with work–family or life–balance issues being taken into account (Tremblay, 2003g).

In short, the concepts of unemployment, inactivity, and active participation are questioned, while a range of employment and unpaid work gain legitimacy. With all these challenges to forms of employment and what is considered real "work," the concept of job security is also in doubt. All this leads to a challenge to the notions of security and insecurity.

---

### Box 4.1: Definitions of security

According to Standing (1999), security involves a sense of well-being or control, or mastery over one's activities and development, as well as the enjoyment of certain self-esteem. Inversely, insecurity involves anxiety and uncertainty (Standing, 1999).

Collective security can also be distinguished from other forms of security or insecurity. Again citing Standing (1999), collective (or societal) security could be seen as the need to identify with or belong to a group, typically to exercise control over the behaviour of others or to limit their control. Security arises from multiple forms of identity, such as class, occupation, and community membership (Standing, 1999), to which we would add territorial belonging (Tremblay and Fontan, 1994), which are also sources of social identity, and therefore, a certain level of security.

# What is security?

The need for security can be defined in different ways, according to the discipline's approach or specific area of interest.

The company can also be considered a source of security, so it is therefore possible to refer to a certain amount of "company security," such as that found within the Japanese company, which generally ensured employees a long term job (Tremblay and Rolland, 1998, 2000, 2003).

There is also individual security; a person's curriculum vitae, skills, and union membership can provide a feeling of personal security (Standing, 1999).

Given this, how can we define security? To return to Standing (1999), security can be defined as a system of defence against the development of a technical division of labour, often through measures that preserve some of the social division of labour or segmentation of the labour process. It is appropriate to wonder if the definition is applicable in the context of the international division of labour.

In the context of mass production and large organizations (Fordism), the stability of employees was considered to be a desirable standard for industrial society. The development of trade unionism and the seniority standard contributed to making it expensive for a person to quit his or her job, which tended to favour job stability and non-mobility of employees. We might wonder why the regulation of the job market occurred. In fact, historically speaking, employment standards, unionization, and unemployment insurance came about as a result of workers' struggles, as a way to compensate for workers' weaker power, but also to ensure stable labour supply for companies who wanted to counter chronic labour instability among farm workers at the beginning of the industrial era.

Over the years, income security became associated with the welfare state. However, benefits were only for full-time workers, and women were frequently dependent on the family benefit coverage of their spouses. We can now discuss the meaning of job insecurity.

# What does job insecurity mean?

Despite the existence of male industrial workers with more or less stable jobs, and despite labour regulations favouring job stability, slow growth in the 1970s resulted in workforce rationalization and layoffs, long-term unemployment, and a reduction in the unemployment insurance benefits offered to jobless people. Today only about one of every two workers is eligible for employment insurance, and in the resource-dependent regions of the country, where unemployment is higher and long periods of unemployment are more frequent, many workers end up excluded from the employment insurance regime. Furthermore, available jobs are often precarious and poorly paid, which leads to lower benefits.

In the current economic environment, companies are in an endless search for improved competitiveness and productivity, which often results in demands for flexibility, diversified types of employment, changed work shifts, and ultimately, insecurity. Globalization and the international division of labour have contributed to the displacement of investment and jobs toward developing countries, which leads to an increased feeling of job insecurity. As discussed above, job insecurity is largely subjective; something an individual feels given his or her job situation and the overall economic situation. Job insecurity can thus be considered a symptom of income insecurity and insecurity about the labour market in general.

This leads us to ask how workers' insecurity can be reduced. This reduction can be achieved in a variety of ways, both direct and indirect. To reduce insecurity directly, one can try to ensure either greater job security or greater coverage of costs (benefits). While the latter approach does not reduce insecurity at its source, increased benefit coverage does make insecurity easier to bear. Insecurity can also be reduced indirectly, by attacking its causes (Standing, 1999).

Another question arises: how can security and insecurity be measured? This is a particularly complex issue which has been the subject of relatively little study.

However, Dasgupta (2001) emphasizes that there are both objective and subjective measures, which brings us to the debate we discussed earlier about labour market indicators, and their validity or relevance. Objective measures are interesting but limited, as we saw earlier. We have already mentioned individual measures: unemployment rates, average length of period of employment vs. unemployment, fixed term contracts vs. indefinite employment, skill transferability, etc. These constitute individual measures of the likelihood that given individuals will maintain ongoing employment and stability and security. There are also contractual measures, such as the rate of non-standard jobs or job status, and institutional measures such as legal protection and collective agreements (Dasgupta, 2001).

As well, there are subjective measures. These may relate to the feelings that one's permanence in employment is guaranteed (by the company, as in Japan) or by society, such

as in Sweden (Tremblay and Rolland, 1998). In order to assess an individual's relative insecurity or security, the following measures would be of interest: the likelihood of losing one's job, the likelihood of finding another, the value of the current job, and the value of the future job or period of unemployment (Dasgupta, 2001).

We may therefore conclude that insecurity is related to the perception of risk. In theory, manual or manufacturing jobs should be associated with greater perceived insecurity, but in fact, this feeling of insecurity rises in countries with higher levels of education. A number of studies on the perception of risk have shown this, in particular those carried out by the Organization for Economic Cooperation and Development (1996). The OECD found an overall increase in perceived job insecurity by individuals. Standing (1999) notes that perceived insecurity does not appear very differentiated by sex, possibly because women have lower expectations regarding security and stability. In fact, as women are more highly represented in part-time and otherwise precarious jobs than men (Tremblay and Chevrier, 2002a), this may affect their expectations of job stability.

Let us examine in greater detail the situation of the Canadian labour market in order to specify to what degree individuals may perceive or experience economic insecurity.

**Unemployment and precarious work in Canada**

In Canada in 2001, women's labour participation rate was 59.7%, while the rate for men was 72.5%. The gap between the rates for women and men are further accentuated if the variables of marital status, sex, and age are taken into account. The largest gaps occur in the groups aged 15–

## Table 4.1: Rates of labour force participation by marital status, sex, and age, Canada, 2001

| Age ranges | Canada Women | Men | Total |
|---|---|---|---|
| **Total** | **59.7** | **72.5** | **66.0** |
| 15–24 | 63.3 | 66.1 | 64.7 |
| 25–44 | 80.4 | 92.1 | 86.3 |
| 45 and older | 41.5 | 57.1 | 48.9 |
| | | | |
| **Unmarried** | **67.1** | **71.3** | **69.5** |
| 15–24 | 61.9 | 64.2 | 63.1 |
| 25–44 | 83.6 | 86.3 | 85.2 |
| 45 and older | 49.7 | 52.2 | 51.0 |
| | | | |
| **Married** | **63.2** | **75.0** | **69.1** |
| 15–24 | 71.4 | 90.0 | 77.6 |
| 25–44 | 79.4 | 94.9 | 86.7 |
| 45 and older | 47.5 | 59.7 | 53.9 |
| | | | |
| **Separated/divorced** | **66.6** | **71.4** | **68.6** |
| 15–24 | 60.0 | 77.3 | 64.4 |
| 25–44 | 82.2 | 90.7 | 85.8 |
| 45 and older | 57.4 | 59.3 | 58.2 |
| | | | |
| **Widows/widowers** | **11.0** | **15.9** | **11.9** |
| 15–24 | - | - | - |
| 25–44 | 69.3 | 83.6 | 71.8 |
| 45 and older | 9.8 | 14.4 | 10.6 |

Source: "Rates of labour force participation by marital status, sex and age, Canada, 2001," adapted from the Statistics Canada publication "Labour force activity (8), age groups (17B), marital status (7B) and sex (3) for population 15 years and over, for Canada, provinces, territories, census metropolitan areas and census agglomerations, 2001 Census—20% Sample Data," Catalogue 95F0377, May 2003.

## Table 4.2: Percentage of persons working part time, according to age, Canada, 1976 to 2001[1]

| | Age Groups | | | | | | | |
|---|---|---|---|---|---|---|---|---|
| | 15–24 | | 25–44 | | 45–54 | | 55–64 yrs | |
| | % Women | % Men | % Women | % Men | % Women | % Men | % Women | % Men |
| 1976 | 25.0 | 18.0 | 21.9 | 1.5 | 24.2 | 1.4 | 24.7 | 3.6 |
| 1981 | 29.4 | 21.6 | 23.4 | 2.1 | 27.6 | 2.1 | 27.7 | 4.4 |
| 1986 | 37.9 | 28.6 | 23.0 | 3.2 | 26.9 | 2.7 | 30.4 | 6.6 |
| 1991 | 45.6 | 36.8 | 22.4 | 3.9 | 24.1 | 3.3 | 32.2 | 8.4 |
| 1996 | 53.4 | 39.0 | 23.2 | 5.1 | 23.3 | 4.2 | 32.4 | 9.8 |
| 2001 | 51.0 | 37.3 | 21.2 | 4.7 | 21.4 | 4.3 | 29.2 | 9.9 |

[1] As a percentage of all occupied persons

Source: Statistics Canada, Labour Force Survey
Source: "Percentage of persons working part time, according to age, Canada, 1976 to 2001," adapted from the Statistics Canada publication "Women in Canada: Work Chapter Updates," Catalogue 89F0133, April 2002, Table 8, page 15.

Social Determinants of Health

24 and 25–44. They are also larger between married women and men compared to single, divorced, and separated women and men. In this regard, we emphasize that the highest participation rate for women was among single women aged 25–44.

The labour force has undergone diversification in types of employment over the last decades, which has especially affected women. Various types of precarious or non-standard employment have increased, amongst them part time work, which mainly concerns women and youth.

It is clear that to varying degrees, those in precarious employment situations perceive a measure of job insecurity due to their employment status. However, we must interrogate the sources of this insecurity and of these diversified forms of employment. We can certainly observe such forms in the job market, but their development should not be seen as a "fact of nature." Thus, many question the contribution of employment policies on the diversification of types of employment.

## Effects of employment policies on security

The contribution of employment entry, employability, social economy and other programs to the de-standardization of forms of employment should be questioned. These programs have, in our view, played a major role in challenging the existing norm of full-time, full-year employment. In some cases, this translates into a simple perception of insecurity, while in others, the de-standardization and insecurity are óbjective: fixed-term contracts, part-time, reduced benefits, etc. (Tremblay, 2003c).

Nonetheless, there is also a subjective dimension associated with these job market entry or short-term employment programs. This dimension can be measured, although not easily. It is linked to various probabilities such as the likelihood of losing one's job or finding another (or, in fact, the perception of such likelihood). The likelihood of finding a job varies by program, but it is generally higher than before taking part in the program, although sometimes participation results in stigmatization of participants, which damages their job possibilities afterward.

Participation in such programs also can result in a reduction of expectations, especially among women. It appears that women lower their employment expectations more readily than men. The value of the current or future job is a further dimension of a subjective nature.

### Comparisons between Scandinavia and North America
The evaluation of the effects of participation in a public job or a job market entry program

---

**Box 4.2**

In Canada, not counting those who are unemployed, only half of all Canadians have a single, full-time job that has lasted six months or more (Lowe, 1999). The current Canadian labour force includes the following:

    16% self-employed workers;
    10% temporary workers;
    11% regular part-time workers;
    6% employed in their current job for less than six months;
    2% are employed in more than one job.

---

also varies according to the place and philosophy reflected in the public policy of the country. Scandinavia provides active support for entry into regular employment. For many years, the nearly full employment situation* in the region made it easier to reintegrate people into jobs after participating in such programs. Job program participants are less under-valued than in other countries of Europe or the Americas, where such programs are less likely to lead to a steady, regular job. Scandinavia also supports integration into work through job training programs, work time adjustment measures, family-friendly policies, and longer family leaves (Tremblay and Villeneuve, 1998). All these policies influence the overall labour market, the chances of finding work, and, accordingly, the subjective assessment of the effects of taking part in a publicly-funded job program.

In contrast, in North America, there is more emphasis on palliative and passive measures such as workfare. There are few alternate work schedule arrangements and little support. In terms of family-supportive policies, there are virtually none in the U.S., and such policies are minimal in English-speaking Canada (although the Federal government enacted a parental leave policy), but slightly more developed in Quebec, where parents have lower costs for State-funded childcare. However, we are still far from the Scandinavian standard.

## Effects of social policy on security

This is a highly complex issue that requires an in-depth analysis. In this chapter, we can only provide an overview of the importance of policy on insecurity.

We can use Esping-Andersen's well-known welfare state typology as a basis for analysis of the different types of social policy and welfare states. According to Esping-Andersen (1985), countries can be divided into three main categories. The first are liberal states based on a laissez-faire approach. The U.S. and Great Britain are the main representatives of this group. The second group includes conservative countries where there is some government intervention of a conservative nature, such as Germany, the Netherlands, and France. The third category includes social-democratic countries, principally the Scandinavian nations of Sweden, Norway, and Denmark. In such countries, the policies are based on revenue sharing at the national level to reduce income gaps between rich and poor. To varying degrees and at different points in their history, such countries have imposed controls on capital exportation and on foreign investment in national sectors, all in aid of full employment. This is what characterizes social and employment policy, although we have seen the typology applied equally well to family policies as well.

From a social policy perspective, the differences translate into major variations in the way unemployed people are considered. In the U.S., an unemployed person is considered to be responsible for his or her condition. Social assistance benefits are seen as a compensation for work. This is laissez-faire economics in which the State sees no need to intervene since individuals are responsible for their lot and the market should allow them to overcome their unemployment, if it is working well. In the U.S. there are the "deserving" poor (disabled persons) and the undeserving poor (those who are considered responsible for their own condition).

In Scandinavia, on the other hand, the accent is on life-long professional develop-ment, labour force integration, and the participation of civil society actors (associations, third-sector, social economy) in the strategies of integration. In Sweden and Denmark, oversight of the compensatory mechanisms is carried out by trade unions, quite a different situation from that of the US.

In France, at least in theory, there is greater emphasis on integration and collective solidarity than on simple compensation benefits for unemployed workers. There is a shared view among a number of researchers that the true results of the minimum integration income, supposedly different from workfare, indicate only a qualified success (Paugam, 1998). There appears to be a gap between the objectives and philosophy and the reality. While the objectives were quite lofty at the beginning of the project, they became decidedly less so over the years. Those who gained the most from the program were those who needed it the least, while at the same time the program was unable to help those with less formal education or lower skill levels escape their dependence (Paugam, 1998; Chapon and Euzéby, 2002).

There is clearly a risk of "downward" convergence and homogenization in the context of the European Union, which many see as being constructed along the lines of the liberal model. The European social models are therefore facing a risk of downward adjustment. The same type of question arises with respect to integration in the Americas (NAFTA, FTAA). Will the liberal model (or U.S./British model) occupy the space of social policy, as many others do? The question is not a trivial one, since such a development could lead to a significant increase in insecurity and relative risk of unemployment and underemployment.

From the perspective of women and their particular situation, social policy has important effects. A first class of policy would favour women's integration into the labour force, with work-family measures, including those that would promote a greater role for men in exercising parenting responsibilities. A second group would support women who choose to remain in the home with their children, through social advantages given to men who support a stay-at-home wife or generous benefits for sole-support mothers.

If we attempt to classify countries by the type of policy they have, we see that the Scandinavian countries favour women's labour force participation and men's role in parenting (although with mixed results). Such politics are based on equality between men and women. They offer women insurance programs created for men, and while failing to be completely appropriate, they consider women as autonomous rather than as a husband's dependent.

Conservative welfare states such as France, Germany, and the Netherlands support men whose wives remain at home (Germany), promote women's part-time work (Netherlands, France), and women's temporary withdrawal from the labour force for the purpose of maternity (Tremblay and Villeneuve, 1998).

Finally, countries with a liberal or laissez-faire approach try to require women to integrate into the labour force (workfare), without providing measures to help work/family balance, nor do they provide for proper wages or working conditions.

There are two major "social risks" for women, namely unemployment and family responsibilities. When there are problems with dependents (children or ageing or ill parents), women tend to reinvest in the family. Very often, there is some reinforcement of women's traditional role, between the private sphere and the labour force, which some call the "gender trap." In fact, since they have not invested enough themselves in the sphere of work, and are often denied their individual rights or benefits due to their limited participation in the labour force, women may become trapped and repressed into a return to the home sphere. We may argue the importance of labour force participation as a source of benefits and income security, which many have done, or argue for citizen's income and other measures of this type (a point to which we will return). However in the current context, it is in the labour market where rights take shape in most countries. It is therefore certainly preferable for women to participate in this market. Failure to participate leads women into the "gender trap."

## Is job security still important?

In light of the reservations set out in the foregoing paragraph about the importance of the labour market as the source of rights, insurance and income, certain questions arise, such as whether job security is still important today, and if so, why, for whom, and how.

From the point of view of employers, job security is a constraint on efficiency and flexibility in adjusting production. Publications of the OECD have shown an inverse relationship between job flexibility and job security. We have seen that in Canada, the various forms of precarious conditions have a tendency to cluster. That is, people working part-time are more likely to be employed in fixed-term and contract positions that do not have benefits. Further, a recent study of several European countries showed that the economic slowdown Europe recently experienced has re-launched the debate about labour flexibility, including precarious forms of employment and wage

reductions (Freyssinet, 2003). Some raise the notion that workers should adapt to having less security. In fact, insecurity or weak job security is becoming the norm in those countries where precarious or non-standard jobs are beginning to outstrip traditional forms of employment.

In defence of job security, some oppose the idea of job security as the main source of income security, especially given the restrictions imposed on the employment insurance regime several years ago in Canada. Job security is considered important for the well-being of workers and their families, as well as being seen as favouring macro-economic stability. Furthermore, it appears that flexibility and wage reductions do not always favour job creation (Freyssinet, 2003).

Also, recent work on business issues indicates that job security is a source of loyalty, commitment, and increased motivation. Furthermore, job security is seen as essential to the interest of both employees and employers in training and skill development. Job security can therefore be seen as positive for business, as it favours productivity and innovation (Tremblay, 2004, 2003a, 2003d).

There are certainly other avenues, and some theorists defend the concept of a guaranteed or citizen's income, mentioned above. While flexibility is necessary, and some consider that job protection works against flexibility, other forms of security can be provided: citizen's income, minimum guaranteed income, etc. Some writers believe that this would simultaneously ensure social justice and efficiency (Standing, 1999).

However, this position is highly contested. It overlooks the non-financial advantages of work, including participation in social life, self-esteem, and personal development. Other critics hold that the cost of providing such a citizen's income at an appropriate level would be extremely high, and that a true minimum income is more realistic. Finally, it is argued that the stigma attached to social assistance would not necessarily disappear by just changing the name of the program, even though some believe that a "citizenship" income, considered the right of every citizen, might change people's perspective (Standing, 1999).

Feminist economists fear a marginalization of women and a return to the home, since a formula providing a minimum integration or citizen's income would compete with the low wages many women earn, and would tend to encourage women to leave the labour force (Tremblay, 2003f, 1997).

Ultimately, security is important for both sides of this debate. On one side, income security is seen as the most important, rather than job security, and providing a decent income for all would solve the problem. In this view, it would be possible to ensure a decent income for many, without affecting low-income earners' interest in continuing to work. On the other side, the expectations of the majority are more along the lines of ensuring a job for everyone, since working is highly valued both socially and as a source of income. We share this position. In this view, it would be impossible to ensure a citizenship income or guaranteed minimum income for more than a small minority of people without levies or taxes that would be totally unacceptable to working people. The debate has been around for quite a few years, but the dominance of the liberal perspective reduces the likelihood of movement toward this option, unless it were to occur in the context of extremely limited programs (both in philosophy and scope), as was the case with the minimum integration income introduced in France.

# How can job security be assured?

This remains the fundamental question of the day. How can we ensure the security of individuals, which we believe must involve job security? In our view, an existence income or citizen's income cannot be a viable solution to ensure income security for all, and such a guarantee would not necessarily ensure job security.

Social security is recognized as a favoured instrument for redistribution of time and money, but it also possesses a symbolic power in the construction of family roles. Social security might therefore be used as a source of redistribution, not just of income, but of societal roles; it could give every person the chance to participate in both spheres, both the workplace and the family.

How can this be done? Women's participation in the labour force must be encouraged through proper measures to help balance work and parenting roles (Tremblay, 2003b, 2003g, 2002c), as well as through high quality jobs and pay equity measures. This can be seen as going beyond social policy, toward essential workplace measures, while social policy can be only a safety net at best. Without such measures, women remain trapped within the family and continue to be their husbands' dependents.

The participation of fathers in parenting and family responsibilities (including caring for ageing or ill parents) must be encouraged. This can be achieved through incentive measures such as those implemented in Sweden, e.g., offering a month of parenting leave only for fathers (Tremblay and Villeneuve, 1998). The extension of parental leave in Canada and the opportunity to share such leave between spouses is not enough to increase the participation of fathers, especially given that women earn on average 70% of what men make.

There will always be a role for social security. More should be done to counteract material or financial insecurity and family instability. The latter is not within the scope of the State, although the government can reduce the costs of such instability to women by ensuring women's autonomous rights. Social security measures should in fact be provided to the dependent person to ensure continuity and a degree of autonomy in decision making. Provision should be made to cover all forms of risks, including the risk of withdrawal from the labour force, loss of a job, illness, and unemployment. There also needs to be more adaptation to the diversity of employment status as applied to self-employed, part-time, and contract employees. Finally, there should be a broad definition of close dependants to ensure coverage of all social risks. Otherwise, there is a risk that women will withdraw from the labour force in order to care for close family, without formal recognition of this responsibility. On the contrary, currently such withdrawal puts the rest of their working lives in peril, and some find themselves permanently excluded from the paid labour force.

Therefore, the key is to ensure income and job security at the same time for both men and women, and above all to avoid trapping women in the private sphere and relegating them to dependence on a spouse. Furthermore, men must not be trapped in the public sphere or labour market, or saddled with the obligation to earn a "family wage" through overtime work that deprives them of essential parenting activities. They should be encouraged to increase their participation in family life and parenting. Financial autonomy of persons with a disability or who are otherwise dependent is also to be ensured.

## Conclusion

It is no surprise that we are putting forward a model similar to the Scandinavian model as one which allows for the economic security of individuals, and that we see a strong association between economic security and job security. In the U.S. and the Anglo-Saxon world, we are seeing the opposite. Their model is based instead on liberal ideology which considers that markets work well and can assume the regulatory role they have been given, and that the free movement of goods around the world is a source of growth, and ultimately, of economic security. Unfortunately, while the model achieves a certain level of economic security, it does not apply to everyone, and certainly does not apply to American women excluded from the labour market or those who earn low wages. However, over the years, the American model has been applied more and more, despite some resistance and opposition. This model appears to be imposed despite our view that it endangers the very objective of economic security, especially for women, which is currently threatened, given the prevailing standards and conditions (unequal wages, discrimination, family responsibilities imposed on women, sole support parents, etc.).

In recent years, the liberal vision has certainly spread, ignoring a number of basic aspects of "economic life." Dominant economic theories are also headed in this direction, which properly gives rise to concern for the economic security of people in the future. This is not the place to expand on the opposite views found within a range of proponents of economic thought (Tremblay, 2002a). Clearly, orthodox theories stemming from the American model, or more generally, Anglo-Saxon models, are based on quantitative and positivist methods, and contribute to the spread of the dominant Anglo-Saxon model. They do not favour the social-democratic visions linked to an alternative role for the State and social policy.

There are three main concerns that should be considered in our search for economic security. First, it is important to contest the dominant economic model in favour of institutionalist theories that are more respectful of the historic, social, and political reality of societies, and more likely to support social democratic policies that provide for true economic security for all. Furthermore, economic security needs to be better defined in the current context. The various types of risk described above must be taken into account, as well as different types of security (food, physical, etc.). Third and finally, the full range of types of work and social situations should be considered; we have progressed beyond the era of full-time work for men and women being assigned to the home. This should be taken into account in any reflection about economic security for men and women.

## Recommended readings

Tremblay, D.-G. (2003e). *New types of careers in the knowledge economy: Networks and boundaryless jobs as a career strategy in the ict and multimedia sector.* Research Note of the Canada Research Chair on the Knowledge Economy No 2003-12A. Online at www.teluq.uquebec.ca/chaireecosavoir

This paper examines career transformations related to the new, knowledge-based economy, particularly in terms of occupational training, mobility, and career development. Learning and training are emphasized.

Tremblay, D.-G. (2003f). *The new division of labour and women's jobs: Results from a study conducted in Canada from a gendered perspective.* Research Note of the Canada Research Chair on the Knowledge Economy No 2003-19A. Online at www.teluq.uquebec.ca/chaireecosavoir.

This paper contains the results of a Canadian study on the division of labour and women's jobs, from a gendered perspective.

Tremblay, D.-G. (2003g). *Working time and work-family balancing: A Canadian perspective.* Research Note of the Canada Research Chair on the Knowledge Economy No 2003-18. Online at www.teluq.uquebec.ca/chaireecosavoir.

This paper examines the increasing difficulty confronting workers who wish to balance working life with family life.

Tremblay, D.-G. and Rolland, D. (2003). *The Japanese model and its possible hybridization in other countries.* Research Note of the Canada Research Chair on the Knowledge Economy No 2003-20A. Online at www.teluq.uquebec.ca/chaireecosavoir

This paper examines the Japanese Human Resources Management policies and considers application beyond the Japanese border.

Tremblay, D.-G., Davel, E. and Rolland, D. (2003). *New management forms for the knowledge economy: HRM in the context of teamwork and participaton.* Research Note of the Canada Research Chair on the Knowledge Economy No 2003-14A. Online at www.teluq.uquebec.ca/chaireecosavoir.

In this paper, the authors present a number of theoretical and contextual elements on the introduction of teamwork and participation in organizations.

# Related websites

Canada Research Chair on the Knowledge Economy—www.teluq.uquebec.ca/chaireecosavoir

The Chair's objective is to re-examine the various theories of the firm, in particular the evolutionary theory according to which, knowledge of an organization is above all, the function of individual knowledge of its members.

Bell Canada Chair on Technology and Work Organization—www.teluq.uquebec.ca/chairebell

Specifically created in order to promote and coordinate scientific research within partnerships between industries and the academic world which it represents, the Network for Computing and Mathematical Modeling (http://www.crm.umontreal.ca/rcm2/rcm2_an.html) signed a partnership agreement with Bell Canada (http://www.bell.ca/) in 1998, thereby creating the Bell University Laboratories. Technology and Work Organization is one of the Research Chairs of Bell University Laboratories.

Interventions Économiques—www.teluq.uquebec.ca/interventionseconomiques

*Interventions Économiques* is a journal that is interested in theoretical debates of a critical nature relating to the political economy and the socio-economic transformation of society. It is a journal devoted to economic interventions and social change. It examines key social issues such as reconciling the family/home life with work, changing work, and workplace trends, etc.

Statistics Canada—www.statcan.ca

From publications to electronic data, census to survey information, the web site is THE official source for Canadian social and economic statistics and products.

Human Resources Development Canada—www.hrdc-drhc.gc.ca

A division of the federal government of Canada, Human Resources Development Canada investigates social development, human resources, labour, and homelessness. The Department of Human Resources Development Canada was recently divided into two new entities: the Department of Social Development and the Department of Human Resources and Skills Development.

## Chapter Five

# LABOUR MARKET FLEXIBILITY AND WORKER INSECURITY

## Michael Polanyi, Emile Tompa, and Janice Foley

## Introduction

Over the past twenty years, the arrangement, content, and organization of work in industrialized countries have been changing. In an effort to remain competitive in the global economy, many firms have adopted flexible production strategies aimed at responding quickly to market signals, in order to increase productivity and decrease costs.

While autonomy and quality of work may have improved for some workers, particularly in the high end service sector, there is evidence that flexible strategies are intensifying work demands, increasing levels of labour-market insecurity, and exacerbating the polarization of wages and working conditions along lines of class, gender, and race.

The purpose of this chapter is to outline some of the direct and indirect health consequences of labour-market restructuring arising from the widespread adoption of flexible production strategies, in particular high-performance work organization and cost-cutting tactics. Based on a consideration of the health consequences of current work practices, we propose rethinking labour-market regulations in Canada, and outline a set of policy initiatives to promote healthy and productive practices.

## Flexible production in the new economy

Technological change, deregulation, intensified international competition and declining productivity gains have combined to stimulate fundamental changes in work systems, employment relations, firm structures, and the labour market experiences of workers in North America and other industrialized countries.

The liberalization of trade and finance has resulted in significant growth in the trade of goods and services and the flow of money across international borders. Meanwhile, technological advancements in computers, telecommunications, and transportation have increased the mobility of physical and financial capital as well as goods and services. Improvements in technology have allowed firms to produce goods more quickly and cheaply, leading to the saturation of domestic markets and exacerbating competition for markets. Technological advancements have also reduced the time it takes to develop new generations of products, thus reducing the shelf life of goods and forcing firms to constantly innovate. Furthermore, technology advancements have allowed consumers fuller access to information about products and the capacity to change brands more readily, again pressuring firms to innovate or reduce prices in order to maintain customers.

Labour market norms and structures have also changed. For example, layoffs are no longer used solely in response to a downturn in the economy; they are also used to rationalize operations in thriving markets. The level of unionization has decreased in many developed countries as has the extent of labour-market regulation. Social safety net programs such as employment insurance have also been eroded in many cases.

In this highly competitive environment, many firms have adopted flexible strategies of production. Two primary forms of flexible strategies adopted by firms have emerged: "task flexibility" (or "functional flexibility") and "numerical flexibility" (Smith, 1997).

Functional flexibility aims to increase productivity and improve profitability and service. It includes practices intended to elicit greater employee commitment and effort by enriching jobs and streamlining production processes.

The economic impacts of such strategies may not be as uniformly beneficial as is sometimes assumed. Reengineering, or redesigning business practices with a focus on outcomes (Hammer and Champy, 1993), can yield performance improvements, but is often unsuccessful (Carter, 1999; Elmuti and Kathawala, 2000). "Lean production," which utilizes problem-solving teams and just-in-time production techniques, has had positive impacts on productivity, quality, and costs, but only by making employees work longer and harder (Fairris and Tohyama, 2002; Yates et al., 2001). Efforts to increase employee commitment—such as employee participation in decision-making, self-directed work teams, and training—can result in improved bottom lines, service, and product innovation (Appelbaum et al., 2000; Varma et al., 1999). However, results have been mixed in terms of productivity, job satisfaction, organizational commitment, absenteeism, and turnover (Farias and Varma, 1998), and are contingent on employee and organizational and intervention characteristics (Belanger, 2000; Morissette and Rosa, 2003; Ramsay et al., 2000; Wood, 1999).

Numerical, or staffing, flexibility is focused on cost reduction. Numerical flexibility is often achieved by reducing labour costs through downsizing, and shifting to short-term contracting and part-time work (see Figure 5.1). It can also be achieved by using overtime as a buffer for fluctuations in demand.

The impact of these practices on the bottom line has also been mixed (Wagar, 1998), beneficial only in the short-term (Appelbaum et al., 1999), and more successful at improving profit than productivity (CFO Forum, 1995). The growing evidence that downsizing does not always achieve its objectives has not halted the trend toward laying off workers in an effort to improve financial performance.

Despite the increased use of contingent workers, there has been little examination of the economic impacts associated with their use. Indeed, costs attached to their use—such as reduced quality of services, reduced employee commitment, increased turnover and training costs—are frequently ignored (Davis-Blake et al., 2003).

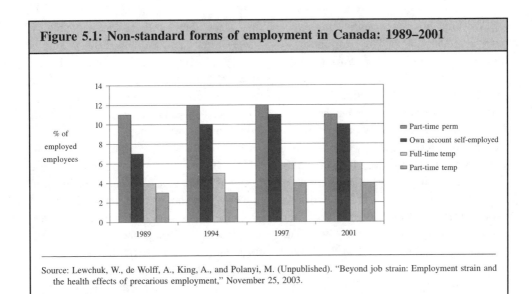

**Figure 5.1: Non-standard forms of employment in Canada: 1989–2001**

% of employed employees

- ■ Part-time perm
- ■ Own account self-employed
- ▢ Full-time temp
- ■ Part-time temp

Source: Lewchuk, W., de Wolff, A., King, A., and Polanyi, M. (Unpublished). "Beyond job strain: Employment strain and the health effects of precarious employment," November 25, 2003.

In sum, the economic impacts of downsizing, re-engineering, and high performance practices have been mixed. The health impacts, however, are of significant concern.

## Flexible organizational strategies and the experience of work

Flexible production strategies have direct and indirect implications for the health and well being of labour-force participants. While it may be that the increased flexibility of labour markets and workplaces has increased autonomy, motivation, and quality of work experiences for some high skilled workers (Applebaum et al., 2000), this appears not to be the case for those who are already disadvantaged in the workplace—low-skilled workers, women, and people of colour (Betcherman and Chaykowski, 1996). While there is some evidence of increases in employee control for standard workers in the United States and Europe (Landsbergis,

2003), there is also evidence in countries such as the United Kingdom of declining employee control (Green, 2002).

In general, studies indicate that work is intensifying, insecurity is growing, and market incomes are stagnating and polarizing.

*Intensification of work:* The intensification of work—or increased effort expended by employees—has been identified as "one of the most significant trends of recent years" (European Foundation for the Improvement of Work and Living Conditions, 2002). Data from the United States (Landsbergis, 2003) and Europe (Burchell et al., 2002; European Foundation for the Improvement of Work and Living Conditions, 2002) show that, since the 1980s, workers increasingly report working at high speed, with high effort and tight deadlines. Data from Europe suggests that the increase in work intensity during the 1990s has been greater for women than for men, closing a gap that had previously existed (Fagan and Burchell, 2002).

Working hours for many employees have also increased. The proportion of Canadian men and women working more than 40 hours a week increased significantly between 1980 and 1995 (Shields, 1999). Similar increases have occurred in the United States (Schor, 2002), and about one in five men, and one in ten women, work more than 48 hours per week in Europe (Fagan, 2003).

Not surprisingly, given the rise in work hours, one in three Canadian workers experiences conflict between work and family (Duxbury and Higgins, 2001), with evidence of similar conflict in the United States (Ferber and O'Farrell, 1991), the United Kingdom (Franks, 1999), and Europe (Fagan, 2003).

*Increased insecurity:* A second trend related to the widespread workplace and societal changes is an expanding and deepening sense of insecurity. Job insecurity has become widespread in Canada and other industrialized countries (Betcherman and Lowe, 1997; Burchell et al., 2002).

Workers are not only more uncertain about the likelihood that they will be retained in their current job, they are also uncertain whether they will be able to find another job that meets their needs (Burke and Shields, 1999; Heery and Salmon, 2000). This is partly a reflection of steady or rising unemployment rates. Finally, there is a broader sense of income insecurity as evidenced in Canada by the low level of confidence workers have in the adequacy of the social safety net (Burke and Shields, 1999). Its inadequacy is corroborated by a rise in the percentage of Canadians living in poverty, and the average depth of poverty, from the 1980s to 1990s (Heisz et al., 2002).

Insecurity is not randomly distributed: women's work in particular has become more precarious in Canada (Cranford et al., 2003), and women are twice as likely as men to work in low-paid jobs (Maxwell, 2002) (See Box 5.1).

*Stagnation and polarization of incomes:* The third key labour market trend is that average incomes have stagnated and compensation for work has become more polarized, particularly among male workers (Beach et al., 2002). Formerly well-paid, unionized, manufacturing sector employees have been forced to seek employment in the expanding service sector, where full-time jobs are scarce, few employees have benefits

---

**Box 5.1: Precarious jobs: A new typology of employment**

- Between 1989 and 1994, the share of the workforce aged 15 and over engaged in part-time work, temporary work, own-account self-employment, or multiple jobholding grew from 28% to 34%. Since then, it has hovered around this level.
- The rise in non-standard employment in the early 1990s was fuelled by increases in own-account self-employment and full-time temporary paid work. Although employees with full-time permanent jobs still accounted for the majority of employment, this kind of work became less common, dropping from 67% in 1989 to 64% in 1994 and 63% in 2002.
- In 2002, women accounted for over 6 in 10 of those with part-time temporary jobs or part-time self-employment (own-account or employers) and for nearly three-quarters of part-time permanent employees.

Source: www.statcan.ca/english/indepth/75-001/online/01003/hi-fs_200310_02_a.html

Social Determinants of Health

or earn living wages, hours are irregular, and many employees hold down multiple jobs in an effort to survive (Broad, 2000). One in six Canadians receive an inadequate wage of less than $10/hour (Maxwell, 2002). While women continue to be paid at lower rates than men at all levels of the hierarchy, and continue to be concentrated in low-end jobs in industrialized countries, the income gap between men and women has lessened somewhat in Canada, as women, on average, experienced better income growth than men during the 1990s (Heisz et al., 2002). Although family disposable income equality remained steady from the 1970s to the mid-1990s, due to government transfers and supports, there is some evidence that inequality had risen by the late 1990s (Heisz et al., 2002). In summary, significant changes to the work landscape are taking place—and these have significant health implications, which we explore below.

## Employer flexibility and employee ill-health

Recent economic and workplace trans-formations have been accompanied by mixed changes in workers' health. The number of work fatalities (Marshall, 1996) and work-related injury and illness claims (Mustard et al., 2001) have decreased substantially over recent decades in Canada and other developed countries.

However, Canada still has the highest work-related mortality rates of Organization for Economic Cooperation and Development (OECD) countries, and is fourth highest in workplace injuries (Osberg and Sharpe, 2003). While this may be attributable in part to different classification criteria and the resource-based nature of the Canadian economy, Canada also performs poorly on within-country trend data. Canada has had

little success in reducing its fatality rate over a 21-year period (only 6.6% compared to Italy's 60% decrease) and only modest success in reducing work-related injuries; six other countries had higher decreases (Osberg and Sharpe, 2000).

While causal connections between changing work conditions and health are difficult to establish, there is reason to believe that both the intensification of work, and rising levels of job, employment and income insecurity are having ill-health effects. There are five potential pathways through which these adverse labour-market experiences may influence health: (1) stress-induced physiological changes, such as increased cholesterol (Kasl et al., 1998); (2) changes in the nervous, immune, and endocrine systems that may have long-term negative health consequences; (3) increased risky health behaviour, such as decrease in physical activity and increase in smoking, drinking, and unhealthy dietary habits (Morris et al., 1992); (4) loss of social support (Gore, 1978); and (5) inadequacy of income. Below we discuss the evidence of negative health implications of intensification of work, non-standard work arrangements, and rising levels of job, employment, and income insecurity.

### Intensification of work and health
European data shows that individuals working continuously at high speeds report roughly twice the rates of stress, injuries and back, neck, and shoulder pain as individuals who never work at high speeds (European Foundation for the Improvement of Working and Living Conditions, 2002). Other unique health conditions arising from work intensification have also been identified. A Dutch study found that "leisure sickness" on weekends and holidays, characterized by headaches, sore muscles,

fatigue and nausea, is common among employees who are perfectionists, carry large workloads, and feel very responsible for their work (Burrell, 2001).

## Non-standard work hours and health

The trend toward longer hours for core employees and people in managerial and professional ranks has been well-established over the past decade. Long hours of work have been directly linked to negative physiological and psychological health symptoms, as well as to family relationship difficulties (Sparks et al., 1997; Landsbergis, 2003). Disturbed relaxation ability, correlated with elevated blood pressure and coronary heart disease, is related to working more than 50 hours per week (Ertel et al., 2000).

Non-standard hours of work (e.g., rotating shifts, compressed work weeks, and irregular hours) have also been linked with ill-health (Martens et al., 1999). However, in general there has been conflicting evidence on the health impacts of non-standard, or "flexible," work hours (Sparks et al., 2001). What seems to be key is whether employees are able to choose, and are satisfied with, their hours and schedules (Ala-Masula et al., 2002; Sparks et al., 2001). Long hours at work may be more detrimental to the health of those workers (most often women) with heavy domestic work loads. The inability to balance work and family, which is exacerbated by long or unpredictable work hours, has also been directly linked with increased stress and negative health symptoms (Duxbury et al., 1994; Ertel et al., 2000; Frone et al., 1997).

## Precarious work arrangements and health

Studies show that temporary and contract workers tend to have poorer working conditions, are more stressed, and are less healthy overall than the rest of the working population (European Foundation for the Improvement of Living and Working Conditions, 2002). Quinlan, Mayhew, and Bohle's (2001) review of 93 studies of contingent work and occupational health in various countries found that a substantial majority of studies showed a negative association between precarious employment and health.

The reasons why non-standard workers experience poorer health are complex. Such workers may face more difficult working conditions, experience higher levels of job insecurity, have lower levels of control over their working conditions and arrangements, experience poorer quality social interactions, or be exposed to particular demands associated with their employment arrangements (Lewchuk et al., 2003).

## Job insecurity and health

In general, studies have found an association between job insecurity and various disease and sickness outcomes (Sverke et al., 2002). A recent review by Ferrie (2001) found a consistent impact of perceived job insecurity on psychological morbidity, and emerging evidence of a relationship between job insecurity and self-reported morbidity. Job-level insecurity—or downsizing—has been associated with increased sickness absence (Kivimaki et al., 2000). Downsizing has been linked to increased workplace fatalities, workplace accidents, musculoskeletal injuries, and psychiatric disorders (Landsbergis, 2003; Probst and Brubaker, 2001). Perceived job insecurity also has negative effects on workers' marital relationships, parenting effectiveness, and their children's behaviour (Nolan et al., 2000).

Turnover and absenteeism rates as well as stress-related disorders increase after downsizing (Applebaum et al., 1999), and Cohen (1997) found that employees who had become disabled after experiencing downsizing took substantially longer to recover. If the downsizing trend continues, the costs associated with employee stress, currently estimated at $200 billion in the U.S. annually (Carter, 1999), will only worsen.

## Employment insecurity and health

The health effects of job insecurity appear to be moderated by the prevailing level of labour market opportunities (Mohr, 2000; Turner, 1995). In other words, job insecurity can be less harmful when there are other employment opportunities available to workers. There is a large literature exploring the mental and physical ill-health impacts of unemployment (Jahoda, 1982; Warr, 1987). Emerging research suggests that there are also negative health impacts of underemployment, although more research is needed in this area (Dooley, 2003).

## Income insecurity and health

The health impacts of employment insecurity and inadequacy are in turn affected by the perceived adequacy and security of income. Price and colleagues (2002) found that "financial strain" explains a significant portion of the relationship between employment status and subsequent depression. In general, income inadequacy,

or poverty, has been clearly established as a predictor of ill health (Raphael, 2001).

Income insecurity—and ill health—is not equally distributed. Women and people of colour are more likely to work in low income jobs, less likely to have benefits, and more likely to live in poverty (e.g., Maxwell, 2002). Finally, there is evidence that the degree of income inequality at the local and national levels is predictive of poorer health outcomes of groups across the income spectrum (Wilkinson, 1996). The polarization of incomes associated with flexible labour markets is hence a health concern.

In summary, there is reason to believe that stress or "strain" in today's flexible economy is related not just to the worker's job, but to the worker's broader experience of the broader organization and arrangements of employment (see Table 5.1 for one depiction of "employment strain"). While further quantitative and qualitative research is needed on the health impacts of cost-cutting and high productivity strategies, there is now enough evidence to initiate action to reduce the negative health effects of neo-liberal, flexible employment strategies, and to promote the adoption of healthier—and more authentically productive—workplace practices and labour market conditions.

## Conclusion: Toward healthy and productive work

While many firms focus on short-term profits and flexibility at a cost to employee health and well being, there are opportunities for firms to adopt a wider array of employee-friendly organizational practices that better balance the dual aims of health and productivity.

### Research and education

Research and education are needed to promote a fuller recognition of the health- and productivity-related impacts of cost-cutting and high performance strategies. There is a

## Table 5.1: Employment strain

| Components | Control / demand | Measured by |
|---|---|---|
| 1. Employment uncertainty | Control over access to work | • average length of contracts<br>• perceived uncertainty regarding current employers offering more work<br>• presence/absence of a union to enforce workplace rights<br>• perceived influence of day to day work performance and attitude evaluations on future offers of work<br>• favoritism in getting new work |
| 2. Earnings uncertainty | Control over future earnings | • presence/absence of written pay records<br>• EI/CPP deductions from earnings<br>• whether employee is paid when sick<br>• whether employee is paid on time<br>• the degree to which employee can plan on future earnings |
| 3. Household precariousness | Control/ demand providing basic needs | • number of dependents in household<br>• individual and household earnings<br>• individual and household benefit coverage |
| 4. Scheduling uncertainty | Control over work schedule and hours | • length of advance notice of work schedule<br>• number of hours to be worked |
| 5. Location uncertainty | Control over work location | • number of work locations<br>• length of advance notice of work location |
| 6. Task uncertainty | Control over use of skills and job assignment | • perceived influence of day to day evaluations of attitude over work tasks assigned<br>• the number of different supervisors and groups of co-employees<br>• frequency of working in an unfamiliar location |
| 7. Employment uncertainty workload | Demand required to manage employment uncertainty | • time spent looking for work<br>• time spent traveling between jobs<br>• conflicts from holding more than one job |

Source: Lewchuk, W., de Wolff, A., King, A., and Polanyi, M. (Unpublished). "Beyond job strain: Employment strain and the health effects of precarious employment," November 25, 2003.

particular need to dispel the assumption that cost-cutting and flexible staffing necessarily lead to economic competitiveness. New forms of knowledge transfer and education are needed. It has become increasingly clear that in order for research to be understood and used, stakeholders must be involved in the research process.

## Culture change

There needs to be a culture change within and beyond organizations. This requires the same kind of sea-change of thinking about work that has taken place on issues of drinking and driving, and smoking, both of which were driven by co-ordinated legal, policy, and community action. Workers, employers, government officials, researchers, and others need to come together to develop a shared vision of healthy and productive work. Developing this shared vision of "good" or "decent" work is the first step towards developing the kind of multi-level strategy that is needed to prevent, hinder and stigmatize unhealthy workplace practices.

To encourage increased social accountability of employer practices, freer and fuller flows of information will be needed. This might include more systematic sharing of good or best organizational practices that have buy-in from both workers and management, as well as the provision of more complete information about the nature of production practices (e.g., some footballs sold in the United States are now certified as not being produced with child labour).

## Institutional change

Countries need to ensure that competitive pressures encourage high-road rather than low-road innovation. This requires that international trade and investment agreements incorporate minimum labour standards. It also requires taxation measures to deter non-productive and destabilizing investments (e.g., financial transfer taxes). It requires moving from a framework of free trade to one of "fair trade" (Mehmet et al., 1999). At the firm level, this requires rethinking corporate governance so that those interested in short term profit alone (i.e., employers or shareholders) do not dictate decisions that impact on workers, families, and communities (Ackerman and Allstott, 1999).

## Policy and legislation

Individual countries and even individual firms have it within their power to react to global economic pressures in a variety of ways, thus suggesting the possibility that policy can be instituted at the national and provincial levels. This can be achieved through a mix of levers such as macroeconomic policy, education and training policy, regulation of workplace practices and benefits, and policies supportive of various forms of unionization.

Particular attention needs to be paid to non-standard forms of work. For example, there could be requirements of prorating retirement, sick leave, holiday, and health care benefits for temporary and part-time workers. Regulation could also extend to training and advancement opportunities, and the requirement that temporary agencies hire staff on a permanent basis after a certain tenure of service. Legislation could also be designed to facilitate collective bargaining for non-standard forms of work through the expansion or reinterpretation of craft-like guilds and unions that cut across several employers. More generally, multi-firm labour and management groups could provide support for workers throughout their careers with services such as career counseling and job referral systems.

Low-paying work systems should be a specific target of public policy, since workers in these systems are particularly vulnerable. Labour-force participants need to be aware of the types of skills demanded by the labour-market, and have access to financing, appropriate training opportunities, and assistance with job search (e.g., access to job banks and career counseling). On the demand side, policy needs to provide a stimulus for firms operating in low-wage systems to raise productivity levels, and in turn, place more value on their human resources. Other policy concerns associated with these work systems are the predictability and length of work hours and autonomy, and control issues related to the pace and intensity of work.

Attention should be paid to enhancing job, employment, and income security of all workers. Job and income security can be promoted by requiring that temporary agencies hire employees after a certain time frame on a full-time permanent basis. Employment insurance premiums can be experience-rated to provide incentives for industries and employers who depend heavily on seasonal, part-time, and short-tenure work to consider a more complete set of costs that arise from these employment practices. Employment security can be promoted through increasing access to training, and by providing further options for reduced—and hence redistributed—work hours. Income security can be promoted by expanding access to employment insurance and pensions (Townson, 2003). Broader income security also requires the protection of public services such as health care, education, and recreation.

Finally, the design of workers' compensation and occupational health and safety regulation need to be revisited. Public policies and programs need to create incentives for firms to safeguard worker health and well-being rather than focus simply on reducing injuries and illnesses. Innovative regulatory practices directed at empowering workplace parties and encouraging firm-level solutions, such as providing employers, particularly smaller ones, with customized training and incentive programs would be helpful, since firms often do not have the knowledge or resources to evaluate the direct and indirect costs of illness and injury and the benefits of investing in preventative measures.

**Power and equity**
The growing power imbalance between employees and employers needs to be redressed. In part this will depend on traditional and new forms of employee representation. In part, it will depend on creating a context of greater employment and income security, so that workers are not forced to choose between poverty and workplace-induced illness.

Inequalities across various labour-force subgroups (along with characteristics such as gender, age, cultural background, and education level) need to be reduced. Indeed, it appears that economically marginalized groups such as women, youth, low-wage, and non-white workers are being disproportionately harmed by flexible workplace strategies. There is a need, therefore, for stronger legislation governing equal opportunity in hiring, pay, training, and career advancement. Consistent with the notion of reducing inequalities, the requirement of certain accommodations for health conditions would allow freer labour-force participation for older individuals and individuals with functional deficits.

This chapter has described labour market and workplace changes that have been shown to impact on health. While some work-related health outcomes, like lost-time work accidents, have shown improvement, other outcomes—like stress and non-acute conditions—seem to be on the rise. Moreover, the outlook in terms of key work-related determinants of health, such as job demands, job control, job security, and income equality, is ominous. Stakeholders concerned about work and health need to better understand the health implications of today's workplace and labour market conditions, and come together to establish a shared vision of, and agenda to create, healthy work for all in the very near future.

# Recommended readings

Broad, D. (2000). *Hollow work, hollow society? Globalization and the casual labour problem in Canada.* Halifax: Fernwood.
> Explains the contemporary casualization of work as integral to global economic restructuring, and explores the human impact of these trends.

Burchell, B., Ladipo, D. and Wilkinson, F. (2002). *Job insecurity and work intensification.* London: Routledge.
> Reviews current research on flexibility, job insecurity and work intensification and examines the impact of these developments on individuals, their families, the workplace and the long-term health of the British economy.

European Foundation for the Improvement of Living and Working Conditions. (2002). *Quality of work and employment in Europe: Issues and challenges* (Foundation Paper). Dublin, Ireland: EFILWC. Online at www.eurofound.eu.int/publications/files/EF0212EN.pdf.
> Reviews challenges and opportunities associated with changes in work based on a multi-country survey of European workers.

Landsbergis, P.A. (2003). "The changing organization of work and the safety and health of working people: A commentary," *Journal of occupational and environmental medicine* 45(1): 61–72.
> Reviews an important new U.S. report on the current state of knowledge on work organization and health.

Quinlan, M., Mayhew, C. and Bohle, P. (2001). "The global expansion of precarious employment, work disorganization, and consequences for occupational health: a review of recent research," *International journal of health services* 31(2), 335–414.
> An important and far-reaching conceptual and review article exploring the health implications of precarious work.

# Related websites

European Foundation for the Improvement of Work and Living—www.eurofound.ie/
> Important and voluminous source of free reports on changing nature of work and health.

International Labour Organization—www.ilo.org/
> Source of leading edge thinking about the promotion of an international agenda for decent work.

Winning Workplaces—www.winningworkplaces.org/
> Range of information, success stories, and research on small and midsize organizations' workplace practices.

# Chapter Six

———●———

# THE UNHEALTHY
# CANADIAN WORKPLACE

## Andrew Jackson

## Introduction

The purpose of this chapter is to provide a broad overview of the state of employment and working conditions to set a context for an analysis of the impacts of the working environment on health. The focus is on the quality of work as opposed to wider conditions in the labour market, and on working conditions as opposed to wages.

The links from employment to health are not examined here in detail, though they implicitly frame the selection of topics. Suffice to say at the outset that research has established strong links from unemployment and precarious employment to poor health outcomes, and from poor employment conditions to poor physical and mental health. Poor employment conditions include: dirty and dangerous jobs, including exposures to harmful substances which pose risks to physical health in terms of injuries and occupational disease; jobs which are stressful by virtue of the pace, demands, or repetitive content of the labour process; jobs which are stressful because of the exercise of arbitrary power in the workplace; jobs which are stressful because they do not meet human developmental needs; and jobs which are stressful because they are a source of conflict with the lives of workers in the home and in the community.

In recent years, health researchers have increasingly emphasized links from work stress to physical and mental health. Stress can arise from many sources, including job insecurity, the physical demands of work, the extent of support from supervisors and co-workers, work–life conflict, and job strain (Wilkins and Beaudet, 1998). High job strain—a combination of high psychological demands at work combined with a low degree of control of the work process—and other sources of workplace stress have been linked to an increased risk of physical injuries at work, high blood pressure, cardiovascular disease, depression, and other mental health conditions, and increased "lifestyle risks" to health.

The well-established linkage from income and social class to physical and mental health outcomes is probably, in very significant part, a product of the work conditions associated with income level and class position. Work poses physical risks, and is clearly a major source of "psycho-social" stress which has been identified as one major cause of increased morbidity and mortality. Gender is, of course, a major intervening variable.

It is ironic, not to say tragic, that the shift to a post-industrial society with an increasingly well-educated and skilled workforce is associated with rising levels of stress rather than increased well-being at work. Research has shown some negative consequences for health to date, but the full impact of current conditions is likely to be slow to appear. Many of today's older workers and retirees were workers in the "Golden Age" of post-War capitalism when working conditions were more closely regulated, and conditions were improving. The health impacts of 21$^{st}$ century work may just be appearing.

This chapter seeks to provide a general overview of current conditions and the overall direction of change, to look at some important cleavages among workers in terms of access to good jobs, and to place the situation in Canada in a comparative context. Comparisons are made with the European Union because better working conditions in the EU along some dimensions do suggest that improvement of the quality of the Canadian work environment is not incompatible with having a highly productive economy.

## What is a "good job"?

An appropriate starting point is to consider what is a "good job" from the perspective of workers. For all of the emphasis which is (rightly) placed on the fundamental importance of waged employment as the critical source of working class income and well-being in a capitalist society, other dimensions of employment are at least as important to workers. On the economic front, non-wage benefits, job security, and opportunities for advancement are as important as wages. The content of work and the nature of the labour process are less tangible and measurable, but count for a lot as well. A major international survey in 1989 found that having an interesting job and being allowed to work independently rank very high as desirable features of employment in all countries (Andrew Clark, "What Makes a Good Job?" www.csls.ca). The recent EKOS/CPRN survey of changing employment relationships in Canada confirmed that a large majority of workers place a high value on having interesting and personally rewarding work, enjoying some

autonomy on the job, and having the ability to exercise and develop their skills and capacities. Jencks (1988) found that there is much more unequal distribution of quality jobs along valued dimensions other than pay, indicating that even large pay differences are an imperfect proxy for large class differences in the quality of employment.

The statement that quality of employment involves much more than pay will come as a surprise only to economists who have been trained to view work as a "disutility" endured in order to gain income. Work is better seen as a potential sphere for the development of individual human capacities and potentials. Production is also a social process. Good workplaces are those in which there are valued relationships with co-workers and some degree of active participation and democratic control of the work process. Bad workplaces, by contrast, are alienating and authoritarian.

For the purposes of this chapter, and recognizing that there is considerable overlap between categories, seven key dimensions of employment with relevance to well-being and health are considered:

- Job and employment security
- Physical conditions of work
- Work pace and stress
- Working time
- Opportunities for self-expression and individual development at work
- Participation at work
- Work–life balance

Before these dimensions are considered in detail, it is useful to briefly summarize some of the wider economic and social forces impacting upon Canadian workplaces.

## Forces shaping workplace change in Canada

In a capitalist labour market, the terms of employment—wages and benefits, hours, working conditions—reflect the relative bargaining power of workers and employers, and the related willingness of governments to establish minimum rights and standards. Over the 1980s and 1990s, the context has been one of high unemployment and underemployment, increased employer ability to shift production and new investments to lower cost regions and countries, and an ideologically-driven retreat from state intervention on behalf of workers.

There has been a pervasive and ongoing restructuring of the labour market and of employment relationships intended to promote productivity and competitiveness, as opposed to promotion of a worker-centred agenda of "good jobs" (Lowe, 2000). The basic direction of change is best understood as a simultaneous intensification and casualization of work by employers. The most common forms of organizational change have been downsizing, contracting-out of non-core functions, and securing

greater flexibility of time worked through a combination of increased overtime and increased part-time and contract work.

The restructuring of work has been driven by employers. Governments mainly have been, at best, passive bystanders. But countervailing forces do exist. The unionization rate has been remarkably steady in the 1990s at about 30% of paid workers, though it has been modestly declining in the private sector. A more extensive discussion of the forces shaping workplace change in Canada is available (Jackson, 2002).

## Dimensions of job quality

### Job security

In considering the linkages from labour market conditions to health, researchers have studied both the availability of work and the nature of work. It is well-established from studies of laid-off workers that the state of unemployment is bad for health for both material and psychological reasons. However, the relatively well-studied transition from stable employment to long-term unemployment is less frequent than alternation between short-term unemployment and precarious employment. Frequent short-term unemployment is also a source of stress and anxiety due to lack of income, uncertain prospects for the future, and its potential to undermine social support networks (World Health Organization, 1999). Workers who must move from short-term job to short-term job are also likely to derive less satisfaction and meaning from their paid work.

Most Canadians are familiar with the national unemployment rate, which is reported monthly and stood at just above 7% in the fall of 2002. Taken at face value, this number considerably understates the true extent of employment insecurity. To be counted as employed, one need only have worked for a few hours in a week, so employment includes temporary employees, part-time workers who want more hours, and people working in low-wage survival jobs while looking for regular jobs matching their skills. To be counted as unemployed, a person has to have been unable to find any work at all, and to have been actively seeking work even if they knew that no suitable jobs were available.

Today, about one-in-five employed Canadians are self-employed, the majority of whom work on their own account (i.e., with no employees) for low incomes, and another one-in-six are in temporary paid jobs. Only two-thirds of the employed workforce are in "standard" paid jobs with no defined end date. Among women part-time workers, about one-in-three would work full-time if they could.

In 1999, when the national unemployment rate averaged 7.6%, just 71% of persons aged 16 to 69 in the workforce were employed all year, and 12% of men and 13% of women who worked at some time in the year were unemployed at least once in the same year. The others worked for part of the year and were not in the work force for another part of the year (*Survey of labour and income dynamics*, ongoing). Earlier in the 1990s, about one-

in-five workers were unemployed at least once in any year. And Statistics Canada reports that no less than one-in-three Canadian families had at least one member of the family unemployed each year in the 1980s and 1990s (*The daily*, September 6, 2000).

Long-term unemployment in Canada is much lower than in other advanced industrial countries. In 2001, just 17% of unemployed workers had been out of work for more than six months compared to a 42% average in Organization for Economic Cooperation and Development (OECD) countries, and 60% in the European Union (EU). However, a lot of Canadians cycle between precarious jobs and unemployment, and precariously employed workers tend to be trapped in low-wage jobs. One recent study found that only one-in-five low-wage workers in 1993 were earning significantly more in 1995 (Drolet and Morrissettee, 1998). Finnie (2000) finds that working poor families tend to stay that way, moving above and below the poverty line as they find and lose jobs, but rarely finding long-term job or income security.

Precarious work in Canada is not only widespread, it is much more precarious than in many other countries. In the EU, a binding policy directive establishes that there should be limits on renewals of temporary contracts and notification of vacancies to temporary

---

**Box 6.1**

As one would expect from the unemployment data, many working Canadians worry about losing their jobs. The Personal Security Index (PSI) of the Canadian Council on Social Development (CCSD) tracks the proportion of persons who think there is a good chance they could lose their job over the next two years. This stood at 28% in 2001, down from a recent high of 37% in 1998. Fear of job loss is slightly higher among men than women, and much higher in lower income households. The PSI also tracks the proportion of workers who are confident they could find an equivalent job within six months if they lost their current job. Thirty percent were not confident in 2001, down from 38% in 1998. Confidence declines significantly with age.

Social Determinants of Health

workers. National laws in EU countries commonly provide for non-discrimination against temporary and part-time workers in terms of pay, benefits coverage, and access to training (EIRO, 2001b). Minimum pay laws and widespread collective bargaining provide a wage and benefit floor to the job market. As a result, there are far larger pay gaps between precarious and core workers in Canada than in most EU countries, though gaps here are somewhat smaller than in the US (Jackson, 2000). For example, one in five Canadians work in low-paid jobs compared to one in four Americans, but just one in twenty Swedish workers. (Low pay is defined as working for less than two-thirds the national median wage.)

Job insecurity in the precarious labour market is heightened by lack of supports and services to promote access to better employment. The dominant ethos is that heavy sticks are needed to drive the unemployed into available low-wage jobs. Hence our minimal and deeply punitive social welfare system which makes even minimum wages look attractive. And, hence, recent cuts to the EI program in the form of higher qualifying hours requirements which effectively cut off the precariously employed workers who need income support the most.

Positive employment measures are undertaken under the EI program and by provincial governments, but the overall training effort is low and has been falling. State labour market training programs for unemployed workers and those at risk amount to just 0.2% of GDP, a fraction of the level spent in some countries. Despite unemployment rates which are lower than in Canada, training spending is 6% of GDP in Denmark and 4% in Sweden (*OECD employment outlook*, 2001, Table 9).

A key difference between core and peripheral workers is access to employer-sponsored health benefits. As shown in Table 6.1, less than half of non-union workers have access to medical, dental and disability coverage compared to about 80% of unionized workers. Access to health-related benefits is much lower for non-professional/managerial non-union workers, particularly in smaller private sector firms. Under the current health care system in most provinces, lack of employer coverage generally means that the costs of prescription drugs outside of hospitals, dental care, and many disability-related supports and services must be paid for from family budgets. There are also large gaps between core and peripheral workers in terms of access to paid sick leave, though here there is at least entitlement to a modest floor through the EI program. Many precariously employed workers thus face directly higher risks to

| Table 6.1: Benefits coverage—union vs. non-union |||||
| --- | --- | --- | --- | --- |
| | Medical plan | Dental plan | Life/disability insurance | Pension plan |
| All employees | 57.4% | 53.1% | 52.5% | 43.3% |
| Unionized | 83.7% | 76.3% | 78.2% | 79.9% |
| Non-unionized | 45.4% | 42.6% | 40.8% | 26.6% |

Source: "Benefits coverage—Union vs. non-union," adapted from the article entitled "Unionization and fringe benefits," published in the Statistics Canada publication "Perspectives on labour and income," Catalogue 75-001, Autumn 2002, 14(3).

health because of the quality of their employment.

Lack of employer-sponsored pension coverage for many precarious workers combined with a relatively ungenerous public pension system implies longer working lifetimes. Many low-wage older workers are significantly better off after they retire at 65 and qualify for the combined Old Age Security pension and Guaranteed Income Supplement, which at least provides an income close to the poverty line.

To summarize, a large minority of workers experience continuing precarious employment and high risks of unemployment. The risks of precarious employment in terms of low income, stress and anxiety are compounded by lack of access to benefits.

**Physical conditions of work**

One might have thought that dirty and dangerous work was a thing of the past, banished along with the dark satanic mills of the Industrial Revolution. But occupational diseases and injuries rooted in the physical conditions of work are very much a feature of the contemporary workplace.

In 1998, there were 793,000 officially recorded workplace injuries, more than three times the total number of traffic injuries. There were 375,000 injuries involving time-loss reported to Workers' Compensation Boards, and 798 workplace fatalities. For every 100 workers in 1998, there were 5.5 injuries, and 2.6 time-loss injuries: 3.4 for men; 1.5 for women; and, 2.9 for young workers (HRDC, 2000). The incidence of accidents and injuries is modestly falling, but still very high. And, there has been a disturbing upward trend in repetitive strain and other soft tissue injuries associated with highly repetitive machine and keyboard work. These account for an upward trend in the proportion of workplace injuries reported by women.

As one would expect, physical injuries—sprains and strains to backs and hands, cuts, punctures, lacerations, fractures, and contusions—are associated with physically-demanding jobs.

Manufacturing and construction account for 20% of employment but about 40% of injuries, explaining the gap between injury rates among men and women. But injury rates are also high in sectors such as retail trade, and health and social services.

Sullivan (2000) argues that workers' compensation practices, which were designed to address physical trauma in a world of manual, blue-collar, male work, have not changed to sufficiently recognize the growing reality of less visible physical injuries which develop over a period of time. Soft tissue injuries, such as repetitive strain injuries affecting women clerical and service workers, are under-reported and under-compensated.

Table 6.2 provides some unpublished data on exposure to physical hazards at work from the *General social survey* of 1991. Astonishingly, no comparable recent information is available. As shown, one-in-three (34.1%) of workers reported some negative health impacts from a workplace hazard exposure, and a significant minority of workers were exposed to dust, dangerous chemicals, loud noise, and poor quality air.

Occupational diseases are, of course, also related to workplace risks and exposures. Lung diseases and cancers are linked to physical risks, including inhalation of toxic fumes, handling of hazardous chemicals, and exposure to carcinogens. In a very limited number of cases, there is a very clear causal linkage from occupational

# Table 6.2: Physical work environment

| | Experienced negative health impact from workplace health hazard exposure | Experienced workplace injury in past year | Risk of injury caused worry | Exposure to dust in air most of the time | Exposure to dangerous chemicals most of the time | Exposure to loud noise most of the time | Exposure to poor quality air most of the time | Negative health impacts from exposure to computer screen |
|---|---|---|---|---|---|---|---|---|
| All | 34.1 | 9.2 | 7.6 | 18.8(45.0)* | 7.5(48.4)* | 15.7(42.1)* | 15.3(70.7)* | 8.5 |
| Men | 36 | 11.9 | 9.6 | 23 | 10.6 | 22.9 | 14 | 6.7 |
| Women | 31.3 | 5.9 | 5.1 | 13.8 | 3.8 | 7.1 | 16.8 | 10.6 |
| Union | 41.2 | 11.5 | 12.7 | 24.4 | 9.7 | 23.1 | 20.8 | 9.1 |
| Non-union | 30 | 8 | 4.8 | 15.9 | 6.4 | 11.8 | 12.5 | 8.1 |
| Managerial/professional | 35.4 | 5.8 | 5.9 | 14 | 5 | 8.3 | 17.6 | 12 |
| Skilled/semi-skilled | 33.1 | 10.5 | 7.8 | 20.9 | 8.8 | 20.4 | 14.6 | 6.7 |
| Unskilled | 34 | 11.1 | 10.2 | 21.5 | 9.4 | 17.7 | 14 | 6.8 |

* Figure in brackets is % of those exposed (most of the time or sometimes) reporting a negative impact on health.

Source: "Physical work environment," adapted from the Statistics Canada publication, "General Social Survey, cycle 6: health (1991)—Custom tabulation service," Catalogue 12C0010, April 2003.

exposure to disease onset which has been recognized by workers' compensation boards. For example, boards recognize that occupational exposure causes asbestosis among asbestos mine workers, and a range of lung diseases among other miners. A handful of highly specific cancers have been demonstrably linked to exposure to specific carcinogens at work. But the overall incidence of occupational disease compared to workplace injuries is extremely low, *if* we go by the official data.

However, a wide range of conditions have been linked to occupational exposures. The workers' compensation system, run by governments and funded by employers, demands high standards of scientific proof of cause-and-effect in order to keep down costs. But, many carcinogens are present in the general environment as well as in the workplace. Experts estimate that anywhere from 10% to 40% of cancers may be caused primarily by workplace exposures, but only a tiny proportion of cancer victims qualify for workers' compensation. Similarly, workplace stress and heavy physical exertion are associated with heart conditions, but only a tiny proportion of heart attack victims (e.g., firemen) qualify. The key point is that occupational diseases due to the physical hazards of work are prevalent, but largely unrecognized. Somewhat ironically, employers end up bearing a large share of the costs anyway through employer-funded, long-term disability plans.

An official European Union institution, the European Foundation for the Improvement of Living and Working Conditions, regularly conducts surveys on European working conditions. The third survey for 2000, followed surveys for 1990 and 1995. It found that "(e)xposure to physical hazards at the workplace and conditions such as musculo-skeletal disorders and fatigue caused by intensification of work and flexible employment practices are on the increase" (EIRO, 2001).

In 2000—defining significant exposure as exposure at least one-quarter of the time—29% of European workers were exposed to noise; 22% to inhalation of vapours, fumes, and dust; 37% reported having to move or carry heavy loads; and, no less than 47% reported having to work in painful or tiring positions. In each case, a little under half of those reporting the hazard were exposed all of the time. Fortunately, given increasing rather than declining exposure to all of these risks (except inhalation exposure), 76% of European workers reported that they had been well-informed of hazards. As one would expect, exposure is greatest in occupations such as machine operators, but the EU data also indicate quite widespread exposure to physical hazards.

The European survey also provides data on the incidence of repetitive work, for which no general Canadian information is available. In the EU, 31% of workers report continuous, repetitive, hand/arm movements, and 23% report working at short, repetitive tasks with cycle times of less than one minute. One-in-four (24%) workers report continuously working at high speed, with the level being highest among machine operators (35%), but still high among clerical workers (20%) and service workers (23%). The incidence of high speed work due to tight deadlines has been modestly increasing, though there is variation between countries and between different categories of workers. The survey found that those working at high speed were much more likely to report negative health effects, such as muscular pain, stress, and anxiety.

To summarize, despite the transition to a "post-industrial society," the risks of occupational injury and disease are still high. Regrettably, little hard data are available on the physical hazards of work in Canada. One aspect of work re-organization has likely been the intensification of physical demands on some groups of workers. Highly repetitive work with short cycle times is likely just as prevalent as in the EU, explaining the sharply rising incidence of repetitive strain injuries among clerical and industrial workers.

## Work pace, control, and stress

Sources of stress at work include the pace and demands of work, and the degree of control which workers have over the labour process. Karasek and others have stressed that jobs are particularly stressful if high demands on workers are combined with a low level of decision latitude with respect to the use of skills and discretion on how to do the job. Stress from high strain jobs (high demands, low control) is greater among women than men, primarily because of lower levels of job control (Wilkins and Beaudet, 1998).

High stress jobs have been found to be a significant contributing factor to high blood pressure, cardiovascular diseases, mental illness, and long onset disability, but the link from stressful work conditions to health is all but unrecognized by workers' compensation boards (Sullivan, 2000). There is a link from low levels of control over working conditions, not only to stress, but also to higher rates of work injuries. Even where work is physically demanding, there is less risk of injury if workers can vary the pace of work, take breaks when needed, and have some say in the design of work stations.

While there have been case studies pointing to high levels of stressful work in many Canadian workplaces, general data are limited. Statistics Canada's *General social survey* provides some information. In 2000, 35% of workers reported experiencing stress at work from "too many demands or too many hours," up slightly from 33% in 1994, and up from 27.5% in 1991. Stress from this source is highest among professionals and managers, at 49% and 48% respectively, but is still high among blue-collar workers (28%) and sales and service workers (29%). By industry, the incidence of stress from "too many demands or hours" is highest in education, health and social services at over 40%. (For 2000 data, see www.jobquality.ca.) As one would expect, there is a strong relationship between working long hours and working in jobs which impose high demands.

Women are more likely than men to report high levels of stress from "too many hours or too many demands": 37% compared to 32%. This partly reflects work–life balance issues considered below. But, it also reflects the high proportion of women working in the high stress educational, health, and social services sectors, as well as in clerical positions which involve highly routinized, fast-paced work.

With respect to job control, data from the *General social survey* indicate that, in 1994, just 40% of Canadian workers reported that they had "a lot of freedom over how to work," down sharply from 54% in 1989. Men generally exercise more control than women (43% compared to 38% in 1994). Professionals and managers predictably report that they exercise much more control than skilled workers who, in turn, have more freedom than unskilled workers (51% vs. 35% vs. 31%, respectively). The same survey indicates that about half of all working Canadians believe that their jobs involve a high degree of skill, with self-reported levels of exercising a high level of skill being a bit higher among women than men.

Data from the *National population health survey* for 1994/95 have been used to construct a measure of decision latitude based on responses to two questions: "I have a lot to say about what happens in my job"; and, "My job allows me the freedom to decide how I do my job." This response is now being used as an official population health indicator. In 1994/95, 48.8% of all respondents, 52.3% of men and 44.5% of women, reported high decision latitude, while 36.6%—30.7% of men and a full 44.0% of women—reported low or medium decision latitude (Statistics Canada, 2001).

To summarize, while we lack detailed information on changes in the overall incidence of work involving high demands and low-worker control, high stress work is common and likely on the increase.

**Opportunities for self-development**

As noted, a valued characteristic of work is the opportunity it provides for the exercise and development of skills and capacities. Most of us welcome the chance to work in interesting, challenging jobs, and the opportunity to learn new things. The data presented above suggest that skilled workers, particularly professionals, are usually able to utilize their skills on the job, and enjoy a fair degree of control over the labour process. Educational credentials are, increasingly, the major requirement to enter these kinds of good jobs. Access to training on the job is also an important determinant of well-being over the course of a working lifetime, since it provides opportunities for further skills development, and for advancement to more challenging and rewarding work.

There is abundant evidence that many jobs are structured to minimize the need for skills rather than to further develop the capacities of workers. The fact that four in ten working-age Canadians have limited literacy skills reflects the fact that the capacities developed in the public educational system are often not used and developed in the workplace, and atrophy from lack of use (Livingstone, 2002; Lowe, 2000). The skills and credentials of many new immigrants are routinely overlooked by employers with the result that they are sidelined into low-pay, dead-end jobs.

Our workplace training system is much less developed than in the Scandinavian countries and Germany, which have long emphasized a "training culture." A survey by the OECD ("Training of adult workers in OECD countries," *Employment outlook*, 1999) shows that the Canadian annual participation rate in adult worker training is, at less than 30% of the employed adult workforce, about 10 percentage points lower even than in the U.S. Not only do less than one in three employed Canadian workers (excluding regular, full-time students) participate annually in job-related learning activities, the rate has been declining in the 1990s (Statistics Canada, 2001).

In summary, employer-provided training is highly concentrated on the "core" workforce in larger firms and in parts of the public sector, while the growing ranks of precarious workers—including many women workers and recent immigrants—are largely excluded. Lack of investment in training, in turn, tends to perpetuate routinized, low-skill employment and poor working conditions.

**Working-time**

An historic goal of the organized labour movement has been to expand free time. Important breakthroughs were the ten- and then the eight-hour working day, the five-day working week and the advent of the weekend, the negotiation of paid days off, and pensioned retirement at progressively earlier ages. By the 1950s, the healthy norm of the standard five-day, 40-hour week with paid annual vacation, and retirement with a decent pension was firmly entrenched.

While progress was made through the 1970s and into the 1980s in terms of reduction of weekly hours, annual hours, and the length of a working lifetime, the past decade has seen an increase in daily, weekly and annual hours for many "core" workers in full-time jobs. Long hours are most prevalent among salaried professional and managerial workers, and among skilled blue-collar workers who frequently work paid overtime. From an employer perspective, overtime helps adjust production to changing market demand, and provides a particularly high-cost saving if the extra hours are not paid for. Even overtime pay premiums are often cheaper than the costs of hiring, training, and providing non-wage benefits to additional workers. Unpaid overtime is increasingly required not just of managers and professionals, but also of public and social services workers attempting to cope with increased workloads. Self-employed workers also tend to work very long hours.

While some workers want to work overtime for higher pay or out of commitment to the job or a career, most have limited ability to refuse demands for longer hours under employment standards legislation and under collective agreements. In most provinces, overtime in excess of 40 hours can be required up to varying maximum levels of up to 50 hours or so, provided an overtime premium is paid. Only 25% of unionized workers have some right (usually conditional) to refuse overtime.

The *Workplace and employee survey* found that 9% of all workers and 12% of workers in firms of more than 500 in 1999 would have preferred to work fewer hours for less pay. This can be considered an underestimate of involuntary long hours to the extent that many other workers would choose to take part of a compensation increase in the form of reduced hours. Reduced work time has recently been emphasized by several major industrial unions. For example, the Communications, Energy and Paper-workers' Union (CEP) have limited overtime in pulp and paper mills, and the CAW have increased paid days off in the auto assembly sector. (On working time issues see *Report of the advisory group on working time and distribution of work*, Human Resources Development Canada, 1997, and Andrew Jackson, *Creating more and better jobs through reduction and redistribution of working time*, available at www.clc-ctc.ca.)

There has been a strong trend to long (and short) working hours for both men and women in the 1980s and 1990s at the expense of the 40-hour work week norm. ("The changing work week: Trends in weekly hours of work," Statistics Canada. *Canadian economic observer*, September 1996.) The proportion of men working more than 50 hours per week in their main job rose steadily from 15% in the early 1980s to about 20% in 1994, and has continued at that level through 2000. Over the same period, the proportion of women working more than 50 hours per week has risen from 5% to about 7% (*Labour force survey* data, available at www.jobquality.ca). About one in three men and one in eight women in paid jobs now work more than 40 hours per week.

As noted above, working long hours is closely associated with working in high demand jobs. While these jobs may be interesting and challenging and give rise to opportunities for advancement, long hours and high demands can be harmful to both physical and mental health. Studies suggest that very long hours are linked to high blood pressure and cardiovascular disease. Statistics Canada has found that moving to longer working hours has some negative impacts on health risks, such as smoking, drinking, and poor diet ("Longer working hours and health," *The daily*, November 16, 1999). Long hours also create a high risk of stress in terms of balancing work with domestic and community life.

The shift of core workers to long daily and weekly hours of work is much more characteristic of the U.S. and Canada than the more regulated job markets of continental Europe. The usual weekly hours of full-time paid workers in the EU are below 40, and falling (EIRO, 2001a). Some countries, notably France, the Netherlands, and Germany, are now close to a 35-hour norm. The proportion of men working long weekly hours is generally very low. For example, just 2% of Dutch men and 8% of German men work more than 45 hours per week (*OECD employment outlook*, 1998, Chart 5.2).

Weekend working appears to be increasing rapidly. The incidence has gone from 11% in 1991, to 15% in 1995, to 25% in 2000 (1991 and 1995 data from the *Survey of work arrangements*. 2000 data from the *Workplace and employee survey* [WES]). Women are more likely to work on weekends than men (28% compared to 21%), reflecting high employment rates in retail and health services. More than one in three production workers work on weekends, reflecting the rising incidence of continuous industrial production.

As noted, regular hours are shorter and jobs are less precarious in most European countries. These countries also provide much more generous paid time off work. In Canada, the minimum vacation entitlement under provincial employment standards is two weeks after a minimum length of service of about one year. (Saskatchewan alone provides for three weeks, after five years.) In collective agreements, the norm is three weeks of paid vacation, rising to four weeks after 10 years. (Seventy per cent of unionized workers qualify for four weeks after 10 years, and 28% qualify after five years.) By contrast, in the EU, the minimum statutory entitlement to paid vacation leave is 20 days or four weeks, and the average provided in collective agreements is 25.7 days, or more than five weeks. German, Danish and Dutch workers get six weeks of paid vacation per year (EIRO, 20001a). Statutory paid holidays on top of paid vacation entitlements are comparable between Canada and European countries.

The average age of retirement in Canada has been steadily falling, but there is generally very limited provision for a phased-in retirement process which would allow older workers to voluntarily reduce their hours of work. Indeed, most defined pension plans create an incentive to maximize earnings (and, therefore, hours) just before retirement. By contrast, most European countries rely more heavily on public than on private pensions, and the tendency in many continental European countries has been to provide more flexible options for older workers.

To summarize, there is a strong trend to longer hours for core workers, as well as to more unsocial hours, and more variable hours. Vacation entitlements and phased-in retirement provisions in Canada are quite limited compared to many European countries. These all have direct implications for stress and for physical and mental health.

## Work–life balance

Longer and more unpredictable hours combined with high and rising job demands are particularly likely to cause stress and anxiety in families where both partners work, and for single-parent families. In both cases, women bear the brunt of the burden. Increased family working-time has been a critical factor in maintaining real incomes in a labour market marked by more precarious employment and stagnating wages. Family work hours obviously determine both income and the time potentially available to spend with family, children, and in the community. While long hours may result in higher incomes, work/family time conflict may affect the physical and mental health of parents and also influence the well-being of children. Much of the burden of caring for elderly parents as well as children is borne by working families. These pressures in terms of balancing work and family are greater than in many other countries because of the relative under-development of publicly financed and delivered early childhood, elder care, and home care programs.

Recent data from the *General social survey* show that time pressures are steadily increasing. Between 1992 and 1998, 25–44 year old parents employed full-time put in an average of two hours more per week in paid work activities. In 1998, fathers averaged 48.3 hours and mothers averaged 38.5 hours per week of paid work and related activities—up 5% for fathers and 4% for mothers from 1992. Lone-parent mothers increased their time in paid work even more than married mothers.

Work/family conflicts arise not just from longer and longer hours, but also from the frequent incompatibility of work schedules with the schedules and needs of children. While a minority of employers do offer flextime arrangements which are responsive to the needs of employees, the great majority of part-time jobs do not offer comparable pay, benefits, and career opportunities.

Reported levels of time stress and work/family stress among parents with children are extremely high. More than one-third of 25–44 year old women who work full-time and have children at home report that they are severely time-stressed, and the same is true for about one in four men. Twenty-six percent of married fathers, 38% of married

---

**BOX 6.2**

There has been a very large increase in the total working hours of two-person families with children since the mid-1970s. This has come through increased work hours for many men, the increased entry of women into the workforce, and the shift of women into full-time jobs. About three in four (73%) of two-person families with children have two earners today compared to one in three in 1975, and three in four (73%) of working women in two-parent families are employed full-time. Thus the majority of women in two-person families with children now work full-time. Six in ten women single parents (63%) with children work, 77% of whom work full-time. Full-time employment rates for women are only slightly lower for those with pre-school children, reflecting maternity and parental leaves taken after the birth of a child (Statistics Canada, Cat. 71-535 MPB #8, *Work arrangements in the 1990s*, Tables 3.1, 3.2.).

---

mothers, and 38% of single mothers report severe time stress, with levels of severe stress rising by about one-fifth between 1992 and 1998. About two-thirds of full-time employed parents with children also report that they are dissatisfied with the balance between their job and home life. Fathers and mothers alike blamed their dissatisfaction on not having enough time for family, which tends to lose out in the event of conflict (Statistics Canada, *The daily*, November 9, 1999).

To summarize, there is strong evidence of mounting work–life conflict and stress. This is driven by mounting demands from work, the still largely unchanged division of domestic labour between men and women, and the failure of the Canadian state to provide caring services on a sufficient scale.

## Social relations and participation at work

Work is a social process, and the social relations of production are an important aspect of the quality of jobs and of working life. But little hard information is available on this relatively intangible dimension. In 2000, 15% of workers reported stress in the workplace from "poor interpersonal relations," down slightly from 18.5% in 1994, but up from 13% in 1991 (*General social survey,* 2003). Women report higher levels of stress from this cause than do men.

About one in three paid workers in Canada are covered by the provisions of a collective agreement. Coverage is highest by far in the public sector and in large private sector firms, particularly in primary industries, manufacturing, transportation, and utilities. By definition, collective agreements give access to a formal statement of conditions of employment, such as hours and working conditions, and access to a formal grievance and arbitration process. A formal grievance system militates against the exercise of arbitrary managerial authority, and against harassment by co-workers. Collective agreements also often provide for joint processes to govern working conditions over the life of a contract, such as labour-management, training, and health and safety committees. While the great majority of agreements contain a management rights clause clarifying the power of management to assign and direct work, the majority also provide for some advance notification of, and consultation over, technological and organizational change. Many collective agreements also feature detailed job descriptions, meaning that changes in tasks are subject to joint agreement.

Most Canadian unions have adopted formal policies relating to workplace health and safety, work/family balance, work reorganization and access to training, and have paid some attention to all of these quality of work–life issues in bargaining. Improvement of the work environment has been on the agenda, and some unions have made gains. However, there are continuous pressures to increase productivity to maintain employment and wages, which tend to militate against an agenda of humanizing work and creating more healthy workplaces.

While some non-union workers also enjoy access to formalized (if non-binding) processes of dispute resolution and collective consultation, worker "voice" in the Canadian workplace is much weaker than in countries where unionization rates are much higher. Moreover, many European countries have legislation providing for joint works councils with powers to at least discuss working conditions. The EU survey shows that 78% of workers believe they have the possibility to discuss working conditions and 71% the possibility to discuss organizational change, most frequently on a formal basis.

John O'Grady (Sullivan, 2000) shows that effective workplace health and safety committees effectively reduce rates of injuries and disability, but are largely absent from the precarious labour market.

To summarize, institutions of collective representation are relatively weakly implanted in Canadian workplaces, undercutting the ability of workers to shape working conditions.

## Conclusion

This overview suggests many grounds for concern over the potential health impacts of trends in Canadian workplaces. Workplace threats to physical health remain significant. Pervasive job insecurity is a source of stress to many peripheral workers. In "core" workplaces, the pace and intensity of work are on the rise, and many are working very long hours in very demanding jobs. The incidence of high-strain jobs which combine high demands and limited control is quite high, particularly among women.

One key conclusion is that we need much more and better information about the level and trends of workplace determinants of health. We lack systematic evidence of the kind collected in Europe. This could and should be remedied by providing sufficient funding to Statistics Canada to conduct regular surveys on the quality of the work environment and working conditions. The new *Workplace and employee survey* (WES) provides only very limited information in this area, and the *National population health survey* provides only very limited information on working conditions.

A second key conclusion is that governments must intervene to help shape and improve workplace conditions. A wide range of relevant recommendations have been made over the years, most recently in the 1990s by two Human Resource Development Canada initiated consultations. These were the Donner Task Force (*Report of the advisory group on working time and redistribution of work*, 1997) and the *Report of the collective reflection on the changing workplace* (1997). The thrust of the first was to regulate working time by limiting long hours and by making precarious work more secure. The thrust of the second—which included a very wide range of options—was to propose changes to employment standards and forms of collective representation. At the end of the day, it is unlikely that there will be significant positive changes in the workplace if everything is left to employers, and if governments do not help equalize bargaining power between workers and employers.

## Recommended readings

Esping-Andersen, G. (1999). *Social foundations of post-industrial economies*. Oxford: Oxford University Press.
  This work provides a detailed account of key institutional differences between advanced industrial countries, showing how the "liberal" labour market of Canada compares and contrasts to the labour markets of "social market" countries like Germany and "social democratic" countries like Sweden.

Jackson, A. and Robinson, D. (2000). *Falling behind: The state of working Canada 2000*, Canadian Centre for Policy Alternatives.
  Contains a wealth of data on income and employment from Statistics Canada sources. (Revised version to be published in 2004.)

Karasek, R. and Theorell, T. (1990). *Healthy work: Stress, productivity and the reconstruction of working life*. New York: Basic Books.

> The classic study of the impacts of workplace stress on health. Stress is seen as the result of high job demands combined with low levels of control.

Lowe, Graham. (2000). *The quality of work: A people centred agenda*. Oxford: Oxford University Press.

> A broad overview of the importance of work to well-being, and a useful introduction to recent trends in Canadian workplaces.

Sullivan, T. (Ed.). (2000). *Injury and the new world of work*. Vancouver and Toronto: University of British Columbia Press.

> Contains recent studies of trends in workplace injuries, showing how "soft tissue" injuries attributable to fast-paced work have grown compared to traditional workplace accidents.

# Related websites

Institute for Work and Health—www.iwh.on.ca

> The leading Canadian research and advocacy organization on issues relating to work and health.

Canadian Labour Congress—www.clc-ctc.ca

> The national umbrella organization for 2.5 million unionized Canadian workers. The Social and Economic Policy sub-site contains many research papers on labour market issues. The site links to the websites of many unions, in Canada and around the world.

Job Quality—www.jobquality.ca

> A sub-site of the Canadian Policy Research Networks that contains a wealth of current data on the quality of jobs in Canada.

European Foundation for the Improvement of Living and Working Conditions—www.eurofound.ie

> Data are available from three European Surveys on Working Conditions, plus many studies of changing workplace conditions.

International Labour Organization—www.ilo.org

> A United Nations organization which promotes "decent work." The site contains many research studies on labour and on working conditions around the world.

# Chapter Seven

———●———

# Understanding and Improving the Health of Work

### Michael Polanyi

## Introduction

The chapters in this book demonstrate that social and economic conditions strongly influence health. This is something that health promotion researchers and practitioners have long recognized. Despite this recognition, we have had only limited success in stimulating action to improve these health-affecting conditions.

Part of the reason for our limited success is that the linkages between social conditions and health are complex. Even as we try to understand these linkages, social and economic conditions are being transformed. There is also a lack of research on what should be done to improve the health of social conditions (MacIntyre, 2003). As well, our *approaches* to research have not always been conducive to stimulating public understanding and action. Conventional scientific research is unlikely to lead to shared understandings of today's complex social problems. Rather, new forms of collective forms of inquiry and dialogue are needed to stimulate understanding and action (Mason and Mitroff, 1981; Shotter and Gustavsen, 1999). As the growing literature on "knowledge transfer" recognizes, researchers need to find ways to involve community members and policy makers in joint processes of inquiry. The opportunities and challenges of collective inquiry have been described elsewhere (e.g., Polanyi and Cole, 2003). Here, the aim is to discuss four steps to addressing key workplace determinants of health: gathering research evidence, undertaking critical reflection and analysis, envisioning a desirable future, and advocating for action. These steps are all important if we are to turn our knowledge of the social determinants of health into actual improvements in health for all (see Figure 7.1).

## Evidence

There is a growing body of research showing that the content, organization, and arrange-ments of work are centrally linked to health outcomes (Polanyi et al., 2000). It is beyond the scope of this chapter to fully review research on such linkages. However, it is

---

**Figure 7.1: A framework for promoting healthy work**

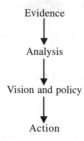

Evidence

↓

Analysis

↓

Vision and policy

↓

Action

---

worth highlighting some key aspects of work conditions that are linked to health (see also Chapter 5).

First, Karasek and Theorell's (1990) research on the negative impacts of a combination of high psychosocial demands and low job control (or high "job strain") provides support for the importance of work pace, participation, and control, and opportunities for personal development, to various health outcomes. High levels of job strain have been found to be predictive of a range of ill health outcomes: mental health, cancer, pregnancy outcomes, periodontal disease (Jones et al., 1998; Ven der Doef and Maes, 1999). Many studies have found relationships between job strain and coronary heart disease (CHD) (Schnall et al., 1994), especially among blue collar workers and men (Theorell, 2001). Research by Johnson and Hall (1988) and others suggests the importance of workplace social support as a moderator of the ill-health effects of job strain.

Second, fairness of rewards is important to health. Workers receiving insufficient recognition and rewards for their efforts have been found to be more likely to experience emotional distress and negative physiological responses (Siegrist, 1996). The "effort–reward imbalance" model (ERI) underlines the health importance of rewards (monetary, esteem, respect from supervisors and colleagues) being in line with demands (time pressures, interruptions, responsibility, pressure to work overtime). Siegrist (2001) reports that there are more than 40 studies of the health impacts of effort–reward imbalance, most with coronary heart disease. Significant relationships between ERI and ill-health have been found for both men and women.

Third, long hours of work have been directly linked to negative physiological and psychological health symptoms, as well as to relationship difficulties with family and others (Sparks et al., 1997; Spurgeon et al., 1997). It is important to bring attention to "anti-social" work hours, given the growing prevalence of work–life conflict and associated mental and physical ill-health outcomes (Frone, 2000).

Work–life conflict can occur when individuals have to perform multiple roles at the same time—as worker, spouse, parent, caregiver, or volunteer. The cumulative demands of multiple roles can result in two types of role strain: overload (having too much to do with to little time to do it) and interference (facing conflicting demands from different roles, such as having to be in two places at the same time). Both have been associated with increased stress and negative health symptoms (Duxbury and Higgins, 2001; Ertel et al., 2000).

Finally, a body of research on the impacts of job insecurity on health is emerging. Wichert (2002), for example, found that job insecurity was related to symptoms of anxiety and depression in a representative sample of British workers. A longitudinal study of U.K. government workers (Ferrie et al., 1998; Ferrie, 2001) showed that those experiencing job insecurity associated with privatization had worse self-rated health and higher rates of longstanding illness, hypertension, mild psychiatric morbidity, and general ill-health symptoms than those not experiencing insecurity.

In summary, there is compelling evidence that the social organization of work matters profoundly to health. Further research is needed to develop a better understanding of the specific dimensions of healthy and unhealthy jobs in order to build support for particular interventions to improve working conditions. Research is also needed to better demonstrate the costs of unhealthy working conditions to companies and to societies in general, since productivity, not health, is the ultimate aim of economic enterprises in capitalist society.

## Analysis

Despite growing evidence of the health impacts of working conditions, so-called high quality employment practices have only been adopted by a minority of companies in Canada (Duxbury and Higgins, 1998; Lowe, 2000). Clearly information and evidence alone do not determine the health of workplace practices. Instead, organizational practices that affect health—for better and

**Table 7.1: Evidence on key work-related determinants of health**

| Work-related determinant of health | Key quantitative studies and review articles | Methodological critiques | Qualitative and policy-oriented studies |
| --- | --- | --- | --- |
| Job strain | (Karasek and Theorell, 1990)<br>(Schnall et al., 1994)<br>(Landsbergis et al., 2000)<br>(Theorell, 2001) | (Kristensen, 1995)<br><br>(Jones et al., 1998) | (Brooker and Eakin, 2001) |
| Effort–reward imbalance | (Siegrist, 1996)<br>(Peter and Siegrist, 1999)<br>(Siegrist, 2001) | | |
| Work hours | (Spurgeon et al., 1997)<br>(Shields, 1999) | | |
| Work–life conflict | (Duxbury and Higgins, 2001)<br>(Frone, 2000) | | (Pocock et al., 2001)<br>(Franks, 1999) |
| Job insecurity | (Wichert, 2002)<br>(Ferrie, 2001)<br>(Ferrie et al., 1998) | (Lavis and Farrant, 1998) | |

for worse—are influenced by an array of factors including technology change, deregulation, declining unionization and international competition, and associated pressures to innovate, improve quality, and increase productivity. Grappling with the complex and conflicting relationship between firm productivity and workplace health is key to the development of strategies to improve the quality of working conditions. One can identify three current analyses of the relationship between workplace health and competitiveness. The first assumes that companies need greater flexibility in order to be able to respond freely and rapidly to changes in consumer preference and demands and thus compete effectively. The policy prescription, therefore, is for governments to pull back from regulation of business employment practices, and to allow a further "flexibilization" of employment contracts. While it is recognized that this may increase job insecurity in the short term, it is argued that the benefits of economic growth and job creation outweigh this cost, and that the emphasis should be on employability rather than job security.

The problem with this view is that it supports the development of work systems which compromise the health-determining conditions discussed above (e.g., jobs with reasonable demands, job control, work–life balance, and job security). It also allows firms to externalize these social costs of production, and provides little incentive for firms to improve working conditions. Moreover, this view rests on the now largely discredited assumption that the benefits of rising profits and economic growth will "trickle down" to all, a claim proved false during the past decade of rising inequality in Canada and the United States.

The second perspective is to suggest that the problem is just the opposite: an *excess* of employer flexibility. This, the traditional left view, is that a shift in the balance of power from workers to management (due in part to declining unionization rates, greater employer ability to relocate to other jurisdictions, and reduced government regulation) has undermined working conditions in general, and job security in particular. The prescription is for a re-regulation of employers, in order to limit their ability to engage in flexible employment practices.

The strength of this view is that it recognizes the serious human problems associated with rising employer flexibility and power. Its limitation is that it fails to acknowledge the legitimacy of employers' need for flexibility in today's global economy, nor the fact that many workers would actually prefer to engage in part-time, flex-time, short-term, and other non-standard working arrangements (Marshall, 2001). In other words, there are positive dimensions to flexibility—*if* it is not simply flexibility for employers at the cost of employees, which has, too often, been the case.

The third view falls in the middle of the previous two. It suggests that there are potential benefits for all to be found in the emerging flexible organization of work (European Commission, 1997). It acknowledges both businesses' need for flexibility *and* employees' (and citizens') need for security. It recognizes that job security, in the form of full-time, permanent employment, is not something that can be retrieved in the new economy. However, it does not hold that *economic* insecurity is either a morally acceptable or an economically positive phenomenon. Instead it aims to forge a new framework of "flexicurity" by accepting the emergence of employment flexibility and short-term jobs, while providing generous social welfare and

Over the past decade, Denmark has experienced a dramatic decline in unemployment. Denmark seems to have created a unique combination of stable economic growth and social welfare since the mid-1990s. The term *flexicurity* is used to characterize this successful combination of adaptability to a changing international environment and a solidaristic welfare system, which protects the citizens from the more brutal consequences of structural change. The recent success of the Danish model of *flexicurity* thus points to a third way between the flexibility often ascribed to a liberal market economy and the social safety nets of the traditional Scandinavian welfare state ...

The Danish "miracle" is not just a trivial mixture of demand-driven growth and the hiding of a large share of the population in various welfare programmes. The relative success of the Danish model in recent years has stimulated ideas about the occurrence of a new employment system model in the form of the so-called "golden triangle," where people are enabled to move between different positions within work, welfare, and active labour market programmes. For instance large numbers of workers are affected by unemployment every year, but most of them return to employment after a short spell of unemployment. Active labour market programmes assist those who do not quickly go back into employment before re-entering a job.

... Due to a non-restrictive employment protection legislation, which allows employers to hire and fire workers with short notice, the Danish system has a level of flexibility. At the same time, through its social security system and active labour market programmes, Denmark resembles the other Nordic welfare states in providing a tightly knit safety net for its citizens.

The Danish model of "flexicurity" ... could serve as a source of inspiration for new ideas about alternative configurations of flexible labour markets and economic security for the individual rather than as a simple scheme that is ready for immediate export.

Source: European Foundation for the Improvement of Living and Working Conditions. (2002a). *Quality of work and employment in Europe: Issues and challenges* (Foundation Paper). Dublin: EFILWC.

unemployment benefits along with active training support for the unemployed (See Box 7.1).

In sum, quite different analyses of the health-productivity dynamic exist. While it is important to be clear about the assumptions that we bring to this complex issue, it is unlikely that a shared analysis is likely to be easily forged. Rather, focussing discussion on developing a shared vision for the future of healthy work may be more likely to stimulate change (Cooperrider and Srivistava, 1987; Weisbord and Janoff, 1995). Hence, while recognizing the importance of delineating and analyzing the

roots of the negative impacts of work on health, it is also important that researchers work to support the development of a shared vision of work, and policy options to achieve it.

## Vision and policy

Given the central focus on work in contemporary capitalist societies, it is astounding how little attention has been paid to the development of broadly shared policy goals with respect to work. In Canada, government committees and commissions have periodically considered aspects of work

(Advisory Committee on the Changing Workplace, 1997; Human Resources and Development Canada, 1994), but there has been no broad-based public visioning process on the desired future role and nature of work in Canada.

There is reason to believe that such a shared vision may be achievable. There is some consistency in terms of what employees, as a group, want from work: jobs that are interesting (something they like to do), jobs that provide opportunities to develop one's abilities, and jobs that allow for freedom to decide how one's job is done (Lowe, 2000; Polanyi and Tompa, 2002).

Research on worker experiences and policy directions suggests four interrelated dimensions of healthy and productive work: *availability* of work; *adequacy* of income from work; *appropriateness* of work arrangements with respect to non-work responsibilities and needs; and *appreciation* or involvement of workers as active workplace participants and valued contributors to society (see Figure 7.2).

### Available work

Work is central to human existence and fulfillment and well-being. It provides us with an income, a sense of worth, and access to social networks. It is not surprising, therefore, that unemployment

and "job creation" have been central public concerns, and important agenda items for politicians and various organizations.

What *kind* of jobs should be promoted? Should we promote only high-paid full-time permanent jobs, as unions often suggest (e.g., Dagg, 1997)? Or should there be an acceptance that the provision of high-paid, full-time jobs to all is neither possible nor desirable, and that a range of work arrangements needs to be promoted? Or, more radically, should we accept that there may no longer be enough paid work for all of us, and instead focus on creating conditions of income security, increasing the viability of a range of citizenship roles (e.g., parenting, caregiving, volunteering as well as paid work)?

It may be right to emphasize waged employment. However, there has been some rethinking of the relative importance of paid work, versus unpaid work, in recent years. This is partly because of the coexistence of chronic unemployment on one hand, and social and community needs going unaddressed on the other. Some question whether it is right that paid work be highly rewarded while unpaid family, community, and civic contributions go largely unrewarded (Brown and Lauder, 2001). The growing importance of early childhood development and social and citizen participation to population health, as explored

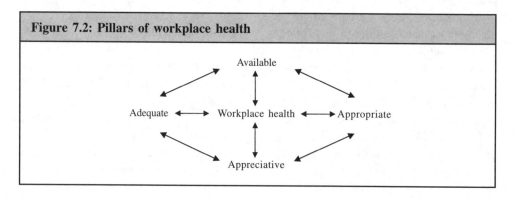

Figure 7.2: Pillars of workplace health

Social Determinants of Health

elsewhere in this book, also suggest a need to rethink the relative importance and rewards given to waged employment as opposed to broader social and civic participation.

Indeed, renewed attention has been directed towards the idea of a basic income policy over the last decade in Canada (Lerner et al., 1999), the United States (Aronowitz et al., 1998) and Europe (Brown and Lauder, 2001; Gorz, 1999). While there are difficulties with this approach, including its economic feasibility, it does merit consideration by those concerned about population health (see Box 7.2).

Increasing income security would prevent workers from being forced to take jobs that are unsafe and underpaid. It would also afford workers greater choice and control over their work content, work conditions, and work arrangements. At the same time, firms would gain a greater degree of flexibility as workers and their representatives would be less economically dependent on long-term job security and more open to a range of different work arrangements.

Providing a greater degree of income security will not necessarily change the fact that bad jobs continue to be disproportionately allocated to women, people of colour, and people with less education and of a lower socio-economic class. Indeed, socio-economic conditions before working life (childhood and adolescence) and outside of work (social networks, education, employability, and financial independence) shape the way that workplace experiences impact on health. Hence a key consideration in all these

---

### Box 7.2: Basic income

**Definition:**
A Basic Income is a regular payment, payable to all, which is sufficient to provide people with a standard of living above the poverty line.
A standard Basic Income scheme has the following features:

- It is a regular cash payment. Services provided in kind may add up to a "social wage" (see www.jrf.org.uk/knowledge/findings/socialpolicy/SP114.asp) but they are not a basic income.
- Neither is it a one-off lump sum such as a stakeholder grant (see www.policylibrary.com/redistribution/stakeholdergrants.htm).
- It is paid to everyone within a nation state or other political unit. If payment is restricted to those who are legal citizens then it is sometimes termed citizen's income. Some variants exclude children, pensioners, and prisoners.
- It is paid to the individual rather than the household.
- It is paid at a flat rate to both rich and poor. There is no means test—Basic income is not withdrawn as other income rises.
- It is paid regardless of employment or family status—to the unemployed, the employed, to the childless and those bringing up children, to students, surfers, and tramps. Proposals have also been put forward to restrict payment only to those engaged in "productive activities"—usually defined as childcare, eldercare, volunteering, and studying—this is termed Participation Income (see www.policylibrary.com/redistribution/participation.htm).

Source: www.policylibrary.com/redistribution/basicincome.htm

---

dimensions of work is to reduce inequalities in the distribution of quality work, by gender (Reskin and Padavic, 1994), class (Johnson and Hall, 1999) and race (Das Gupta, 1996).

## Adequate work

Most would agree that those who work should earn an adequate income to meet their needs. However, minimum wages have stagnated and fallen in Canada and the United States, to the point where a full-time employment at minimum wage often leaves individuals and families well below the poverty line (Maxwell, 2002).

Numerous authors in Canada and the US call for increases in, and better still, an indexing of, minimum wages for both social and economic reasons (Bluestone and Harrison, 2000; Goldberg and Green, 1999). Wage levels are a "health" issue: Maxwell (2002) indicates that wage supplements, the living wage, and individual development account strategies in both Canada and the U.S. "can have significant positive effects on the well-being of beneficiaries" (p. 11).

There is also a widespread view that there is a need to extend and enforce adequate wages, benefits, and rights to non-full time workers. Books and reports from both the U.S. (e.g., Herzenberg et al., 1998; Skocpol, 2000) and Canada (Betcherman and Lowe, 1995; Advisory Committee on the Changing Workplace, 1997) recommend the extension of pro-rated benefits, pensions, and health insurance to part-time workers. Others suggest that temporary workers should be treated more like permanent workers with their placement agencies (European Foundation for the Improvement of Working and Living Conditions, 2002a), with agencies being obliged to provide benefits (King et al., 2000).

Requiring employers to provide pro-rated benefits to part-time workers would help to address the further problem of fixed costs and perverse incentives that deter the hiring of additional employees and instead encourage firms to ask or demand overtime work, which is often unpaid (Advisory Committee on the Changing Workplace, 1997). Finally, it should be made easier for workers to transport their pensions from employer to employer (so-called "portable pensions") (Advisory Committee on the Changing Workplace, 1997; Herzenberg et al., 1998).

## Appropriate work

Contemporary work and family (or home) lives are highly interdependent as workers—a growing proportion of whom are now women—are increasingly combining paid work with family and home responsibilities. We have already seen the health importance of ensuring a fit between the demands of paid jobs and non-work interests and responsibilities. It is of fundamental importance, therefore, to increase workers' control over their time—how much they work, when and where.

A first step to increasing worker control over hours is to ensure that even the lowest paid workers make a living wage (Schor, 2002). A second step is to increase the rights of workers to choose and control their hours of work, by providing them with the option of taking time off in lieu of overtime pay, increasing vacation entitlement, increasing parental and care-giving leave, making it easier for workers to change from part-time to full-time and vice versa, and giving employees the right to voluntarily reduce work time (Duxbury and Higgins, 2001). Again, enhancing income security by providing a basic income would ensure that workers are in a better position to negotiate and enter into working arrangements that fit with their non-work lives (Gorz, 1999).

## Appreciative work

Finally, new efforts are needed to ensure that workers are appreciated as actively contributing members of workplaces. If there are to be more open and flexible legal frameworks surrounding employment arrangements, "the role of workers in decision-making and the need to review and strengthen the existing arrangements for workers' involvement in their companies will also become essential issues" (European Commission, 1997). Proposals for improving democratic voice in companies include elected single- or multi-employer worker committees established on a voluntary basis, mandated employee participation councils, and greater worker, consumer, and community representation on company boards (Herzenberg et al, 1998; Vail et al., 1999).

Appreciative work also means providing work that is linked to workers' interests, is meaningful to workers, and that encourages learning and growth (Polanyi and Tompa, 2002). Here again, the importance of increasing worker choice over the content of their work is central.

In summary, a range of policy directions seem to offer the possibility of creating social and economic conditions conducive to improved population health. However, it is important to recognize that different workers in fact want different kinds of jobs, working conditions, and arrangements, depending on their interests, life situations and responsibilities, skills, values, personalities and so on (Polanyi and Tompa, 2002). Workers may be more or less able to deal with difficult working conditions, depending on the level of social support, financial independence, employability, and education outside of work. This is not to excuse poor working conditions for people who have minimal skills or awareness of other opportunities. Rather, it is to say that workers need the opportunity to choose and engage in work that fits with their desires, interests and needs.

In sum, work is complex, and people are diverse, so researchers should not expect, on their own, to be able to identify the desirable dimensions of work. The specific policies at this point are less important than underlining the need to generate a broad-based dialogue on policy options conducive to healthy and productive work. There is a need for all stakeholders to collectively develop, in dialogue, a shared vision of the future of work, and a program to achieve it. There are promising methodologies for engaging stakeholders in future visioning processes.

Policies are also influenced by and reflective of the power distribution among various interest groups. Given that labour market changes have reduced the power of workers and unions in may places, we need to focus on strategies to re-balance the distribution of power in workplaces.

This could be done by expanding opportunities for representation among high-skilled and autonomous workers, and developing new forms of representation such as sector-based representation systems and multi-employer bargaining systems for smaller service sector firms (Advisory Committee on the Changing Workplace, 1997; Herzenberg et al., 1998).

In part, changing power relations requires changing the structures of decision-making and the opportunities that are provided to influence decisions in various institutions. We have already spoken of the importance of creating increased opportunities for worker participation at the workplace level. However, there is also a need to create opportunities for broader democratic participation in social and political institutions (government, media, schools, community-based organizations). There is reason to believe that enhancing democratic participation will lead to more equitable decisions, build social cohesion, increase social support, and develop a greater sense of power and capacity among citizens—all of which are key to health.

## Conclusion: Advocating for action

There is a need to strengthen evidence of the links between work and health, to better grapple with the complex relationship between worker health and firm competitiveness, and to articulate a shared vision for work and set of policy options conducive to healthy work. The above issues are important, but if they do not lead to action, they will have failed.

In our pursuit of action, those of us who are concerned about population health can learn from the successes—and failures—of health promotion. One of the great successes of health promotion has been to make a strong argument for broadening participation—of communities, professionals, and policy-makers—in processes of social and political change. Specifically, the case has been made that those whose health is affected by research and policy have a right to participate in these endeavours; that involving those affected by issues will lead to better understanding of health issues; and that involving those whose health is at stake is more likely to bring about change. Today, there is still a need to open up the research and policy process to meaningful involvement of these players.

We also need to learn from the failure of health promotion to shift attention and resources from health care to the social determinants of health. "Failure" may be too strong a word—for this is a monumental task, when the vested interests of professional groups and other political and institutional barriers to change are taken into account. Yet it does suggest that new kinds of efforts are needed to place the social determinants onto the political landscape.

Some modest proposals are worth mentioning. First, population health researchers and professionals need to pay more attention to the constraints under which policy-makers function if we are to expect action on the so-called determinants of health. Government structures militate against the kind of future-oriented, cross-sectoral policy analysis and development that action on social determinants of health requires, and policy-makers' time is often consumed by fighting today's fire, protecting the programs and services they currently run, and wresting money from the finance department.

This means ceasing to lament over-simplistically that policy-makers and bureaucrats are "too political" and pay insufficient attention to population health research evidence. It means starting to provide clear and manageable policy options that resonate with specific policy-makers. It means shifting from "research transfer" and "knowledge dissemination" to processes of interactive policy development.

It is correct that policy making is influenced as much by public pressure as it is by "evidence." Hence, those concerned with population health need to build a constituency supportive of action. To do so, we can work through existing national health-*care* coalitions (e.g., Canadian Healthcare Association, The Health Action Lobby, and the Canadian Health Coalition), encouraging them to go beyond their focus on health care into upstream social and political determinants of health. As well, we can also work with numerous national,

Social Determinants of Health

regional, and local social policy and community organizations concerned with social determinants of health (even though they do not use that terminology), learning from their social policy analysis and experience in advocating for improvements to social and economic conditions. Finally, now may be the time to develop our own national network to put the social determinants of health on the political landscape. Such a network or coalition could articulate a vision for population health and a set of principles and specific policy options for its achievement. We could identify the core social determinants of health, and raise a strong population health-based voice for income, employment, labour, child care, housing, and welfare policies conducive to meeting these core determinants of health.

Above all, we should build on the revived interest in democratizing policy-making processes and providing citizens with opportunities for meaningful engagement in "democratic deliberation." People often have a better sense than we acknowledge of what makes them and their communities healthy or sick. Pushing for meaningful citizen involvement in the development and implementation of social, economic and political policies and practices that impact on their well-being may be the best thing we can do to improve population health.

## Acknowledgements

Thanks are given to Tom McIntosh, Peter Smith, and an anonymous reviewer for helpful comments on an earlier draft of this paper, and to Ann Bishop for editorial assistance.

## Recommended readings

Dunham, J. (Ed.). (2001). *Stress in the workplace: Past, present, future*. London: WHURR Publishers.
Collection of writings by key authors offering various perspectives on the relationship between working conditions and health.

Karasek, R. and Theorell, T. (1990). *Healthy work: Stress, productivity and the reconstruction of working life*. New York: Basic Books.
Classic book on psycho-social demands at work and health that outlines the theory and evidence of the job strain model.

Lowe, G.S. (2000). *The quality of work: A people-centred agenda*. Toronto: Oxford University Press.
Review of organizational research and proposed pathways to improving the quality of work.

Peter, R. and Siegrist, J. (1999). "Chronic psychosocial stress at work and cardiovascular disease: The role of effort-reward imbalance," *International journal of law and psychiatry, 22*(5-6), 441–449.
Readable review of the theory and empirical evidence underlying the effort-reward imbalance model.

## Related websites

Institute for Work and Health—www.iwh.on.ca
Canadian research organization focused on preventing and treating work-related injuries and illness.

National Institute for Occupational Safety and Health—www.cdc.gov/niosh/homepage.html
U.S. Federal agency responsible for conducting research and making recommendations for the prevention of work-related injury and illness.

# Part Two

—————◆—————

# FOUNDATIONS OF
# LIFE-LONG HEALTH: EDUCATION

A CONSISTENT THEME in the social determinants of health literature is the importance of early experience. Hertzman outlines three health effects that have their origins in early childhood. *Latent effects* are biological or developmental early life experiences that produce health effects later in life. Low birth-weight, for instance, is a reliable predictor of incidence of cardiovascular disease and adult-onset diabetes in later life. *Pathway effects* are experiences that set individuals onto trajectories that influence health, well-being, and competence over the life course. As one example, children who enter school with delayed vocabulary are set upon a path that leads to lower educational expectations, poor employment prospects, and greater likelihood of illness and disease across the life-span. *Cumulative effects* represent the accumulation of advantage or disadvantage over time that manifests itself in incidence of a range of indicators of poor health. These involve the combination of latent and pathways effects. Education and literacy are important not only for providing children with key experiences that may have life-long effects but for setting individuals on a life-course trajectory for either health or illness. In this section, authors outline the importance for health of early childhood education and care and education and literacy.

**Martha Friendly** makes the argument for early childhood education and care (ECEC) as a crucial determinant of health for Canadians in general and children in particular. She provides an overview of what is known about what constitutes quality ECEC and its health effects upon both children and their families and for society as a whole. She then describes the current state of ECEC in Canada and compares this to developments in other nations. Canada's ECEC policies are woefully inadequate for the needs of Canadian families. Despite numerous governmental commitments to ECEC, only a small minority of Canadian families have access to quality regulated childcare. Numerous policy lessons are provided and steps for the future described.

**Gina Browne** outlines how integrated children services—including quality ECEC— significantly reduce the incidence of behavioural and emotional problems that originate in childhood. Basing her analysis on recommendations of the Organization for Economic Cooperation and Development for ECEC, she reviews studies that demonstrate not only the economic efficiency of establishing such programs, but also their social and educational benefits to families and society. Browne provides numerous Canadian examples of research that documents the value of such an integrated approach towards children's services.

**Charles Ungerleider and Tracey Burns** review the state of public education in Canada. The importance of education to Canadian society is argued. After providing a snapshot of some of the factors that determine educational success, they show how changing Canadian values are influencing the perceptions of the Canadian educational system. The authors argue that public education is doing well by Canadians as our children perform very well in international comparisons of achievement. But commitment to shared communal institutions such as public education is wavering, threatening public education and our futures.

**Barbara Ronson and Irving Rootman** detail the pivotal importance of literacy for health across the life-span. Literacy has direct and indirect effects upon health. The mechanisms by which this occurs are presented. Factors that support or hinder literacy such as income and its distribution, culture and gender and the interaction among these and other social determinants of health are considered. Recent governmental actions to address problems of literacy among Canadians are reviewed. Since governmental policies are crucial influences upon literacy attainment, policy directions to improve literacy and current research needs are provided.

# Chapter Eight

———●———

# EARLY CHILDHOOD EDUCATION AND CARE

## Martha Friendly

## Introduction

It is widely recognized today that early childhood experiences have a long-term effect on physical and mental health. As the 1996 *Report on the health of Canadians* noted, "there is strong evidence that early childhood experiences influence coping skills, resistance to health problems and overall health and well being for the rest of one's life" (Federal Provincial Territorial Advisory Committee on Population Health, 1996). Early childhood development provides a platform for adult employment, education, income, status, and lifestyle and these, in turn, are linked to adult health.

Early childhood education and childcare (ECEC) outside the family is only one of a number of factors known to have an impact on children during early life. A sufficient income, adequate food and good nutrition, a healthy environment, housing, and educational early childhood programs all have an effect on children's development and health here-and-now, then on the young school-aged child, and on into the child's development into an adult. Some of these factors (such as a healthy environment and good nutrition) affect children directly and some (such as adequate income) have their main impact more indirectly, through their effect on the child's first and primary environment, the family. Although these factors are all important, there is strong research support for the idea that ECEC programs are an important—even a determining—factor that affect children both directly and more indirectly, through their impact on their parents.

More than 30 years ago, a landmark report from the Royal Commission on the Status of Women first recommended a national childcare program to support women's equality. Since then, the labour force participation rate of mothers has risen above 70%, child development research has demonstrated that high quality ECEC is developmentally beneficial and Canada has become one of the most pluralistic countries in the world. Today what was customarily called "daycare" in the 1970s, then "childcare" in the 1980s and 1990s, is commonly called "early learning and care" or "early childhood education and care." The term "early childhood education and care" or ECEC is now used internationally to describe inclusive, integrated services that play multiple roles for children and families. A 2001 international study uses the term ECEC to:

> Reflect the growing consensus in OECD countries that "care" and "education" are inseparable concepts … this term describes an integrated and coherent approach to policy and provision which is inclusive of **all** children and **all** parents regardless of employment or socioeconomic status. This approach recognizes that such arrangements may fulfill a wide range of objectives including care, learning, and social support (Organization for Economic Co-operation and Development [OECD], 2001).

In Canada, the term ECEC encompasses childcare centres and other care services like family childcare in private homes whose primary aim is to allow mothers to participate in the paid labour force. It also includes kindergartens and nursery/preschools whose primary purpose is early childhood education. However, while well-designed ECEC programs enhance child development and simultaneously support parents in a variety of ways in and out of the paid workforce, Canada has barely even begun to develop policy and programs that meet the OECD's definition.

The first part of this chapter reviews how ECEC is linked to a number of social domains that play a role in determining health over the life course. The second part describes the current state of Canadian ECEC using a policy framework for effective programs derived from an international comparative policy analysis of ECEC.

## ECEC as a social determinant of health

That child development is complex is more than an overworked cliché. Research identifies many factors that contribute to whether children develop into healthy, competent adults—innate or genetic characteristics, prenatal conditions, the physical environment, nutrition, family attributes and interaction, peers, the community, schools, civil society, and the larger social-economic environment. Many of these have an impact on one another, combining in intricate ways to produce children who are successful, confident, content, competent, and resilient, or, conversely, who lack these attributes. Among these factors, there is considerable research that supports the idea that ECEC programs

are a key—even a central—factor in child development and, ultimately, in life as a successful, healthy adult. As we shall see, ECEC programs are an especially good social determinant of health because if they are well designed, they can fulfill multiple goals at one and the same time.

### Policy goals for ECEC
Over the past two decades, shifting Canadian rationales for ECEC have included life-long learning, school readiness (or "readiness to learn"), child development, parents' employability, women's equality, balancing work and family, anti-poverty, alleviating at-risk status, and social integration. Some of these (school readiness, lifelong learning) are focused on children. Others—women's equality and labour force participation, alleviating poverty and unemployment——are

more focused on families or parents. Others are associated with the community or the larger society. These rationales fall into four policy goals that are explored in the following section.

*Goal 1: Enhancing children's well-being, healthy development and lifelong learning*
That ECEC programs play an important role in child development is well supported by research. High quality ECEC programs provide intellectual and social stimulation that promotes cognitive development and social competence. These effects persist into the school years to establish a foundation for later success. The benefits of ECEC programs pertain regardless of social class (although poor children may derive more benefit) and whether or not the mother is in the workforce (see Shonkoff and Phillips, 2000, for a comprehensive review of this literature).

There is overwhelming evidence that the positive effects of ECEC programs occur only if they are high quality and that, indeed, poor quality programs may have a negative effect, especially for children from low-resourced families. Thus, it is the *quality* of ECEC programs that is critical in determining how developmentally effective they are, not merely whether children participate in them.

Although there are many definitions of high quality in ECEC, generally, the term is used as shorthand for characteristics of ECEC programs that go beyond basic health and safety requirements to those that support children's development, learning and well-being. From this perspective, studies show that high quality ECEC services:

- Employ staff who are well educated for their work and have decent working conditions and wages.

- Organize children into groups of manageable size with adequate numbers of adults.
- Provide challenging, non-didactic, play-based, creative, enjoyable activities.
- Ensure consistent adult and peer groups in well-designed physical environments.

High quality ECEC services are also responsive to diverse populations of children and parents, include children with disabilities in a meaningful way, have a connection with the community, and involve and support parents both as workers and in the parenting role.

Good evidence shows that the positive effects of high quality ECEC persist into later life. This is especially—but not exclusively—true for low-income children. A longitudinal study of very low income American children who attended high quality childcare in infancy found that participants had lower juvenile crime and school dropout rates and much higher earnings as adults (the earnings of their mothers became much higher than those of a control group as well) (Masse and Barnett, 2003). This study of full-day infant childcare reinforces research on ECEC's long-term benefits to low-income American children in part-day programs that began between two and three years of age (Schweinhart and Weikart, 1993). A study of children in Sweden's universal high quality childcare centres found that entry sometime around the first birthday meant that children performed better in school at 8 and 13 years regardless of family income and received more positive socio-emotional teacher ratings than children who began childcare later or were in family day care (Andersson, 1992).

There is good evidence, then, that high quality ECEC contributes to a platform of healthy child development that can have effects over the lifespan. In this way, ECEC programs can be conceptualized not only as reducing risks or deficits but also as playing a positive role in ensuring that opportunities are not missed.

*Goal 2: Supporting parents in education, training, and employment*

In Canada, labour force participation of mothers of young children has risen steadily so that by 2001, 73.4% of mothers with a youngest child 3–5 years worked outside the home, up from 68% in 1995. As financial pressures on families began to mount in the 1980s, it became the norm for affluent and middle class as well as poor families to have both parents (if there are two parents) in the labour force. At the same time, paid employment and careers have become appropriate and desirable roles for women. A third motivation for employment, especially for lone mothers, is associated with Canada's diminished social safety net and the introduction of mandatory workfare programs in the 1990s.

Whatever the motivation, dependable care for children is essential if mothers who would have been expected to provide it a generation ago are to participate in the workforce, training or education. ECEC services are fundamental if mothers are to be employed or train for employment; without access to child-care, women may be compelled to remain out of the labour force, work at poorly paid part-time employment, or may be forced to rely on social assistance. While a low-paid insecure job is not necessarily a route out of poverty, without child-care, poor women and their families lack even the possibility of escaping poverty.

ECEC as it supports parental employment and training is linked to social determinants of health such as family income and poverty that are both directly experienced by the child and mediated through the family. Thus, children benefit in the short and longer term if child-care that helps sustain their families economically is accessible. However, as described in the previous section, if the quality of child-care upon which parents rely so they can go to work or training is not high enough to support healthy development, children may not benefit.

*Goal 3: Fostering social cohesion*

ECEC programs can be focal points for parents and children, child-care providers, health and social service professionals, and community volunteers that exemplify and build social cohesion in a number of ways. As early childhood is a critical period not

| Table 8.1: Mother's labour force participation | | | |
|---|---|---|---|
| Labour force participation of women with children 0–15 years (rounded) | | | |
| | 1995 % | 1998 % | 2001 % |
| With youngest child less than 3 years | 62 | 64 | 65.8 |
| With youngest child 3–5 years | 68 | 70 | 73.4 |
| With youngest child 6–15 years | 77 | 78 | 80.7 |

Source: Friendly, M., Beach, J. and Turiano, M. (2002). *Early childhood education and care in Canada 2001*. Toronto: Childcare Resource and Research Unit, University of Toronto.

Social Determinants of Health

only for language learning but also for the early stages of establishing the basis for tolerance and acceptance of difference, inclusive ECEC programs can enhance social solidarity over the long-term. At the same time, neighbourhood ECEC programs that are community institutions can facilitate parents' participation in common activities related to the well-being of their children, strengthening solidarity within a geographic community as well as across class, ethnic, and racial boundaries. Community-based ECEC programs that are holistic, welcoming and well-connected to other community supports, reinforce social integration for parents, especially those who are immigrants or refugees or new to a neighbourhood. As Canada's pluralistic society has become even more diverse and mobile in the 1990s, universal ECEC programs that operate with the goal of fostering social cohesion should be of particular interest.

*Goal 4: Providing equity*
ECEC contributes to equity for multiple groups in society, but for two groups in particular—children with disabilities and women—access to ECEC is a particularly important equity and social justice issue. Ensuring the rights of children with disabilities is a matter of basic social justice. For children with disabilities and their parents, the opportunity to participate in early childhood programs with typical children is critical for child development, for supporting parents as parents and as workers, and for normalizing their lives.

From a feminist perspective, that universal child-care is critical for women's equality is certainly not new. As an equity issue, this goes beyond pragmatic considerations of access to employment and training as discussed in a previous section. That ECEC is a basic citizenship right for

women is associated with the idea that social rights constitute a key element of citizenship and go way beyond training or employment. Putting it simply, equality for women cannot be a reality without full access to child-care.

## How does Canada measure up?

Canada's ECEC programs have developed as a hodgepodge of separate programs and policies. Its limited public funding has led to scarcity of opportunity. This has in part been shaped by two key Canadian realities. The first is linked to the nature of Canadian federalism in which responsibility for social programs is primarily provincial/territorial. Within this political reality, the respective roles and responsibilities of the two orders of government——federal and provincial/territorial—have shifted and changed over the years. Compared to the 1960s/1970s when the modern social safety net was created, Canada underwent a deconstructing trend in the 1990s. In this environment, developing a national approach to a social program like ECEC is not straightforward. This has had profound implications for the fragmented way ECEC has developed in the modern era. (For further discussion of this, see Friendly, 2001 and White, 2002.)

Second, a further reality is that Canada is a liberal democracy with a relatively weak welfare state. As Meyers and Gornick's (2000) comparative application of Esping-Anderson's typology of welfare states to childcare points out, Canada's ECEC provision relies on "market-based solutions and means testing, mak[ing] only limited public investments in ECEC" (p. 23). In this analysis, the liberal (Canada, the U.S., the U.K.) regimes are distinguished by their reliance on the marketplace for child-care— high use of informal care, reliance on parent fees with subsidies for those who can qualify and private, sometimes for-profit provision—compared to the stronger role for the state that characterizes ECEC in continental Europe. Perhaps the clearest symbol of Canadian child-care's private nature is that almost all responsibility for developing and managing it (even finding capital funds) is assumed by the private sector—parent groups, voluntary organizations, or entrepreneurs. It is interesting to note that while Canadian responsibility for child-care is primarily private, kindergarten under public education is a public responsibility. This is consistent with Meyers and Gornick's description of the liberal regimes' strong commitment to public education.

Through the absence of comprehensive public policy development, Canadian ECEC has developed so incoherently that although each province/territory has multiple programs, only a small minority of children and families has access to needed services. ECEC services are either in short supply, inaccessible for many because user fees are too high, of mediocre quality or—like kindergarten—not sensitive to the labour force needs of parents. And although a majority of young Canadian children have mothers in the labour force, most rely on unregulated arrangements privately arranged by parents.

In contrast, almost all continental European nations have developed publicly funded systems that provide developmental early childhood programs with reasonable sensitivity to parents' labour force needs. Although different countries have different approaches to program delivery, generally, ECEC programs become available to all children by between the second and third birthday, and a number of countries have relatively broad coverage for infants and toddlers as well.[1] European ECEC programs

are generally complemented by family policy with decently paid maternity and parental leaves and child benefits. These models are noteworthy because they show that—although no country is entirely "perfect"—ECEC programs can be organized to be relatively seamless and universal.

## What we can learn about Canada using the OECD's eight policy lessons

Thus far, this paper has discussed how ECEC is linked to four social goals—healthy child development, family income, strong communities, and equity—that contribute to health in the broad sense. But these links are in place only if certain characteristics of public policy and service delivery are present. An international policy study conducted by the Organization for Economic Co-operation and Development (OECD) provides a good basis for examining the enabling conditions for ECEC programs and their implications for public policy. One of the study's key findings is that eight interrelated aspects of policy and program are the *"key elements … that are likely to promote equitable access to quality ECEC"* (OECD, 2001, p. 125). These form a useful framework for examining Canadian ECEC.

### Policy lesson 1

Policy lesson 1 stresses the value of a systematic and integrated approach to policy development and implementation including a co-ordinated policy framework and a lead ministry. That Canada does not have a systematic approach to policy and services was discussed previously. Canada has neither a national approach to ECEC nor is the approach in most of the provinces/territories—the level of government with the jurisdictional responsibility—coherent or integrated either (Friendly et al., 2002). The absence of coherent policy at the two senior levels of government not only has negative implications for accessibility and quality but also means that public financing and other resources are used ineffectively.

At the service delivery level, each province/territory has a program of regulated child-care and separate kindergarten for five year olds; in each, there are child-care centres, kindergartens, nursery schools/preschools, regulated family child-care, parenting programs, and an array of funding arrangements. However, at a practical level, although each province/territory has a tangle of programs, only a minority of children and families has services that provide the reliable care that parents need or the early childhood education programs that benefit child development.

*Policy lesson 2*

Policy lesson 2 is that a strong and equal partnership with the education system is valuable. It suggests a lifelong learning

approach to encourage smooth transitions for children and recognize ECEC as a foundation of the education process. Although care and early childhood education are inevitably tied together, Canadian ECEC generally does not blend these two functions. Kindergarten as part of the education system is regarded as a foundation for lifelong learning and treated as a public good. While provinces/ territories regulate some elements of child-care services such as staff training and ratios that research links to child development, child-care programs are of such uneven quality it can be questioned as to whether they are "educational." Although Quebec has taken a positive step to reinforce the partnership between education and

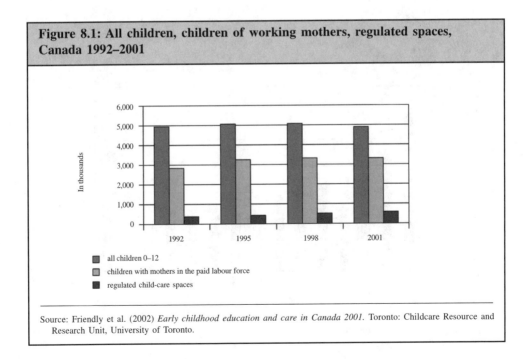

**Figure 8.1: All children, children of working mothers, regulated spaces, Canada 1992–2001**

Source: Friendly et al. (2002) *Early childhood education and care in Canada 2001.* Toronto: Childcare Resource and Research Unit, University of Toronto.

childcare by publicly funding childcare for all 0–4 year olds—not just for those whose mothers are in the labour force—the overall partnership between child-care and the education system in Canada is limited, not "*strong and equal.*"

*Policy lesson 3*
Policy lesson 3 calls for a universal approach to access to high quality ECEC regardless of family income, parental employment status, special educational needs or ethnic/language background with particular attention to children in need of special support. To be accessible, ECEC must be available, affordable, and appropriate. This requires an adequate supply of services, affordable parent fees (either free, very low cost, or geared to income) and services that fit the needs and characteristics of the family and the child (for example, they must be responsive to parents' work schedules).

Few Canadian children under the age of five have a chance to participate in high quality ECEC programs that benefit their development and only a minority of parents can rely on the care they need to train or work. In 2001, there were only enough regulated child-care spaces (including both part-day and full-day) to accommodate 12.1% of children aged 0–12 (or approximately 15% of 0–6 year olds), an increase from 7.5% of 0–12 year olds in 1992 (and it should be noted that much of the increase in coverage can be attributed to a shrinking child population). Over the 1990s, expansion in child-care slowed dramatically compared to the previous decade. While between 1992 and 2001, regulated child-care spaces grew from 371,573 to 593,430, most of this was in Quebec. Child-care spaces in Quebec grew 156,517 spaces (from 78,388 in 1992 to 234,905 in 2001) while in the rest of Canada the growth totaled 65,340 spaces (from 293,185 in 1992 to 358,525 in 2001). In comparison, in the 1980–1990 decade, regulated child-care spaces outside Quebec grew by 160,980.

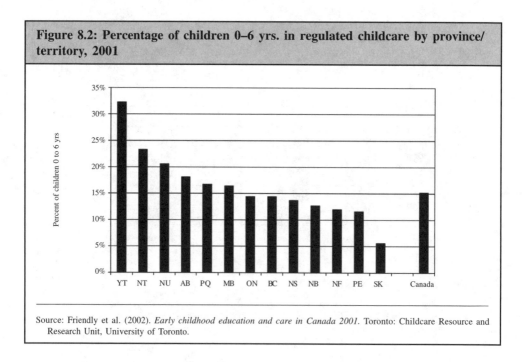

**Figure 8.2: Percentage of children 0–6 yrs. in regulated childcare by province/territory, 2001**

Source: Friendly et al. (2002). *Early childhood education and care in Canada 2001.* Toronto: Childcare Resource and Research Unit, University of Toronto.

Social Determinants of Health

From 1992 to 2001, the percent of children for whom a regulated space was available dropped only in Alberta, but the percentage increases in the other provinces were almost all less than +3%. By province, in 2001, the percent of children for whom there was a regulated space ranged from 4.2% in Saskatchewan to 21.1% in Quebec; 40% of regulated spaces were in Quebec (Friendly et al., 2002).

The way ECEC is financed also makes it inaccessible to many families. Parent user fees in childcare programs create barriers to access for poor, most modest, and many middle-income families. While fee subsidies targeted to low income families are available in all regions (outside Quebec which began providing regulated childcare at $5 a day in 1998[2]), modest and middle-income families are usually not eligible for them; under-funding often means that subsidies are not available even to families who qualify. In addition, subsidy eligibility levels (in constant dollars) dropped between 1992 to 2001 in seven of nine provinces/territories for which data were available. Indeed, most improved their eligibility levels very little (if at all) during the past decade (Friendly et al., 2002).

Generally, Canadian childcare is characterised by eligibility based on narrow categories, scarcity, children in need of special support being left unserved, and extensive targeting to selected populations. It cannot be said that it is moving towards *"a universal approach to access with particular attention to children in need of special support."* Indeed, with the exception of public kindergarten and Quebec's developing universal childcare program, Canada has not defined universality as an objective.

*Policy lesson 4*
Policy lesson 4 calls for substantial public investment in services and infrastructure.

| Box 8.2 |
| --- |
| • Universal approach to access<br>• Substantial public investment |

Substantial government investment is required to support a sustainable system of quality, accessible services. In ECEC programs, financing is directly linked to accessibility and quality. Canadian ECEC has multiple policies and programs associated with multiple funding sources, most of them provincial/territorial. Altogether provinces/territories spent an estimated $1.5 billion on kindergarten in 2001.[3] With regard to childcare, there are multiple sources of funds—fee subsidies, capital, operating and wage grants, tax measures, and vouchers. Overall, however, regulated child-care is largely a user pay program; cross-Canada data show that 49% of an average child-care centre's revenue came from parent fees in 1998 (Goelman et al., 2000). By 2001, Canada-wide spending on regulated child-care reached $1.9 billion; of this total, 58% was spent by Quebec (Friendly et al., 2002). While Quebec's spending on child-care increased dramatically over the past decade, total spending in the rest of Canada dropped about $70 million in constant 2001 dollars.

There was considerable variation in provincial/territorial spending for childcare over the 1990s with several provinces increasing spending considerably and two (Ontario and Alberta) reducing spending. From the perspective of per child spending, the jurisdictions range from a low of $91 (Nova Scotia) to $980 (Quebec) in 2001 (Friendly et al., 2002). In comparison, the European Union Childcare Network has proposed national spending on ECEC of at

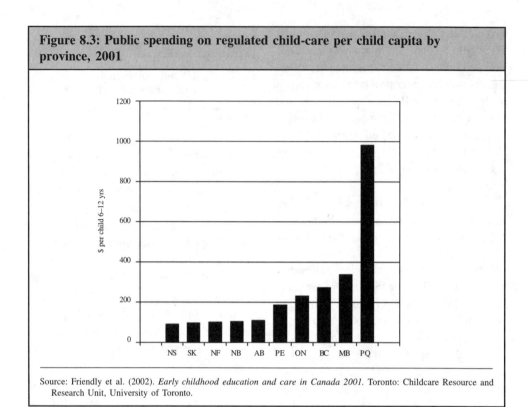

**Figure 8.3: Public spending on regulated child-care per child capita by province, 2001**

$ per child 6–12 yrs

Source: Friendly et al. (2002). *Early childhood education and care in Canada 2001*. Toronto: Childcare Resource and Research Unit, University of Toronto.

least one percent of GDP for children aged 0–5 years (European Commission, 1996). Canada's GDP was somewhat more than $1 trillion in 2002; 1% of that would be about $10 billion annually.

*Policy lesson 5*

Policy lesson 5 recommends that all forms of ECEC be regulated and monitored and suggests that pedagogical frameworks focusing on children's holistic development and strategies for ongoing quality improvement are key. As described earlier, the characteristics of ECEC services that determine whether they are likely to meet not only basic health and safety requirements but also provide environments that ensure development and learning have been well documented in research. Two structural elements have been shown to be key in

determining the likelihood that high quality will occur in an ECEC program. The first of these—financing—was discussed in the previous section.

While the second—regulation—has been shown to be linked to quality through the form and content of programs, especially staffing (Gallagher et al., 1999), regulation does not guarantee quality. Several Canadian studies have identified concerns about quality in regulated childcare services. *You bet I care!* (YBIC!) a cross-Canada study of process quality (that is, derived from structured observations of multiple program activities and elements) in child-care found that:

Fewer than half of the preschool rooms (44.3%) and slightly more than a quarter of the infant/toddler

Social Determinants of Health

rooms (28.7%) are providing activities and materials that encourage children's development. Instead, the majority of the centres in Canada are providing care that is of minimal or mediocre quality. The children's physical and emotional health and safety are protected but few opportunities for learning are provided. (Goelman et al., 2000)

The YBIC! study of regulated family childcare showed similar results (Doherty et al., 2000). Analysis of the YBIC! data confirms that significant provincial differences in process quality scores are linked to strength of regulation (as well as whether the centre is for-profit or non-profit) (Doherty et al., 2002). At the same time, the unregulated child-care—unregulated family or in-own-home child-care—that provides care for most Canadian preschool age children while mothers work are outside systems of quality assurance altogether. While research on the precise details of these arrangements is sparse, enough is known to suggest that the majority of preschool-age children whose mothers work outside the home spend a good deal of time in child-care arrangements that are lacking as early childhood enhancing environments.

*Policy lesson 6*
Policy lesson 6 suggests that appropriate training and working conditions for staff in all forms of provision is a foundation for quality ECEC services which depend on strong staffing and fair working conditions. Strategies for recruiting and retaining a qualified, diverse, mixed-gender workforce and for ensuring that a career in ECEC is satisfying, respected, and financially viable are essential. As human interaction makes up the substance of a child's ECEC experiences, staff are the essence of ECEC programs. Research shows that adequate training and fair working conditions—wages and benefits, working environments, turnover, training, and morale—are all strongly and directly associated with the quality of a child's experience and development (Goelman et al., 2000; Whitebook et al., 1990).

While public school teaching credentials are required for kindergarten teachers in all provinces/territories, training in early childhood education is not. At the same time, there is strong agreement that Canadian ECEC provides inadequate working conditions and training requirements in regulated childcare (Environics Research Group, 1998). A 1998 national study of the child-care workforce found that Canadian caregivers receive little public support, few resources, and unacceptably low wages, that education in the field is poorly coordinated and there are many gaps in training. It concluded that Canadian society places little value on the work and skills of the women who care for young children (Beach et al., 1998).

At the same time, requirements for staff to have training in early childhood education are weak—no jurisdiction requires all staff in a child-care centre to have post secondary ECE training. Overall, requirements to work in a child-care center range from no training requirements to a community college diploma (one to three years). Generally,

---

**Box 8.3**

- Regulation, monitoring, and strategies for improvement key to quality
- Appropriate training and fair working conditions for staff

---

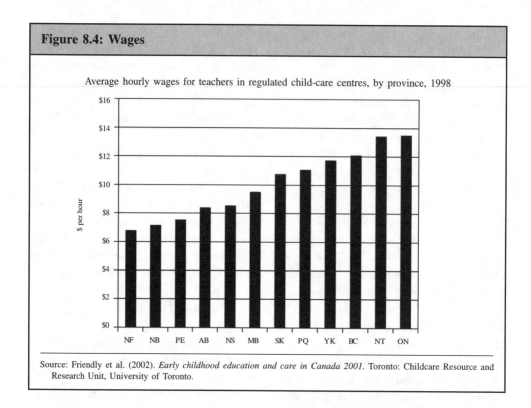

**Figure 8.4: Wages**

Average hourly wages for teachers in regulated child-care centres, by province, 1998

Source: Friendly et al. (2002). *Early childhood education and care in Canada 2001*. Toronto: Childcare Resource and Research Unit, University of Toronto.

regulated family day care has no minimum educational requirements and providers earn low wages.

*Policy lesson 7*
Policy lesson 7 calls for systematic monitoring and data collection with coherent procedures on the status of young children, ECEC provision, and the early childhood workforce. An analysis of Canadian ECEC data needs concludes that Canada essentially has no reliable, consistent, comparable data on various aspects of ECEC that can inform policy or improvements to service provision, or assess changes and effects on children and families over time (Cleveland et al., 2003).

*Policy lesson 8*
Policy lesson 8 suggests that a stable framework and long-term agenda for

**Box 8.4**

- Systematic data collection
- Sustained support for research and evaluation

research and evaluation requires sustained investment to support research on key policy goals and is a necessary part of a process of continuous improvement. While some research and evaluation studies—mostly conducted through a series of federal funding programs—have yielded valuable information, there has not been a *stable framework and long-term agenda*. The systematic data collection discussed in the previous section is linked to this research agenda; basic data to provide public accountability should be a complement to a research and evaluation agenda that can help provide answers to more complex questions.

# First steps and next steps

One concern about Canada's approach to ECEC has been that the process of establishing a coherent, sustained system of ECEC has not even begun. In the years between the 1970 recommendation of the Royal Commission on the Status of Women for a national childcare program and the present, there were four efforts to begin this process by three successive federal governments. Each announced that a national strategy for childcare would be developed but each of the first three attempts failed to materialize. However, the most recent effort, the Multilateral Framework on Early Learning and Care (March 2003) broke through the "anything but child care" approach of the last decade and may now have begun to establish the shape of a national strategy. This agreement, supported by all provinces/territories except Quebec (which had already begun to put its own program in place) was characterized by Human Resources Development Canada Minister Jane Stewart as "the first step to a national child care program." The agreement restricts use of federal funds to regulated childcare and commits to public reporting in a number of key areas. There are, however, no national goals, objectives, legislation, targets, and timetables, or implementation plans.

In Canada, addressing social policy issues that are within provincial/territorial jurisdiction requires both federal leadership, resources and vision, and the collaboration of provinces/territories. Progress in fundamental areas such as quality, access, planning, and human resources will require federal/provincial/territorial co-operation. Federal financing will be important in leveraging provincial/territorial willingness to collaborate. Most observers—even the strongest advocates for ECEC—would agree that building a universal system of high quality ECEC programs across Canada will take some years. A key question is: If the Multilateral Framework is the "first step to a national child-care program," what are the next steps?

An important first next step would be a national statement that a system of universally accessible high quality ECEC is a goal to be developed across Canada within 10 or 15 years. To be effective, a national goal statement would need to be accompanied by a policy framework with stated principles; federal ECEC legislation; quantifiable short and medium-term objectives; and implementation plans with targets and timetables including program development, quality improvement and data, research, and evaluation. As governments have already committed themselves to ensuring that children get the best possible start in life by signing the National Children's Agenda and the Early Childhood Development Initiative, designing an ECEC policy framework has a head start.

A second important signal about serious intentions to take the next steps would be for the federal government to establish a "home" for ECEC—a directorate or secretariat within the federal government as was proposed by Brian Mulroney's Special Committee on Child Care back in 1987. Setting up such an administrative structure would be fundamental to being able to carry out the intergovernmental policy and reporting work that a national ECEC strategy would entail. The Directorate's responsibilities would include (in collaboration with provinces/territories) designing national guidelines and principles, spearheading the policy process, defining roles and responsibilities for the various stakeholders, facilitating intergovernmental work on best practices, setting targets and timetables for improving accessibility and quality, ensuring that data, research, and evaluation are in place, and ensuring accountability for effective use of public resources.

A third step in ensuring that the Multilateral Framework moves from a "first step" toward a national ECEC program is a fiscal one. ECEC has not yet had serious consideration within federal budget priorities. As federal budgets now commonly set out 4 or 5 year budget commitments, a first phase of developing accessible, high quality ECEC programs across Canada would command a budget that would "ramp up" as province/territorial capacity improves. The Social Policy Committee of the Federal Liberal Caucus (2002) has proposed a first phase budget of $1 billion (Year 1), $2.2 billion (Year 2), $3.8 billion (Year 3), and $4.5 billion (Year 4). This commitment of new dollars should be on top of existing spending and depend upon provincial/territorial willingness to use federal funds within agreed-upon terms.

## Conclusion

ECEC programs are an important social determinant of health through their impact on children, their families, and communities. This chapter has argued that although ECEC outside the family is only one of a number of factors that have an impact on children during early life, it is known to provide a platform for adult employment, education, income, status, and lifestyle. These are, in turn, well linked to adult health. Some would argue— given our knowledge today about their multiple impact—that ECEC is so fundamental to well-being that it should be a human right. In addition to including early childhood education and child-care in such United Nations' compacts as the Convention on the Rights of the Child, the Convention on the Elimination of All Forms of Discrimination Against Women, and Education for All, UNICEF, the United Nations Children's Fund calls on world government leaders to take action on ECEC in order to "make children—the youngest especially—the priority at all policy tables ... and to ensure that this has the necessary political and financial support" (UNICEF, 2001). For Canada, this will require the mustering of vision, commitment, and political will to ensure that the "first step" leads to the next steps and, ultimately, to the goal of high quality early childhood education and care for all.

## Notes

1. It should be noted that these services are all publicly funded although—with the exception of full school-day programs for children aged 2.5 to 6 which are usually free to the user—there are parent fees in most cases. However, affordability isn't a significant issue in most countries even outside the older preschool group.
2. The $5 a day fee was increased to $7 a day for all income groups in the fall of 2003.
3. The availability of figures for kindergarten spending varies by jurisdiction. This is a very rough estimate based on figures found in Friendly et al., 2002.

## Recommended readings

Cleveland, G. and Krashinsky, M. (Eds.). (2001). *Our children's future: Child care policy in Canada*. Toronto: University of Toronto Press.

Social Determinants of Health

Cleveland and Krashinsky have assembled many of the key experts and activists in the area of Canadian child care policy, and asked them to consider a number of crucial questions.

Friendly, M., Beach, J. and Turiano, M. (2002). *Early childhood education and care in Canada 2001*. Toronto: Childcare Resource and Research Unit, University of Toronto.
   The Childcare Resource and Research Unit has periodically assembled pan-Canadian data to produce a national snapshot of child-care and early childhood education. The fifth edition of Early childhood education and care in Canada presents 2001 data.

Mahon, R. (2001). *No small matter: Child care policy research*. Ottawa: Institute on Political Economy, Carleton University.
   The author establishes three reasons why we need to pay attention to policies directed to children. She then establishes two dimensions of social policy that allow us to put Canada's response to these challenges into a larger context.

Organization for Economic Co-operation and Development. (2001). *Starting strong: Summary report of the thematic review of early childhood education and care and education*, online at www.childcarecanada.org/pulstudies/int/oecdstrong.html.
   Comparative report on early childhood education and care carried out by the Organization for Economic Co-operation and Development. *Starting strong* summarizes the findings of a two year analysis of ECEC in 12 OECD countries.

Social Policy Committee, Federal Liberal Caucus. (2002). *A national child care strategy: Getting the architecture right now*, online at www.childcarecanada.org/pulstudies/can/godfrey-arch.html.
   This paper provides the framework for a National Child Care Strategy as outlined in the August 2002 report of the Social Policy Committee of the National Liberal Caucus. This report identified the rationale for action on a national child-care strategy: The August Social Policy Committee report argued that the single most important investment our government can make at this time to address child poverty is to invest in a national child care strategy.

## Related websites

Childcare Resource and Research Unit (CRRU), University of Toronto—www.childcarecanada.org
   The Childcare Resource and Research Unit focuses on early childhood care and education research and policy. The comprehensive web site includes links to a wide range of documents on the topic, online versions of CRRU reports and current developments in ECEC in Canada.

Thematic Review of Early Childhood Education and Care, Organization for Economic Co-operation and Development—www.oecd.org/linklist
   Invited by participating countries, OECD expert teams review policy, programmes, and provision for children from birth to compulsory school age, including the transition period from ECEC to primary schooling.

Childcare Advocacy Association of Canada—www.childcareadvocacy.ca/
   The Child Care Advocacy Association of Canada (CCAAC) is dedicated to promoting quality, publicly funded child-care accessible to all.

Campaign 2000—www.campaign2000.ca/
   Campaign 2000 is a cross-Canada public education movement to build Canadian awareness and support for the 1989 all-party House of Commons resolution to end child poverty in Canada by the year 2000.

# Chapter Nine

———●———

# EARLY CHILDHOOD EDUCATION AND HEALTH

### Gina Browne

## Introduction

The Organization for Economic Co-operation and Development (OECD) recommendations are key elements likely to promote equitable access to quality early childhood education and care (ECEC). These OECD recommendations are to provide:

1. A systematic and integrated intersectoral approach to policy development and implementation.
2. A strong and equal partnership with the education system and ECEC.
3. A universal approach to access with particular attention to children in need of special support as a result of family income, parental employment status, special education, and/or ethnic/language background.
4. Substantial public investment in services and infrastructure.
5. Regulation and standardization of all forms of ECEC.
6. Appropriate training and staff working conditions.
7. Systematic attention to monitoring and data collection re: the status of young children, ECEC provision, and required human resources.
8. A framework and agenda for research and evaluation as a necessary part of continuous quality improvement.

There are a number of reasons to focus attention on integration of existing human services for children. Twenty five percent of children and youth have one or more treatable behavioural problems (emotional, conduct, hyperactive). Only 16% of these receive any treatment (Offord, 1987). The vast majority of children's problems go unrecognized and often are inappropriately, incompletely, or reactively treated with school expulsion, dropouts, and/or incarceration. There is a growing recognition that problems in children and youth (depression, anxiety, and substance abuse) coexist with other risk circumstances (poverty, inadequate parenting) and risk conditions (learning disabilities, poor social environments, gangs, and/or drug trafficking) (Byrne et al., 2003).

## BOX 9.1: The health of Canada's children: A CICH profile

### Income inequity

Research demonstrates that wide disparities in wealth are intricately connected with the health of a population. The greater the level of income inequity, the poorer the population health. Those with the lowest incomes have the worst health outcomes, but the negative impact of inequity is felt among all.

### Poverty

The after-taxes poverty rate for children is significantly higher in Canada (14%) than in countries such as Sweden (3%), the Netherlands (6%), France (7%), Germany (7%), and the United Kingdom (10%). The after-taxes poverty rate for children is significantly lower in Canada than in the United States (22%).

The number of children living in poverty (below the Statistics Canada Low-Income Cutoffs) in Canada grew by over 700,000 between 1981 and 1996. One in four children lived in poverty in 1996 compared with one in eight in 1981.

In all provinces, younger children are at greater risk of poverty than older children. The national poverty rate for children under the age of 7 climbed to 25% in 1996. It was 13% in 1981 and 21% in 1991. For children between the ages of 7 and 17, the poverty rate in 1996 was 19%.

### Social assistance and minimum wage

In 1998, across Canada, social assistance provided lone-parent families with one child with an income that amounts to between 50% (in Alberta) and 69% (in Newfoundland) of the poverty line. Social assistance, therefore, did not provide these families with adequate incomes to ensure that they could meet their needs. Housing and food security is jeopardized for these families.

To reach the Statistics Canada low-income cut-offs, families working for minimum wage must work long hours. This is true for lone-parent and two-parent families. Depending on the province, lone-parent, one-child families needed to work between 61 and 80 hours per week in 1996. Two-parent, two-child families needed to work between 89 and 118 hours per week. Research shows that families working under these conditions can experience extreme stress that may compromise family functioning.

### Risk factors

Living in a lone-mother family is a risk factor for poverty. Between 1981 and 1997, the rate of poverty for children in lone-mother families was dramatically higher than the rate for children in two-parent families. In 1997, the rate of poverty for children in lone-mother families was 60%—for children in two-parent families it was 13%.

Children who are from visible minority groups are at elevated risk of living in poverty. 43% of children under 15 years of age who belonged to visible minority groups lived in poverty in 1995.

Aboriginal children are at increased risk of poverty. 52% of Aboriginal children under the age of 15 years lived in poverty in 1995. Children under the age of 15 years who have an activity limitation are more likely to live in poverty than children of the same age with no activity limitation (37% compared to 23%). The families of children with activity limitations must often reduce or modify their workforce participation in order to care for their children in the absence of appropriate child care, respite, and family responsibility leave policies.

con't

**Inequity and child health**

Children who live in poverty encounter more hurdles to healthy development and are, consequently, at an elevated risk for a wide range of negative health outcomes.

Babies born to low income parents are at an increased risk for low birth weight. In 1994–95, where the household income was less than $30,000, the low birth weight rate was 7%. Where the household income was greater than $60,000, the rate of low birth weight was 4%.

Income and injury are inversely related for boys. Males from birth to 19 years of age in the poorest quintile had an injury death rate of 22/100,000 compared to 15/100,000 for male children in the richest quintile. The higher rate of injury death among male children in low income families may be attributable to unsafe housing, a lack of safe play spaces and limited access to supervised recreation and sports. The poorest 20% of children are at greater risk of dying in a fire or a homicide than other children. The rate of death in fires was 1.7/100,000 for the poorest children compared to 0.4 to 0.1 for other children. The rate of homicide death was 2.5/100,000 for the poorest 20% of children compared to 1.1 to 0.5 for other children.

Children living in households with incomes less than $20,000 per annum are at considerably elevated risk of "hyperactivity" and "delinquent behaviours."

Source: Canadian Institute of Child Health. (2002). *The health of Canada's children: A CICH profile, 3rd edition*, Ottawa: CICH, online at www.cich.ca/income.htm.

Agencies have been historically funded to address, on-demand, slivers of a young person's predicament (Schorr, 1988). This contributes to ineffective programming and children and youth who "fall through the cracks." A review of elements of effective health promotion programmes to be achieved within existing budgets compels us to consider the integration of services for children, especially those of school-age.

## Elements of effective health promotion programs

While research continues on how best to promote mental health and reduce negative risky behaviours in children and adolescents, a sizable body of evidence has already accumulated that identifies common elements of effective programming to reach those ends based on the recognition that a complex web of factors influences child development (Catalano and Berrglund, 1999; Durlak and Wells, 1997; Greenberg et al., 1999). The realization that effects of those factors may be altered by what society does

to protect and assist children has informed a variety of innovative programs, particularly for young children, e.g., "Sure Start" in the U.K. and "Healthy Babies, Healthy Children" in Canada. This chapter considers how best to converge theory and practice around the issue of incorporating best practices into an integrated service structure extended toward school-aged children and youth.

A mix of protective and risk factors (biological and environmental) work in concert to lay the framework for a child's emotional/psychological functioning (Boyle and Offord, 1987a; Bennett and Offord, 1998); thus, a range of potential developmental problems can be addressed by enhancing protective factors and minimizing risk factors. Earlier studies by the author and colleagues, among others, provide evidence for both the effectiveness and efficiency of certain fundamental elements of universal and early intervention youth services (Browne et al., 1999a; Browne et al., 1995). Primary among these are the need for: (1) early and long-term interventions, with periodic follow-up and reinforcement; (2) interactive, positive, non-didactic programming; (3) the inclusion of families, community involvement, and/or direction; (4) cultural, age, and gender sensitivity; (5) appropriate, continuing adult training and staffing; (6) a holistic or ecological context for services; (7) services that emphasize competencies or skills development. To expand on the last point, interventions seem most often effective when they include comprehensive, integrated strategies that affect more than one of a child's social environments, i.e., family, school, and community (Catalano et al., 1999; Greenberg et al., 1999).

These strategies seem to be effective because they address the multi-faceted, contextual origins of multiple emotional and behavioural problems and competencies that protect children in the face of problems. Children with identified disorders tend to have clusters of more than one disorder (Anderson et al., 1987; Browne et al., 2002). Risky negative behaviour (e.g., substance abuse or unprotected sex), which has ramifications for individuals, families, and the wider society, has also been associated with underlying mental health disorders (Browne et al., 2002). Integrated programming that touches the multiple domains of a child's life in and outside school stands a greater chance of addressing

these clusters of problems via likely risk factors and behaviours (Boyle et al., 1987b; Browne et al., 2001a; Boyle et al., 1987a; and Browne et al., 2002, "Convergence" Working Paper on the website).

## Integration of services

Integration is a key strategy for extending the coverage, as well as effectiveness, of children's services, according to key informants in the child care sector (Browne et al., 2001b). Intersectoral integration may present the greatest challenge to implementation, among the various elements identified as components of effective children's services. Currently only a portion of children and youth who could benefit from help receive appropriate formal care and treatment (Briggs-Gowan et al., 2000). Likely factors that hinder appropriate care include incomplete screening and diagnosis, as well as unwillingness to receive treatment and non-compliance on the part of youth and/or their parents. Mental health advocates point to a fear of being stigmatized as a serious limiting factor for access to care (Ontario Association of Children's Mental Health Centres, 2001).

Youth services employ a range of selective or targeted programs oriented toward children because of their behavioural or risk profile, yet targeting selective groups based on presence of specific risk factors is a less than perfect exercise. Although research has been able to identify particular factors such as family breakdown and socio-economic disadvantage that are associated with later mental health problems, each particular variable explains only a small portion of the known variance (Boyle and Lipman, 2002). Ongoing comprehensive longitudinal contextual studies such as

Canada's National Longitudinal Study of Children and Youth (NLSCY) may more fully explain variable interactions (Boyle et al., 1987a; Human Resources Development Canada/Statistics Canada, 2000). At present, because of the small percentage of children with identifiable risk factors in the population, most children with emotional/behavioural problems fall outside the confines of a high-risk profile. With selective programming, children who might in the long term benefit from mental health initiatives are not exposed to them (Mustard and McCain, 1999). Universal programs aimed at the full spectrum of community children would extend the net to enhance the development of children and adolescents with unrecognized or hidden risk factors. These programs can carry their own limitations such as high cost and the inability to provide intensive initiatives, however recent evidence documents that these programmes can pay for themselves in the same year in publicly funded systems of National Health Insurance by averting the use of more expensive services (Browne et al., 1999a; Browne, et al., 2001a). An integrated framework could accommodate a combination of clinical, targeted, and universal programs, which has been suggested as an optimal approach (Offord et al., 1999).

Children who have problems at home often "act out" at school. Symptoms may also appear more visible in venues outside a family environment. Providing services across home, school and community domains increases the likelihood of reaching more children who would benefit from interventions, sewing up the gaps in the social safety net. In an integrated model, child-care and recreation workers, caregivers, educators, social service, and juvenile justice employees would receive training to recognize indications of mental health problems and be linked to a system for early professional identification and referral of children and adolescents. Using a measure piloted in Ontario to assess all young children's readiness for school, some teachers have already been able to rate young children on age-appropriate emotional functioning and behaviour (Applied Research Branch Strategic Policy, 1998).

In addition to increasing numbers of children assisted by mental health services, integration can address existing gaps in knowledge about programming, dissemination of information and accessibility to services (Fonagy, 2000). For example, in Ontario there are no systematic links among shelters, hostels, and schools to connect street kids to school-based programs. As well, due to the transient nature of many high-needs, homeless, or low-income families, agencies lose track of youth who need help, even within the same community. Since many programs are developed and operated on a neighbourhood basis, transiency results in children dropping out of programs, which reduces their effectiveness, and often necessitates costly and inefficient reassessment of children and families at subsequent sites (Browne, 1999b; Catalano et al., 1999). A program to assist street youth may concentrate on job skills or substance abuse counselling without addressing availability of housing, welfare regulations, mental and physical health problems, family counselling, police procedures, community bylaws, or stigmatization, all areas that may need to be considered in crafting a multi-dimensional care strategy. An integrated system could provide such a proactive, comprehensive approach to reach and maintain contact with reluctant or recalcitrant older youth, reconnecting them with school and community programs. Integrating services across domains would help close service gaps by emphasizing a holistic focus on the child and family.

## Effectiveness and efficiency of universal integrated health promotion services for vulnerable families and children

The advantages of an integrated strategy can be successfully argued from an economic perspective, since the input of resources for developing healthy children is a societal investment that can reduce massive future outlays for social ills such as crime, poverty and substance abuse, and will pay dividends in increased education and productivity levels (Browne et al., 1999b). Studies of direct and indirect costs for youth mental health problems are consistent in finding contemporaneous savings as well from the delivery of appropriate services (Browne et al., 1999a). People who fail to find appropriate services use other and often more expensive, publicly funded services over the same time period as those receiving appropriate care. These studies show consistently that coordinated or integrated service delivery is more effective, efficient, and less costly than single-focus initiatives (Browne et al., 1999b; Browne et al., 2001b). For example, the cost of treating adolescents with mental health problems by a co-ordinated program of health, social, and educational school-based services was compared to the cost of hospital and specialist care for matched teens eligible for, but not yet enrolled in, the program. Troubled adolescents not enrolled in the coordinated program used health and social services worth twice as much ($10,000 per year per person) as those in the program ($5,000 per year per person) while

evidencing poorer emotional health outcomes (Browne et al., 1995).

The study entitled "When the bough breaks" was a randomized trial of the effects and expense of 5 social policy directions for single parents and children on social assistance. It compared the value of:

1.  Ontario's 1995 on-demand health and social care for this group;
2.  proactive age appropriate quality child care for all children and youth in the household provided by NGO services alone;
3.  proactive publicly funded professional employment retraining for parents on social assistance previously classified in 1995 as unemployable, and therefore never offered this service, alone;
4.  proactive and publicly funded professional nurse in-house visits to help the parent solve the mix of her health, child-care, youth, financial, housing, and domestic problems, alone;
5.  a combination of all three proactive services representing some integration of separately financed, regulated and organized services from three sectors.

The findings from the article "Evidence that informs practice and policy: The role of strategic alliances at the municipal, provincial, and federal levels" (Browne, 1999) were as follows:

The studies, "When the bough breaks" (2001) and "Benefiting all the beneficiaries" (Browne et al., 1999a), concluded that providing additional health and social services to mothers of social assistance families and making quality child-care and recreation services available pays for itself in a relatively short period, and produces more permanent beneficial outcomes in families at risk. The methodology of the two studies is more completely dealt with in the reports and their abstracts, but the research consisted of examining 765 households comprising 1,300 children aged 0–24. The research project, headed by Dr. Gina Browne, made a number of key findings:

- Half of the heads of sole-support families suffer from mental health problems. Assisting clients with depression and other disorders gives them the self-esteem and confidence they need to contemplate exiting social assistance.
- Offering a full range of services to families—such as public health nurse visits for mothers and subsidized recreation for children—produced social assistance exit rates of 25% compared to 10% for those receiving no supplementary services.
- The cost of provision of additional public health nurses was more than offset by a reduction in the use of less appropriate and more expensive medical services by subjects who sought out help for themselves; i.e., emergency visits, specialists, hospitalization.
- Offering recreational services helps psychologically disordered children achieve social, physical, and academic competence at a rate equal to a non-disordered child. Recreation paid for itself through reduced use of social and health services—probation, child psychiatry, child psychology, social work, and emergency services.

- Age appropriate quality child-care and/or recreation and skills development services for children and youth produced reductions in parental nervous system, anxiety and sleep problems, and less use of the food bank.
- Even providing a partial menu of proactive supplementary services produced greater social assistance exit rates compared to parents who did not receive the service:
  - subsidized recreation alone; 10% greater exit rate.
  - public health visits alone; 12% greater exit rate.
  - employment retraining alone; 10% greater exit rate.

These results illustrate a number of things that can be used to inform the ECED agenda.

Age-appropriate arts and recreation services (an intervention aimed at the child/youth):

1. was acceptable to 75% of families and more acceptable than either of the professional services that unwittingly insinuate people have problems.
2. was necessary to produce an effect in child/youth competence. In children with a behavioural disorder it had a protective effect, maintaining their academic, interpersonal and social competence to be equal to that of a child with no disorder.
3. in and of itself, produced positive results in the parents, of reductions in anxiety, sleep, nervous system problems and use of the food bank services.
4. facilitated children with a behaviour disorder to use other therapeutic

services appropriately in comparison to children with a disorder without these services.

5. paid for itself within a year by reduction in publicly funded children's aid, physician specialists, emergency services, probation, psychology services, social workers, and physiotherapy services.

6. was no more expensive than usual care or publicly funded professional care.

7. was equivalent to professional services in doubling the exit from social assistance within a year, amounting to a $200,000/yr savings for every 100 mothers offered the program.

These examples of cost-savings highlight a major impediment to development of program integration in that cost savings are often realized in sectors other than those operating the various youth services. For example, savings in use of physician or

---

**BOX 9.2: Investments in comprehensive programming for families with children on welfare: Services for single parent mothers and children on welfare pays for itself within one year**

Overwhelming evidence points to the importance of childhood experiences in determining health and social success throughout a person's life. All families need support in raising their children, but some parents face greater obstacles in establishing the environment that will help them to provide the best possible experiences for their children. Poverty—and especially the deep poverty of families on welfare—has extremely detrimental effects on children's development. Many studies have shown that families benefit from the supports of good social and health programs. Emerging evidence also suggests that what works best with high-risk, low-income families are comprehensive, coherent and integrated programs that see the child in the context of family and the family in the context of its surroundings.

Two parallel studies titled "When the bough breaks" and "Benefitting all the beneficiaries" showed that it is equally effective, but less expensive, to respond to the needs of mothers and children on welfare with services that are comprehensive and supportive. Proactive, comprehensive health and social services for mothers and quality child-care or recreation services for children produce more impressive results than services that leave families to direct and try to finance their own opportunities. Proactive services for mothers and children pay for themselves in reduced use of other (public) services. In addition, there are important short-term financial gains (for the mothers and children and for the public nurse) along with long-term societal benefits in the form of earlier exit from social assistance.

Most effective of all the programs tested are age appropriate child care and recreation. Services work even better when they also provide employment supports that help mothers on welfare to re-enter the work force and the support of nursing services. Good, integrated services that provide several types of support for mothers and children are far more effective—both for families and for taxpayers—than leaving families to cope on their own with the existing welfare and social services system.

Source: Browne, G., Roulston, J., Ewart, B., Schuster, M. Edwardh, J. and Boily, L. (1999). System-Linked Research Unit Working Paper Series #99-02. Hamilton: System-Linked Research Unit on Health and Social Service Utilization, online at www.fhs.mcmaster.ca/slru/paper/wp9902.htm

Social Determinants of Health

corrections services may be reinvested in education or recreation programs. However, there is currently no easy provision for compensating programs that generate cost savings in other service areas.

## Implementation model

The task of implementing an integration model seems daunting, if only because of the proliferation of services, with differing bureaucratic structures, objectives, mission statements, levels of staff expertise, professionalism, and funding mechanisms. In developing a model of integrated, school-linked children's services, Volpe et al. (1999) identified requirements for organizational change: supportive policies and funding, institutional leadership and a climate of trust to overcome parochialism. As well, community leadership and support from families, business, political interests, and other community organizations were integral factors.

Figure 9.1 offers a three-dimensional model of integration among service agencies that could be used to foster continuity of care within a sector, intersectoral approaches to a comprehensive menu of services and the pooling of public, private, and not-for-profit financing and resources.

This three dimensional matrix of services proposes stronger linkages between health, education, social, and child-care sectors; between the universal, early intervention and remedial continuum of care; and between public, private, and not for profit funded services. The framework also allows one to critique the extent of integration of children's services in a given province such as Ontario or its regions.

Integration for the purpose of screening, case-finding and continuity of care refers to a network of organizations within a sector, e.g., health that: (1) provides a co-ordinated continuum of services (prevention, detection, early intervention, support, and remediation) and (2) is accountable for

Figure 9.1: Scope of human services

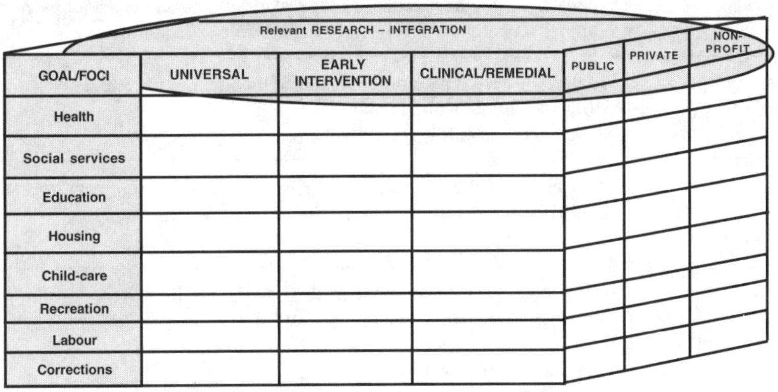

| GOAL/FOCI | UNIVERSAL | EARLY INTERVENTION | CLINICAL/REMEDIAL | PUBLIC | PRIVATE | NON-PROFIT |
|---|---|---|---|---|---|---|
| Health | | | | | | |
| Social services | | | | | | |
| Education | | | | | | |
| Housing | | | | | | |
| Child-care | | | | | | |
| Recreation | | | | | | |
| Labour | | | | | | |
| Corrections | | | | | | |

Relevant RESEARCH – INTEGRATION

Source: Browne, G., Byrne, C., Roberts, J., Gafni, A., Majumdar, B., and Kertyzia, J. (2002). "Convergence: Why Ontario should develop community-based models of integrated service for school-aged children," System-Linked Research Unit Working Paper Series #01-02. McMaster University, Hamilton, Ontario, online at www.fhs.mcmaster.ca/slru.

resulting health status by tracking, follow-up, and systematic evaluation of client outcomes. Ontario's Healthy Babies, Healthy Children universal and early intervention program is but one example. Intersectoral integration refers to a collaboration of disparate agencies covering health, education, social services, corrections, and recreation (physical and cultural). Each sector contributes services that promote healthy child development and parent productivity. Financial integration refers to the sharing or amalgamation of private and not-for-profit resources in publicly funded systems. Savings that result from, and enhance integration, of service delivery can be reinvested in services/activities that further promote healthy development and productivity.

Table 9.1 provides a set of variables that serves as indicators of the scope and depth of integration as well as outcomes this integration of services could have on children's function in a given community. A combined community planning and administrative group could collaborate to co-ordinate school-based universal screening as well as service responses to local needs, assess benefits, and track cost-savings across different sectors from these collaborative efforts.

Some recent publicly funded initiatives in Canada integrate services from two or more domains and several incorporate an ecological perspective involving the child, family and neighbourhood, e.g., Ontario's *Integrated services for Northern children*, *Better beginnings, better futures* (Health Canada, 2000); *Growing together* (Growing together short-term evaluation, 2001) in Toronto and Halifax, and *1,2,3,GO* in Montreal (Bouchard, 1999). The current emphasis in Ontario on admittedly vital pre-school initiatives (Figure 9.2), combined with reductions in school recreation and

| Table 9.1: Measures of system integration | |
|---|---|
| **Program variable** | **Measure** |
| Scope | • Number of and type of member organization |
| Outreach | • Numbers of youth screened by type of health, social, academic screening<br>• Number of parent/child meeting to link to opportunities |
| Integrative mechanisms | • Number of Steering Committee and Sub-committee meetings decisions, actions (communication, planning)<br>• Shared accountabilities, service agreements |
| Percent uptake of opportunities: early intervention (services) | • Number of children engaged in number of activities (services) directed by the number of parent child planning meetings |
| Impact of child engagement in opportunities and early intervention services | • annual competency scores for grade 3 and grade 6<br>• youth volunteerism and employment<br>• youth school completion rates<br>• reductions in untoward events<br>   – CAS placements<br>   – teen pregnancy<br>   – rates of youth school dropouts/suspensions<br>   – risk behaviors<br>   – rates (costs) of use of remedial/therapies, custodial, probationary services. |

music programs, special needs resources, counselling services, and extra-curricular activities resulting from government funding changes, has perhaps left school-aged children more vulnerable than younger children.

An integrated, school-based delivery model would: provide (1) both universal and targeted services, and (2) a common set of available initiatives from elementary through secondary school levels, ensuring the possibility for effective, long-term programming. There would also be an increased likelihood of earlier identification and referral of at-risk children and youth to appropriate remedies and skills development community recreation programs. Comprehensive plans for children at risk for, or identified with, a disorder could be provided by year-round community-linked programming co-ordinated by the school and by the department of public health. The issue of labelling, false positives, and

confidentiality are a consideration for non-universal school-based programs and perhaps to a lesser extent for recreation centre and health centre-based services (Greenberg et al., 1999). Special attention would be needed to resolve these issues and as well, provision would have to be made for children not attending school.

For example, the circles in Figure 9.2 labelled HBHC identify that universal and early intervention, publicly funded health and social services for children under six years, are encouraged in each region of Ontario in the Healthy Babies and Healthy Children (HBHC) universal programme. But it also points out that this circle, or scope of intervention is often not well integrated with remedial publicly funded children's services such as children's mental programs, nor with not-for-profit child-care and recreation services.

Similarly, the program circle labelled LEAP (Learning, Earning, and Parenting) for

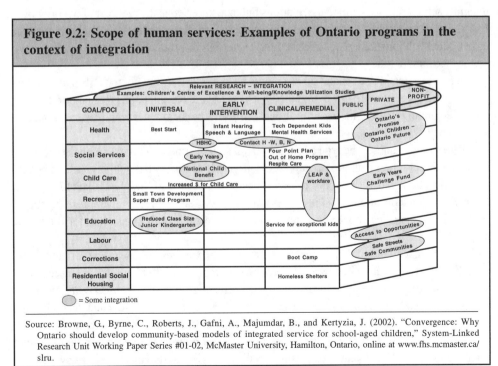

**Figure 9.2: Scope of human services: Examples of Ontario programs in the context of integration**

○ = Some integration

Source: Browne, G., Byrne, C., Roberts, J., Gafni, A., Majumdar, B., and Kertyzia, J. (2002). "Convergence: Why Ontario should develop community-based models of integrated service for school-aged children," System-Linked Research Unit Working Paper Series #01-02, McMaster University, Hamilton, Ontario, online at www.fhs.mcmaster.ca/slru.

pregnant adolescents connects publicly funded remedial, social, education, and child-care services, but it is not connected to publicly funded health services, mental health services, nor to NGO child-care services.

In summary, as a universal programme, Early Childhood Education and Care would enhance its effectiveness and produce more savings if it were also linked to other universal health, social, and recreation services and where pluralism of funding sources were encouraged as well as links to remedial services.

Next steps regarding implementing integration of human services include development of an integration mechanism such as a local office of integrated services that could (1) review incentives and disincentives for collaboration among agencies and professionals, (2) provide a systematic assessment and evaluation system that could quantify the extent/scope and depth of service integration before and after local initiatives that require agency collaboration (Browne et al., 2003), and (3) facilitate integrated service responses to the local needs of children and youth. We are heartened by the initiatives to develop a comprehensive perspective for child-oriented services, yet additional potential cost-savings are being neglected and, more importantly, children and families continue to be failed by a haphazard patchwork of well-meant but uncoordinated services that could be melded into a more effective service delivery framework such as we envision.

## Conclusion

The OECD recommendations assume that a considerable investment in ECEC is required to integrate services, however their calculations fail to acknowledge the real cost of not providing ECEC and ongoing child and youth arts and recreation services, both immediately (in systems of national health insurance), and in the long term (loss of productivity of parents and youth as they become adults).

While provincial and federal governments have a role, they are not the only stakeholders of resource. There is a role for national NGOs and private organizations to push for political will, recognizing that the necessary political will is at the local level with respect to making a vision reality.

When one examines the type of savings from an investment in proactive age appropriate NGO quality child-care and/or arts and recreation that accrue to the publicly funded health, social, education, and correction services, it becomes possible to find the dollars to invest in these prevention/education and skills development quality services for vulnerable populations. Indeed, NGO agencies should be compensated for the savings they generate for the whole system.

The evidence that quality of children's recreation services enhanced identification and referral of children with a behaviour disorder to appropriate early intervention and remedial services, supports the need to further integrate universal programs with early intervention, health and social remedial services. Children with a behaviour disorder not receiving the proactive recreation received no more services than children without disorder.

Offering age appropriate children's services to all children and youth in a family rather than only those under six years of age supports the ecological notion that a child's environment

Social Determinants of Health

plays a big role in his/her development. Children under six are influenced by older brothers and sisters in trouble with the law, using drugs and precipitating family disharmony. In summary, we currently pay for children's services in the same year one way or another. Prevention is cheaper than remediation.

# Recommended readings

Hewlett, S.A. (1991). *When the bough breaks: The cost of neglecting our children.* New York: Harper Perennial.

"Across the face of America, children are failing to flourish. Rich kids, middle-class kids, poor kids—all deal with risk and neglect on a scale unimagined in previous generations," writes Sylvia Anne Hewlett in this compelling, meticulously researched study. *When the bough breaks* doesn't just identify the problems, though; it outlines a multifaceted action plan encompassing parenting leave and child-care policy, tax reform, family-friendly workplaces, volunteer efforts, and more.

Hofrichter, R. (Ed.). (2003). *Health and social justice: Politics, ideology, and inequity in the distribution of disease: A public health reader.* San Francisco: Jossey-Bass.

*Health and social justice*, a collection of reprinted and new articles, assembles a broad range of contributors in different fields to explore particular political and ideological aspects of health inequities among different population groups. Its purpose is to extend public debate about the ways in which the sources of health inequities derive from injustices associated with class, race, and gender relations and to encourage questioning of contemporary approaches, in theory and practice, in addressing them.

Hartwell, S.W. and Schutt, R.K. (Ed.) (2001). *The organizational response to social problems: Research in social problems and public policy, volume 8.* New York: Elsevier Science.

From the de-institutionalization of psychiatric hospitals to the privatisation of prisons, the dramatic public policy changes of the last three decades have been, to a large extent, changes in organization. We learn how organizations shift strategies, create alliances, cross boundaries, and react to incentives as they respond to changing environmental pressures. We learn about the complex relationships between organizations and their clients and how these relations can be altered in response to environmental change.

# Related websites

System-Linked Research Unit on Health and Social Service Utilization—www.fhs.mcmaster.ca/slru

This website is the author's, and lists numerous studies on the effects and expense of proactive comprehensive care for vulnerable populations. Each has been published and requests for publications can go to browneg@mcmaster.ca

Centre of Excellence for Early Childhood Development—www.excellence-earlychildhood.ca

The Centre identifies and summarizes the best scientific work on social and emotional development of young children and makes this information available to service planners, service providers, and policy-makers. The bulletins are a publication of the Centre of Excellence for Early Childhood Development which is one of four Centres of Excellence for Children's Well-Being funded by Health Canada.

Children Fare Better with Work Supports for Low-Income Families—www.researchforum.org

In this report, the Research Forum describes findings from the New Hope program in Wisconsin that demonstrate the importance of stable work supports and flexibility for welfare-to-work families. The program increased both the well-being of children and the work participation among welfare-to-work families, although there were some scattered negative outcomes for teens in these families.

Chapter Ten

# THE STATE AND QUALITY
# OF CANADIAN PUBLIC EDUCATION

## Charles Ungerleider and Tracey Burns

## Introduction

Since its inception in the late 19th century, universal public schooling in Canada has responded to forces arising beyond its borders as it has prepared the young for the responsibilities of adult citizenship. This chapter explores the impact of recent demographic, social, and political forces on the state and quality of Canadian public elementary and secondary schools.

Notwithstanding their considerable successes, Canadian public schools today struggle to respond to the challenges posed by changes to Canadian society. Failure to respond to the challenges puts public schools at risk. In turn, because of the centrality of public schooling in the transmission of core Canadian values, the failure of public schooling puts Canada at risk.

## Canada transformed

Social, demographic, and economic changes have transformed Canada and Canadian families with consequences for the education and educability of school age children. People are marrying later in life, having fewer children, and delaying childbirth (Lochhead, 2000). High rates of separation and divorce have created new family relationships: common-law marriages, single-parent, step-families, and blended families have brought about changes affecting the education of the children living in those families.

## Children from more advantaged families perform better in school

Those who delay parenthood tend to have more formal education and higher family incomes. The reverse is true for those who have children early. Children living in families with two-parents have more favourable behavioural, psychological, and school outcomes than children living in lone-parent or step-families, even when socio-economic conditions are controlled (Kerr and Beaujot, 2001). But more than one-third of all marriages end in divorce. Children of families that have experienced disruption are more likely to leave home at an earlier age because of family conflict and less likely to return home after they have left (Ravanera, 2000). Adolescents whose parents divorced were more likely to remain unmarried, and, if they did marry, were likely to marry later and have their own marriages end in divorce or separation (Corak, 1999).

Child poverty remains a significant Canadian problem. Over the past quarter century, income inequality between families with children has worsened:

> In 1973, the poorest 40 percent of families with children earned only 18.8 percent of all market income—that is, earnings from employment and private invest- ments. By 1997, that percentage had dropped to 13.6 percent. At the same time, the top 40 percent of families with children saw their share of market income rise from 62.6 percent to 68.2 percent. Stated another way, families in the top two quintiles had about three times the market income of low-income families in 1973, increasing to five times by 1997 (Ross et al., 2000, 51–54).

Recent estimates indicate that 22% of the approximately 1.4 million children 15 years of age or younger in Canada were living in low-income families in 1996 (Canadian Education Statistics Council, 2000).

Socio-economic status has a direct impact on higher levels of achievement and superior academic focus. Young children who live in families with lower incomes and children living in single parent families face more challenges than older children and children in two-parent families. Children living in poor families have higher rates of emotional and behavioural disorders, are less likely to perform well in school, and may experience a lower level of social acceptance by others (Canadian Education Statistics Council, 2000). For children living in single-parent families, the situation is considerably worse—more than half live below the Statistics Canada low-income cut-off.

When one considers young families— those in which the eldest person is 30 years of age or younger—the rate of poverty has doubled over the past ten years. Children in low-income families differ from children in moderate or high income families in ways that affect their socialization and education both directly and indirectly. They are more likely to: live in poorly functioning families; live in neighbourhoods where drug use and alcohol consumption is prevalent; be in the top 10% in terms of frequency of delinquent behaviours; have high delinquency scores; have a problem with one or more basic abilities such as vision, hearing, speech, or mobility; and to exhibit delayed vocabulary development (Ross et al., 2000). In addition, socio-economic status has an indirect influence on achievement. Higher socio-economic status is correlated with lower levels of parental depression which, in turn, diminishes the incidence of family dysfunction, lowering the amount of hostile parenting. Lower levels of hostile parenting contribute to better academic focus, which, in turn, influences higher achievement (Ryan and Adams, 1999).

## Changing patterns of socialization

Schools attempt to address problems that have their origin in unsuccessful socialization prior to the youngster entering school. More Canadian children have relatively little

## Box 10.1: Participation in post-secondary education and family income: 1998

Young people from high-income families were 2.5 times as likely as those from low-income families to have participated in university education in 1998 or before, according to data from the Survey of Labour and Income Dynamics (SLID). Individuals aged 18 to 21 who came from low-income homes were less likely to have ever enrolled in any form of post-secondary institution by 1998. But the gap was particularly pronounced for university education.

The analysis divided the 18- to 21-year-old population into four equal quartiles, or quarters, according to family income when they were aged 16. Among those from families in the highest quarter, about 40% in 1998 had attended university at some time in their life.

Post-secondary education participation and family income, 18- to 21-year-olds: 1998

| | Family income at age 16 | | | |
| --- | --- | --- | --- | --- |
| | Lowest quartile | Middle half | Highest quartile | Average |
| Highest level of education participated | | | | |
| All post-secondary[1] | 48.8 | 61.4 | 71.0 | 60.7 |
| University | 16.3 [2] | 26.1 | 39.6 | 27.0 |
| College[3] | 26.7 | 29.5 | 28.2 | 28.5 |

1  Includes university, community college or institute of applied arts and technology or CEGEP, and trade/vocational schools, but excludes business/commercial schools.
2  Estimates with relatively high sampling variability.
3  Includes community college or institute of applied arts and technology or CEGEP.

This rate of university attendance was about 2.5 times that of individuals in the same age group from the lowest one-quarter of incomes (16%). In comparison, about 26% of young people from families whose income was in the middle two quarters had attended university.

Among the families in the highest quarter, more than 70% of young people by 1998 had at some time in their lives participated in some form of postsecondary education-university, college or trade, or vocational schools. Among families in the lowest quarter, 49% of young people had done so. In the middle two family income quarters, 61% had participated in postsecondary education of some sort. The gap between young people who came from the highest and lowest levels of income in 1998 was narrowest for participation in college—either a community college or CEGEP.

On average, almost 29% of young people aged 18 to 21 had attended college, but never university. The differences in college participation rates across family income groups were not statistically significant; thus it is impossible to reject the hypothesis that there is no real difference in college participation among the 18- to 21-year-olds by family income.

Among young people aged 18 to 21 from low-income families who had pursued any post-secondary education, the majority went to college. Among those from high-income families who had pursued any post-secondary education, the majority went to university.

Source: "Participation in postsecondary education and family income: 1998," adapted from the Statistics Canada publication *The daily*, Catalogue 11-001, December 7, 2001.

## Box 10.2: Factors related to adolescents' self-perceived health: 2000/01

While the majority of Canadian adolescents considered themselves to be in "very good" or "excellent" health in 2000/01, nearly one in three 12- to 17-year-olds rated their health as no better than "good," according to a new study. Adolescents who considered their own health to be poor, fair, or good were more likely to smoke, drink, or be obese. They were also less likely to live in a relatively high-income household. The study also found that the lower the educational level is in the adolescent's household, the worse his or her self-rated health is likely to be.

Boys' self-perceived health tends to be better than that of girls. According to data from the 2000/01 Canadian Community Health Survey (CCHS), girls' perceptions of health become less favourable in mid- to late-adolescence. At ages 12 to 14, 73% of boys and girls reported very good or excellent health. But by ages 15 to 17, the proportion for boys remained about the same, while it dropped to 66% for girls.

### Girls vulnerable to depression

Mental health is a major factor in overall health. Previous studies have shown that adolescents, and girls in particular, are vulnerable to depression. According to the 2000/01 CCHS, nearly 6% of 12- to 14-year-old girls had a high risk of having had a major depressive episode in the year before the survey, compared with 2% of boys the same age. Among 15- to 17-year-olds, the proportion of girls who had had such an episode was much higher (11%). By contrast, 15- to 17-year-old boys were no more at risk of depression than those aged 12 to 14.

Depression was significantly associated with reduced odds of reporting excellent or very good health for both older and younger adolescents, even accounting for other factors such as chronic conditions, socio-economic status, obesity, and health behaviours.

### Knowledge of risks doesn't prevent smoking and drinking

Smoking and drinking were associated with the way that adolescents rate their health. Even after accounting for other contributing factors, the 15- to 17-year-olds who were daily smokers or episodic heavy drinkers had lower odds of reporting very good or excellent health, compared with those who did not drink or smoke. "Episodic heavy drinking" is defined as having five or more drinks on one occasion at least once a month.

Other studies have suggested that adolescents may be aware of the health effects of smoking and excessive drinking. Nonetheless, 14% of 15- to 17-year-olds were daily smokers, with girls slightly more likely than boys to smoke daily. About the same proportion of adolescents in that age group also reported episodic heavy drinking, although in this case, the practice was more common among boys.

### Obesity also key factor in self-perceived health

Being obese lowered the odds of an adolescent reporting very good or excellent health, even when the effects of other potential factors were taken into account. The study also found that adolescents who reported relatively low fruit and vegetable consumption or being physically inactive had lower odds of reporting very good or excellent health.

con't

supervision than at any previous time. Initial socialization that was once provided directly by family members is now provided by a combination of parents, caregivers, a child's peers, and the media. Access to media has exposed them to values and experiences that children a half-century ago would not have acquired until they attended school for some time. Though still eager to learn when they come to school, today's youngsters are equally eager to be entertained.

## The aggression trap

Aggression between young people is creating stress in schools. Although they are reputed to under-report, about 15% of Canadian students say their peers abuse them. This figure is consistent with reports from other countries. In 1997, The National Crime Prevention Council of Canada interviewed 6,000 Canadian students from grade one to eight. Six percent of the students admitted to bullying other children more than once or twice in the previous six weeks. Twenty percent admitted to being involved as either a bully or victim more than once or twice during the school term (Pepler, 1997).

Richard Tremblay, Chair of Child Development at the University of Montreal, points out that children who do not learn alternatives to physical aggression early in life are more likely to be: hyperactive and inattentive; less likely to respond when others need help; often rejected or isolated by their classmates; more disruptive in school; more likely to leave school before graduation; more likely to have serious accidents; more likely to engage in violent behaviour; and more likely to be charged under Canada's Young Offenders Act. Such children have lower grades, are more susceptible to substance abuse, and have sexual intercourse earlier and more frequently than children who have learned to solve conflicts peacefully (Tremblay, 2000).

According to Tremblay (2000), studies following aggressive children into their adult years have shown that there are extremely negative consequences for the aggressive individuals, for their mates, their children, and for the communities in which they live. These consequences include early parenthood, unemployment, family violence, and poverty. "From this perspective," says Tremblay, "failure to teach children to regulate violent behaviour during the early years leads to poverty much more clearly than poverty leads to violence."

School academic and social factors are not the only things leading to delinquent and aggressive behaviour. Risk factors in the family and environment are also associated with such behaviours. Basically, the more risk factors children and youth face, the more likely they are to say they are engaged in aggressive and delinquent behaviours.

## Demographic changes

Changing sources of immigration, increasing linguistic diversity, growing numbers of Aboriginal children, the survival of low birth weight babies, and a growing proportion of children with special needs make demands upon public schooling that were less evident fifty years ago. The number of children with learning disabilities is increasing. New medical technologies have saved the lives of children who, even a decade ago, would not have survived birth, resulting in a dramatic increase in the number of the children with severely impaired cognitive abilities entering public schools. De-institutionalization in the health and social services sectors has resulted in retention in the community of students who, in previous generations, would have been "out of sight, out of mind." More sophisticated diagnosis of learning and behavioural problems has led to higher expectations on the part of parents that the diagnosed conditions will be addressed.

In 1994–1995, Canadian teachers reported that one-tenth of students received some form of special education because of learning disabilities, emotional or behavioural problems, problems at home, speech impairment, intellectual or physical disabilities, language problems, or other problems that limited their ability to do schoolwork. Children living in low income families are more likely to receive special education. Children living in single parent families are twice (17%) as likely as children from two parent families (9%) to receive special education assistance and to have "problems at home" (63% vs. 37%). Children receiving special education are more likely (24%) to have a parent who did not finish high school than children who are not receiving special education (14%) (Bohatretz and Lipps, 1999).

Over the course of the past twenty-five years Canadian students have also become more diverse in terms of their ethno-cultural backgrounds. At any given time, Canada's population includes 15% born elsewhere. Diversity is also evident in the presence of languages other than French or English. Linguistic diversity poses challenges to public schools. Because immigrant integration depends upon the education of children and youth, public schools play a central part in helping those who do not speak English or French to acquire one of Canada's official languages and in ensuring that children learn about respectful treatment of persons from backgrounds different from their own. Once ignored, addressing the differences between students from differing backgrounds and the challenges those differences sometimes produce is central to the success of public schooling.

## Aboriginal and First Nations learners

Persons of Aboriginal ancestry make up approximately 4.4% of the Canadian population. The birth rate among Aboriginal Canadians exceeds that of non-Aboriginals. The birth rate for Status (i.e., registered) Indians was 28/1000 population in 1993, compared to 13/1000 for the Canadian population as a whole. Status Indians have a median age of 25 compared with a median age of 35 for the Canadian population as a whole.

The First Nations population in Canada is young, growing, and moving more towards band-centred education. The proportion of children enrolled in band-operated elementary and secondary schools is increasing (from 44% in 1990–91 to 61% 2000–01). The remaining 39% of children are enrolled in schools under the jurisdiction of provincial (37%) or the federal (1%) governments (Department of Indian Affairs and Northern Development, 2002). The decline in attendance at federal and provincial schools signals a change in the role of the band in First Nations education. While this trend is positive in terms of band self-determination and identity, it also raises the possibility of greater variance in the quality of instruction and education between schools of different bands and social circumstances. Lowering the variance among band schools becomes crucially important in light of Chandler's findings that the prevalence of adolescent suicides and other correlated social variables were directly (and inversely) linked to the level of band self-determination across B.C. communities (Chandler and Lalonde, 1998).

Graduation rates (and rates of post-secondary attendance) for Aboriginal and First Nations are well below levels for the rest of Canada. Although the graduation rate has remained relatively constant over the last three years, it is only 32% of those enrolled. Aboriginal students attending provincial public schools are much less successful than their non-Aboriginal classmates. The significant gap between Aboriginal and non-Aboriginal students is evidence that public schools have not addressed racism toward Aboriginal Canadians and attests to low expectations that affect their school success.

Until recently, public schools have done relatively little to address racism, low expectations, and the neglect that produces low academic achievement, poor grade-to-grade transitions, and abysmal failure rates—especially for Aboriginal learners. One of the consequences for a society in which the gap between its values and its achievements remain wide for an identifiable segment of the population is a demand for separate institutions. Over the course of the past two decades there have been calls for schools exclusively for girls, Black Canadians, and Canadians of Aboriginal origin.

## Canadian attitudes toward and expectations for public schooling are changing

Guppy and Davies (1999) examined Canadians' confidence in public institutions to provide a context for their analysis of Canadians' confidence in public education. They found that between 1974 and 1995, there was widespread erosion of confidence in modern institutions. They observed that, while there was a decline in school confidence, "compared with other institutions, schools fared quite well," ranking behind church and the Supreme Court, and ahead of the House of Commons, newspapers, labour unions, large corporations, and political parties (Guppy and Davies, 1999). Unlike some critics of public schooling who attribute the decline to poor system performance, Guppy and Davies attribute it to a gap between the performance of the educational system in relation to heightened public expectations:

> We argue that this gap between reality and expectations is what underlies declining confidence. Our interpretation is premised on a changing cultural context. Greater uncertainty in society coupled with a more knowledgeable public has generated a "malaise of modernity," seen most directly, perhaps, in greater public cynicism about core institutions. This cynicism, however, is coupled with higher expectations for institutions,

particularly education which, we argue, is increasingly criticized because the public deems it increasingly crucial for individual and societal well-being. (Guppy and Davies, 1999, p. 277)

Like Guppy and Davies (1999), Bricker and Greenspon (2001) describe a new "mindset" about education, one that demands "tougher standards, greater discipline, and heightened accountability."

Most Canadians continue to place primacy on schools preparing students for work. However, it isn't surprising that political differences are manifest in the importance that voters of different parties assign to various dimensions of public schooling since division is the most apparent characteristic of the Canadian electoral landscape.

Divided politically, Canadians are also becoming increasingly self-centred and individualistic:

Since Sept. 11 [2001], more than ever, people long to slow things down and escape from the constant onslaught of bad news. As fearful Canadians feel the need to "Look out for Number 1," Environics has seen a decline in Canadians' interest in others and willingness to entertain different points of view. Whether it is Canada's poor, Native Canadians on remote reserves, or Afghans who end up as "collateral damage" in the war against terrorism, we are less willing to listen, imagine, and empathize. (Adams, 2001, A13)

For example, in a recently published essay, Fred McMahon (Schachter, 2002) of the Fraser Institute argues that "poverty is largely a voluntary choice." McMahon articulates the view that the poor, the unskilled, and teenage mothers are autonomous moral agents who are

| Table 10.1: Educational purpose by political party affiliation | | | | | | | |
|---|---|---|---|---|---|---|---|
| | Percent | | | | | | |
| Educational purpose | Overall | Liberal voters | Alliance voters | PC voters | NDP voters | Bloc voters | Other voters |
| Training youth for the work world | 32 | 36 | 35 | 26 | 19 | 41 | 16 |
| Creating good citizens | 23 | 23 | 15 | 31 | 38 | 11 | 35 |
| Creating inquiring minds | 17 | 16 | 15 | 25 | 33 | 8 | 14 |
| Creating happy people | 7 | 5 | 7 | 3 | 4 | 22 | 6 |
| Teaching ethics | 7 | 6 | 15 | 6 | 4 | 14 | 6 |
| Teaching religious values | 4 | 5 | 5 | 2 | 0 | 0 | 4 |
| Producing good parents | 3 | 3 | 3 | 3 | 0 | 3 | 4 |
| Encouraging people to question authority | 2 | 4 | 0 | 0 | 0 | 3 | 4 |
| None of the above (unprompted) | 1 | 1 | 2 | 2 | 0 | 0 | 4 |
| Don't know (unprompted) | 5 | 3 | 3 | 3 | 2 | 0 | 6 |

Question: "Which of the following eight purposes of education is most important or valuable in your judgement [ROTATE] ..."

Source: COMPAS/National Post, 2001.

Social Determinants of Health

responsible for the consequences that befall them because of the decisions they make. Canadians appear increasingly accepting of inequality and put greater emphasis on the individual's own resources and resourcefulness rather than other factors.

## Changing conceptions of public schooling

For much of their history, Canadian public schools were seen as serving the needs of the larger society through the development of citizens. A vibrant balance was achieved and maintained over most of the history of the public school. But Canada's emergence as an advanced industrial society and the changes concomitant with that transformation have upset the balance in favour of the individual.

## Canadian public schools teach the "basics" well

Notwithstanding the tensions produced by changing values and the impact of demographic and structural changes, Canadian public elementary and secondary students do well. The educational attainment of Canadians has risen steadily over the years. According to Statistics Canada more Canadians are graduating from high school (Statistics Canada, January 23, 2002), and continuing on to post-secondary education (Statistics Canada, April 14, 1998). In 1990, one-fifth of Canadians between the ages of 25 and 29 had less than a grade twelve education. By 1998, the percentage had declined to 13%. During the same period, the percentage of Canadians in this age group who had earned university degrees rose from 17% to 26% (Statistics Canada, February 21, 2000).

In 1995, Canada had the highest percentage of the population (48%) with some postsecondary education compared with an average of 23% for the member nations of the Organization for Economic Co-operation and Development (OECD). And, although most Canadians have completed their formal education by the time they are 24, there has also been an increase in the full-time attendance rate among those between 25 and 29 years of age (Statistics Canada, April 14, 1998).

Over the course of the last fifty years, the proportion of Canadians with less than Grade 9 education declined from 51.9% in 1951 to 14.3% in 1991 and the proportion of Canadians who had earned university degrees increased five fold (Statistics Canada, 2003). Nevertheless, Canada's ratio of graduates to population aged 18 (75%) is the second lowest among G-7 countries. Another troubling statistic is the number of years Canadian children expect to stay in school. Among all the countries surveyed by the OECD from 1995 to 2002, only Canada showed a decrease in the number of expected years in school across the time period (Canadian Education Statistics Council, 2000).

One of the many success stories of Canadian education is the improvement Canadian women have made in educational attainment in the past several decades (Statistics Canada, September 4, 2000). In fact, among the population between the ages of 25 to 29, women now achieve higher levels of educational attainment than men (Canadian Education Statistics Council, 2000).

Canadian students perform well in reading, mathematics, and science, according to OECD study that assessed the performance of 15-year-olds in these subjects. Canadian students ranked second in reading, fifth in science, and sixth in mathematics among the 32 countries that participated in the OECD's Programme for International Student Assessment (PISA) (Council of Ministers of Education Canada, et al., 2001).

There are, however, sizable differences among the provinces, with Alberta, Quebec, and British Columbia obtaining significantly higher scores than other provinces and territories. In addition, Canada was one of only three countries (along with Germany and France) where gender was significant in the performance on the math test (with boys outperforming the girls in all three countries). The Third International Mathematics and Science Study (NCES, 1999) reveals similar results.

Across Canada, scores on the School Achievement Indicators program (SAIP) 2001 have remained generally steady from 1997–2001. As with many similar findings, gender differences are not present in 13 year old performance but are in 16 year olds. Again, of the provinces Alberta had the best overall performance on all tests, with significant differences among the provinces (School Achievement Indicators Program, 1996, 1997, 1998, 1999, 2001, 2002).

Canada as a whole performs well on national and international assessments, but disparities exist between populations and regions that do not seem to be diminishing with time. Inter-provincial performance, for example, is a continuing problem, with sizeable differences in performance among provinces. In addition, gender differences persist in older children, with girls outperforming boys in reading and boys outperforming girls in math. The PISA data indicate that the male advantage in math is not a worldwide trend and thus cannot be dismissed as a result of "gendered abilities." Along with the rest of the world, Canada

shows a significant difference in performance on PISA literacy tests as a function of socio-economic status and English and French Second Language, with lower socio-economic status and second language students performing significantly worse. Although Canada does not do significantly worse than the other countries surveyed by the OECD, the difference in performance is worrisome. Although Canada is a nation of immigration and has long-standing English and French Second Language programs, the result of the PISA literacy tests indicate that we are not at the forefront of countries that can accommodate different background factors, at least not in our teaching of reading skills.

## Graduation and drop-out rates

Across Canada, the 1999 graduation rates were 84.6% of students enrolled in their last year of post-secondary study. Drop-out rates (self-report) are higher for men than women (14.7 vs. 9.2%), and vary dramatically across provinces (from a low in Saskatchewan of 7.3% to a high in Prince Edward Island of 16.4%). Overall, the drop-out rate for 20 year olds in Canada in 1999 was 12%, down from 18% in 1991. It is asserted that this figure will decline with time as over-20 year olds take advantage of "second chance" education initiatives (Bowlby and McMullen, 2002).

Despite the reduction in the drop-out rate, it is still high in some populations. The Youth in Transition Survey provides a relatively comprehensive profile of dropouts and graduates. Drop-outs are more likely than graduates to live in "mixed" (vs. nuclear) families and single parent families. Twice as many graduates (57% compared to 28% of dropouts) had at least one parent who

## Table 10.2: Selected findings from the Youth in Transition Survey

| | Graduates | Drop outs |
|---|---|---|
| **Family structure** | | |
| Two parent family | 81% | 66% |
| Single parent family | 16% | 33% |
| **Parental education** | | |
| University degree | 31% | 11% |
| Post secondary certificate or diploma | 26% | 17% |
| High school | 45% | 34% |
| Less than high school | 9% | 27% |
| **Father's occupation** | | |
| Management | 17% | 9% |
| Business, finance, and administration | 9% | 4% |
| Health, natural and applied science | 12% | 6% |
| Social science, government, art, culture and recreation | 9% | 4% |
| Sales and service | 13% | 13% |
| Trades, transport, and equipment operators | 25% | 41% |
| Primary processing, manufacturing and utilities | 16% | 23% |
| **Academic grades (overall gpa final year)** | | |
| 80–100% A | 42% | 13% |
| 70–79% B | 43% | 35% |
| 60–69% C | 14% | 35% |
| 50–59% D | 1% | 14% |
| < 50% F | - | 4% |
| **Hours worked for pay each week during the last year of high school** | | |
| 0–No job | 37% | 48% |
| 1 to 9 | 17% | 11% |
| 10 to 19 | 23% | 13% |
| 20 to 29 | 17% | 16% |
| 30 or more | 5% | 13% |
| **Peer influence and behaviours** | | |
| Most or all close friends planning to further education or training beyond high school | 79% | 52% |
| Skipped class once per week | 21% | 58% |
| Drank alcoholic beverages one a week or more during the last year of high school | 29% | 38% |
| Used marijuana or hash once a week or more during the last year of high school | 9% | 28% |
| **Educational aspirations** | | |
| University degree | 65% | 23% |
| College, CEGEP, trade, vocational, or business school | 26% | 45% |
| Some post-secondary | 1% | 4% |
| High school completion | 2% | 20% |
| Less than high school completion | - | 4% |
| Undecided | 6% | 6% |

Source: Developed from Bowlby, J.W. and McMullen, K. (2002). *At a crossroads: First results for the 18 to 20 year old cohort of the youth in transition survey*. Ottawa: Human Resources Development Canada, online at www.hrdc-drhc.gc.ca/sp-ps/arb-dgra/publications/research/2002docs/YITS/yits-encov.pdf

completed post-secondary education; and three times as many graduates had at least one parent who completed a university degree.

In terms of work, there is a bimodal distribution for drop-outs. They were both less likely than graduates to have worked in their last year of high school and more likely to have worked at a job more than 30 hours a week. Drop-outs are also more likely to have children (14% of drop-outs vs. 2% of graduates). For women, 28% of all drop-outs had children (compared to 5% of male drop-outs). More than half of the female drop-outs with children were single.

Overall, the data on graduation rates are positive in that they show declining rates of dropout over the last ten years. However, they also reveal that students in danger of dropping out generally fit a well-established demographic profile. They exhibit readily identifiable behaviours at school and in the community which are characterized primarily by non-involvement. These patterns of behaviour have remained constant in the last ten years. Most troubling is the finding that over a quarter of female dropouts had children, and half of those were single parents, making the possibility of returning to school less likely. These data suggest that more resources for at-risk adolescents and teen parents would further decrease the dropout rate and increase drop-outs' likelihood of returning to complete their studies.

## Gender and educational achievement

Recent reports indicate that there is still a trend for girls to encounter difficulties when transitioning between elementary and high school, and for boys to have more difficulty transitioning between high school and post secondary education. There are also continuing differences in academic achievement in math and reading related to gender and age, as discussed above (McCall, 1998).

In addition, teachers had higher expectations of future educational attainment for girls compared to boys. The role of teacher expectation and behaviour is highlighted here, as there is an urgent need for more research into how teacher's expectations translate into behaviour in the class. We need clearer data on the correlation between teacher evaluation, parent evaluation, and future academic and workplace performance.

## Immigration

Data from the 1994–1998 *National longitudinal survey of children and youth* indicate that (1) children born in Canada of immigrant parents do at least as well as the children of Canadian-born parents; (2) children born in Canada of immigrant parents whose language is either English or French have especially high outcomes; (3) children born in Canada of immigrant parents whose language is neither English or French have problems in kindergarten, although by elementary school these problems remain only for reading. As would be expected, the longer the child stays in the school system the less the difference between children of native and non-native born Canadians. Children born in Canada of immigrant parents perform at least as well as children of Canadian-born parents by the age of 13 (Lipps and Yiptong-Avila, 1999).

However, this analysis does not include data on children who themselves are immigrants to Canada, nor those who enter the Canadian school system after the age of

11. Given what we know about increasing difficulty of language acquisition after puberty, there exists a real possibility that students who speak neither English or French who enter Canadian schools after their elementary years will continue to have problems in scholastic performance, especially in reading and writing. The OECD 2002 data on literacy support this (Lipps and Yiptong-Avila, 1999).

## Conclusion: The vulnerability of public schools and students at risk

Canadians can take pride in the accomplishments of their public schools. At the same time, they should be worried about their vulnerabilities and about the inequalities among students distinguished by socio-economic, ethno-cultural, and gender differences.

Most of human history is the story of political, social and economic inequalities based upon accidents of birth or group membership. While there was gradual improvement in equality over time—largely following the industrial revolution—most of the significant improvements occurred after the Second World War. The depression and the Second World War made Canadians conscious of the importance of fairness, human rights, and the need to diminish inequalities.

People who had suffered the privations of the depression helped to forge policies that would ameliorate the most severe consequences of the accidents of birth, place of residence, or plain bad luck. People who had survived the nationalisms that permitted the extermination of people on the basis of their group membership helped to create institutions to protect human rights. People who had fled societies in which basic human rights and well-being were primarily determined by economic and social standing helped to create institutions that tempered the most egregious consequences of inequalities. But these changes, largely occurring after the Second World War, seem to have been relatively short lived.

Today, strong forces are at work to alter the relationship between citizens and government in order to diminish the part that government plays in our lives. The still malleable citizenship that was created in the post-war period is devolving into something "old" and "worn out." Canada is becoming a country that wants to make individuals responsible for looking after themselves, rather than a country that says we create institutions to look after each other.

From Whalley to Whitehorse, from Hazelton to Halifax, and from Sannich to St. Johns the trends are the same: as the bulk of the population ages, concerns have changed. Interest in childcare and education and the part that education plays in ameliorating inequalities has been replaced by interest in pension protection and health care. For those who have remained interested in childcare and education, orientations have shifted. The balance between concern for the well-being of one's own children and for children generally has shifted to an emphasis on one's own children to the exclusion of other children. The delicate equilibrium between means and ends that we have tried to achieve has given way to a preoccupation with competition, ends, outcomes, and the bottom line.

Public schools are the institutions that we rely upon to bind us together as Canadians. They do it by communicating the values—fairness, respect for persons, and a sense of social justice—that Canadians share.

At a time when selfishness and individualism are increasing; ethnocentrism and alienation are growing; petty regionalisms divide us; politicians describe concerned citizens as "special interests" and are capable of uniting only in opposition to their central government, we need an institution that can remind us of the values that we share and can help us to preserve our communities and our country.

Our public schools are not perfect. There are many ways in which they can be and should be improved. But, like Canadian singer-songwriter Joni Mitchell wrote " ... you don't know what you've got till it's gone." If we allow public schools to fail those most in need of their services, it won't be long before our communities disintegrate and Canada comes undone. Make no mistake about it: if our public schools fail, Canada fails.

## Recommended readings

Bowlby, J.W. and MacMillan, K. (2002). *At a crossroads: First results for the 18 to 20-year-old cohort of the Youth in Transition Survey*, online at www.hrdc-drhc.gc.ca/sp-ps/arb-dgra/publications/books/yits-encov.pdf

The Youth in Transition Survey (YITS), designed to collect a broad range of information on the education and labour market experiences of youth, is a longitudinal survey developed by Human Resources Development Canada and Statistics Canada. *At a crossroads* presents findings from the first cycle of the YITS 18- to 20-year-old cohort, a survey of more than 22,000 Canadian youth conducted between January and March 2000.

Statistics Canada, Census Operations Division. (2003). *Education in Canada: Raising the standard.* Online at www12.statcan.ca/english/census01/products/analytic/companion/educ/pdf/96F0030XIE2001012.pdf.

*Education in Canada: Raising the standard* provides information on the changes in the education profile of the Canadian population over the past ten years.

Stroick, S.M. and Jenson, J. (1999). *What is the best policy mix for Canada's young children?* Canadian Policy Research Networks, online at www.cprn.com/en/doc.cfm?doc=178

This report is the result of a three-year multi-staged project which asked *What is the best policy mix for Canada's children?* The study—a synthesis of research, policy, current thinking, and data about the outcomes achieved by children in Canada—shows how inter-sectoral policies can improve child outcomes.

Ungerleider, C. (2003). *Failing our kids: How we are ruining our public schools.* Toronto: McClelland and Stewart.

Drawing on the latest research and using examples from across the country, Ungerleider describes what's right and what's wrong about our public schools system and provides solutions for making them a lot better.

Wiegers, W. (2002). *The framing of poverty as "child poverty" and its implications for women*, online at www.swc-cfc.gc.ca/pubs/0662322177/index_e.html cfc.gc.ca/pubs/0662322177/index_e.html

*The framing of poverty as "child poverty" and its implications for women* examines the sources and implications for women of a focus on "child poverty" in discussion of Canadian state policy.

## Related websites

Statistics Canada—www.statcan.ca

Canada's central statistical agency publishes a variety of documents and reports about nearly every facet of Canadian society, including demographics, health, education, resources, economy, and culture.

The Vanier Institute for the Family—www.vifamily.ca/

The Mission of the Vanier Institute for the Family is "to create awareness of, and to provide leadership on, the importance and strengths of families in Canada and the challenges they face in their structural, demographic, economic, cultural, and social diversity." The institute provides information and analysis based research, consultation, and policy development "to elected officials, policy makers, educators and researchers, the business community, the media, social service professionals, the public and Canadian families themselves."

Canadian Policy Research Networks—www.cprn.com/

Canadian Policy Research Networks is a Canadian "think tank" specializing in social and economic policy issues affecting Canada and Canadians. The research conducted by CPRN is organized under four networks: Family, Work, Health, and Public Involvement.

Institute for Research on Public Policy—www.irpp.org

The mission of the Institute for Research on Public Policy, an independent, national, nonprofit organization is "to improve public policy in Canada by generating research, providing insight and sparking debate that will contribute to the public policy decision-making process and strengthen the quality of the public policy decisions made by Canadian governments, citizens, institutions and organizations."

Canadian Centre for Policy Alternatives—www.policyalternatives.ca/

The Canadian Centre for Policy Alternatives describes its mission as offering "an alternative to the message that we have no choice about the policies that affect our lives." The CCPA produces research reports, books, opinion pieces, fact sheets, and other publications about issues of social and economic justice.

## Chapter Eleven

# LITERACY: ONE OF THE MOST IMPORTANT DETERMINANTS OF HEALTH TODAY

### Barbara Ronson and Irving Rootman

## Introduction

Literacy skills predict health status even more accurately than education level, income, ethnic background, or any other socio-demographic variable (Grossman and Kaestner, 1997; Weiss, 2001; OECD and Statistics Canada, 2000). In international studies, this determinant is often estimated by years of schooling, or highest grade level achieved. However, there is potential for serious error bias in literacy estimates based on years of schooling that do not control for a wider set of socio-demographic factors and the quality of years of schooling (Charette and Meng, 1998). There are many examples of discordance between years of schooling and literacy at the individual level.

For example, before the new policy of literacy test achievement as a prerequisite for high school graduation, one in five high school graduates tested as functionally illiterate (Calamai, 1999). As our education system undergoes profound changes and opportunities for learning outside school increase, there is little certainty that literacy levels and years of schooling will remain comparable. Literacy skills needed to function in society have greatly increased over the past century or more. As a result, the definition of literacy has evolved. Because of recent developments in defining and measuring literacy and recent technological and social trends, this construct has become equally if not more important than years of education as a determinant of health. As the definition of literacy becomes more refined, its measurement and study promise to shed light on the best ways that public education efforts can enhance the health of populations.[1] In the meantime, this chapter presents empirical evidence regarding the importance of literacy as a social determinant of health and considers the role of policy in determining the level of literacy within jurisdictions.

**Box 11.1**

**Relative importance of education/literacy as a determinant of health**
A number of statistical analyses which have controlled separately for the effects of education and of income indicate that, while both are associated with ill health, lack of education is the predominant factor. For example, an analysis of the Health Promotion Survey found that when controlled for education, the initial relationship between income and self-reported health drops out. In other words, apparent effects of income on self-reported health in this survey are actually a result of education/literacy. Similarly, a re-analysis of Statistics Canada's 1976 Survey of Fitness, Physical Recreation and Sport found that education accounted for a much larger share than did income or other factors of the differences in physical activity rates. In other countries Slater and Carlton (1985) have indicated that "the education differentials probably provide more reliable indicators of socio-economic differentials in mortality in the United States than do income differentials." Grossman (1987), following a review of a variety of studies, concluded that "schooling is a causal determinant of the two other components of socio-economic status: income and occupation" and cites 10 separate studies in the United States that all indicate that "schooling is a more important correlate of health than occupation or income."

Source: Perrin, B. (1989). *Literacy and health-making the connection: The research report of the literacy and health project phase one: making the world healthier and safer for people who can't read.* Ontario Public Health Association and Frontier College, online at www.opha.on.ca/resources/ literacy1research.pdf.

## Empirical evidence regarding the importance of literacy as a social determinant of health

### Direct effects of literacy on health

There is evidence in the research literature that literacy is directly related to both overall health status and to mental health status (Baker et al., 1997, 2002; Roberts and Fawcett, 1998) as well as co-morbidity burden (Guerra and Shea, 2003) and life expectancy (OECD and Statistics Canada, 2000). In addition, there is evidence that low-literate consumers and their families are at risk of harm due to their difficulty reading medication prescriptions, baby formula instructions, and other written material (Kalichman et al., 1999). The direct effects of literacy on health are a matter of concern for all health care providers. If their communications and instructions are not helpful and are potentially harmful for up to one half of their clients, addressing the problem should be a priority. Concerns relate not only to health service providers' professional effectiveness but also to the costs to the system of drug benefit plans and medical insurance when prescription drugs are misused and patients are unable to follow directions properly (Friedland, 1998). Particularly unsettling is the fact that seniors are among the least literate groups in society and also the most heavily dependent on medications and health services (Roberts and Fawcett, 1998).

Literacy should also be of concern to employers, manufacturers, and retailers who handle potentially dangerous products and processes. Direct effects of literacy on health also occur in workplaces and other settings where safety may be dependent on one's ability to read rules, signs, and manuals.

Social Determinants of Health

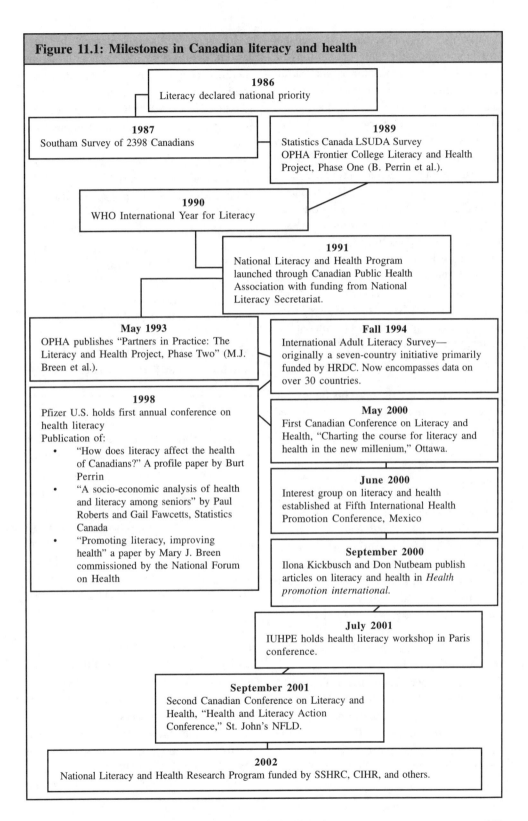

**Figure 11.1: Milestones in Canadian literacy and health**

**1986**
Literacy declared national priority

**1987**
Southam Survey of 2398 Canadians

**1989**
Statistics Canada LSUDA Survey
OPHA Frontier College Literacy and Health
Project, Phase One (B. Perrin et al.).

**1990**
WHO International Year for Literacy

**1991**
National Literacy and Health Program
launched through Canadian Public Health
Association with funding from National
Literacy Secretariat.

**May 1993**
OPHA publishes "Partners in Practice: The
Literacy and Health Project, Phase Two" (M.J.
Breen et al.).

**Fall 1994**
International Adult Literacy Survey—
originally a seven-country initiative primarily
funded by HRDC. Now encompasses data on
over 30 countries.

**1998**
Pfizer U.S. holds first annual conference on
health literacy
Publication of:
- "How does literacy affect the health
  of Canadians?" A profile paper by Burt
  Perrin
- "A socio-economic analysis of health
  and literacy among seniors" by Paul
  Roberts and Gail Fawcetts, Statistics
  Canada
- "Promoting literacy, improving
  health" a paper by Mary J. Breen
  commissioned by the National Forum
  on Health

**May 2000**
First Canadian Conference on Literacy and
Health, "Charting the course for literacy and
health in the new millenium," Ottawa.

**June 2000**
Interest group on literacy and health
established at Fifth International Health
Promotion Conference, Mexico

**September 2000**
Ilona Kickbusch and Don Nutbeam publish
articles on literacy and health in *Health
promotion international.*

**July 2001**
IUHPE holds health literacy workshop in Paris
conference.

**September 2001**
Second Canadian Conference on Literacy and
Health, "Health and Literacy Action
Conference," St. John's NFLD.

**2002**
National Literacy and Health Research Program funded by SSHRC, CIHR, and others.

Literacy: One of the Most Important Determinants of Health Today 157

A Manitoba study for example, indicated that "difficulty comprehending precautions on farm and recreational machinery such as all-terrain vehicles, watersleds, snowmobiles and farm equipment of all sorts, makes rural life more dangerous" (Sarginson, 1997). The Canadian Business Task Force on Literacy (1987) estimated that of the $4 billion lost by business due to literacy problems, $1.6 billion is attributable to workplace accidents (Canadian Business Task Force on Literacy, 1986). Edwards (1995) found that the Workplace Hazardous Materials Information System (WHIS) consists of text often written at the college level. In addition, there is evidence that occupational injuries, the degree of awareness of the dangers in the workplace, and installation of home safety features are associated with limited literacy (Health Canada, 2003).

**Indirect effects of literacy on health**

Research also suggests that literacy is related to lifestyle practices. For example, an Australian study of students in primary schools found that low literacy predicted tobacco use among both boys and girls and alcohol use among boys (Hawthorne, 1997). Similarly, a study in the United States found that low literacy was associated with choice of contraceptive methods as well as knowledge about birth control (Gazmararian et al., 1999). In addition, there is much evidence that education has a powerful influence on a range of personal lifestyle choices. The higher the level of education, the less likely Canadians are to smoke or be overweight (Federal, Provincial, and Territorial Advisory Committee on Population Health, 1999).The higher the literacy levels, the more likely people are to participate in voluntary community activities and the higher the representation of females in government (OECD and Statistics Canada, 2000).

People with limited literacy also have less knowledge about medical conditions and treatment (Parker et al., 2003) and they have trouble understanding health issues generally (Rudd et al., 1999). They also have more difficulty with verbal communications from practitioners (Schillinger, 2002) and they tend to have higher stress levels and feelings of vulnerability (Health Canada, 2003). People with lower literacy levels also tend to be less aware of and make less use of preventive services (Scott et al., 2002). They are also less likely to seek care (Scott et al., 2002), but have higher rates of hospitalization (Baker et al., 2002) and experience more difficulties using the health care system (Davis et al., 1996).

## Mechanisms and pathways by which literacy influences health

It is conceivable that literacy is a marker variable for other determinants of health such as income and social status, quality of living and working conditions, personal health practices and coping skills, and healthy child development. These other determinants, moreover, directly affect the quality of housing, food security, and to some extent health care services. Undoubtedly, health has a strong impact on literacy just as literacy impacts on health. Children who are hungry, tired, and stressed by poor or abusive home lives do not learn well (Anderson, 2003). They are absent more often and leave school earlier. Much recent research illuminates the inextricable relationship between health and learning, and the World Health Organization has made much progress with its Global School Health Initiative and its support for Health Promoting Schools and/or Coordinated School Health initiatives around the world (WHO, 2003). The link between literacy and the following other determinants of health will be discussed below: income, living and working conditions, culture, gender, and early life.

## Income

Literacy is clearly linked to income. People with limited income are more likely to have limited literacy skills (Weiss et al., 1994). The larger the proportion of adults at the highest literacy levels, the larger the GDP per capita; and the higher the proportion of adults with the lowest literacy levels, the lower the GDP per capita (OECD and Statistics Canada, 2000). Furthermore, in the latest International Adult Literacy Survey (IALS), literacy skills were highly correlated with wages in 22 of 23 countries who participated. The data suggested that the role literacy plays in the determination of wages is greater in economies that are more flexible and open (e.g., U.S. and Canada), i.e., the economic returns of literacy (when controlling for education) are largest in open economies. As well, in all participating countries in the Programme for International Skills Assessment (PISA) study, students from higher socio-economic backgrounds performed better than those from lower

socio-economic backgrounds. People with limited literacy are more likely to be unemployed and to be working for minimum wage in unskilled jobs (Statistics Canada, 1996). They are also more likely to be working in older industries (Statistics Canada, 1996). Literacy is also related to type of employment. Highest literacy levels in the *Survey of literacy skills used in daily living* (LSUDA) study were found in the teaching, science, engineering, social science, and managerial professions. The greatest proportion of respondents testing at the lowest levels were in the product fabricating, service and farming sectors (Statistics Canada, 1991).

There is evidence that countries with a wide gap between income levels of the rich and the poor also have the widest gaps between highest and lowest literacy levels of the top and bottom quarter of the population. In Denmark the range of scores between 5th and 95th percentile is 120 points. In the U.S. it is almost twice as large (231 points). In Canada the range of scores between the 5th and 95th percentile is also large on all three IALS scales (prose, document and quantitative). On the prose scale it is 219 points (the 3rd largest

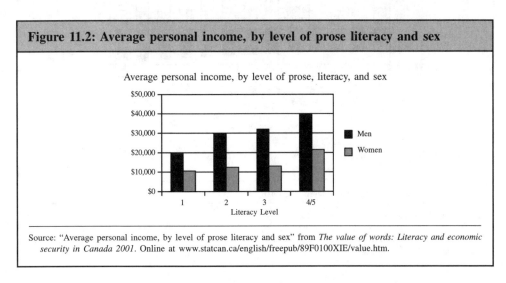

**Figure 11.2: Average personal income, by level of prose literacy and sex**

Average personal income, by level of prose, literacy, and sex

Source: "Average personal income, by level of prose literacy and sex" from *The value of words: Literacy and economic security in Canada 2001*. Online at www.statcan.ca/english/freepub/89F0100XIE/value.htm.

Literacy: One of the Most Important Determinants of Health Today

### Figure 13.3a: Percentage of adult population aged 16–65 at each *prose* literacy level, 1994–1995

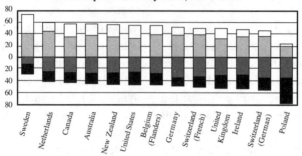

### Figure 13.3b: Percentage of adult population aged 16–65 at each *document* literacy level, 1994–1995

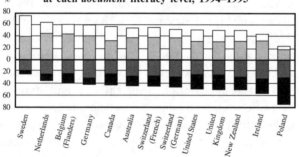

### Figure 13.3c: Percentage of adult population aged 16–65 at each *quantitative* literacy level, 1994–1995

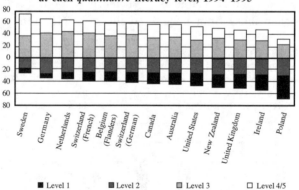

■ Level 1          ■ Level 2          ▨ Level 3          ☐ Level 4/5

Countries are ranked by the proportion in levels 3 and 4/5.

Source: International adult literacy survey, 1994–1995.

Figure 11.3 shows the proportion of adults at each level of literacy for each country. Level 1 is the lowest; level 5 is the highest..

discrepancy of all IALS countries). A similar range is found in the U.K., Poland, Portugal and Slovenia as well as the U.S.

The fact that literacy outcomes vary in some countries by socio-economic status more than in others suggests that the problem can be addressed through policy and quality of the education system. For example, Sweden, which has a strong income security system, also has the highest scores on all three IALS scales, ranging from 301–306 points for each out of 500. Chile has the lowest (from 209–221 points). Canada ranks 5th on prose (279) behind Sweden, Finland, Norway, and the Netherlands; the U.S. ranks 10th; and the UK 13th. On the document scale, Canada ranks 8th (279) and on the quantitative scale Canada is 9th with 281 points. In Sweden even those who did not complete secondary education do better than their counterparts in other countries with 59% scoring above level 2 compared to 27% without secondary education above level 2 in Canada, and 51% in Germany (OECD and Statistics Canada, 2000).

Further evidence that policy may affect literacy levels comes from the PISA study. Students in Canada from the 25% of families with the lowest SES scored above the average for all students in OECD member countries with an average of 503 compared to the overall average of 500. This contrasts to the U.S. where the poorest quartile averaged 466. The wealthiest quarter of students in both countries scored more comparably: 568 on reading, math and science for Canadians and 554 for U.S. students (Totten and Quigley, 2003).

**Living and working conditions**
Between 22% and 50% of adults with lower levels of literacy live in low-income households, compared with only 8% of those with high-level literacy skills (Roberts and Fawcett, 1998). Violence and abuse are key threats to learning capacity. Women in literacy programs have identified men's violence (or its threat) as the greatest barrier to their learning (Davies, 1995). Violence and abuse undoubtedly affect children's capacity for learning as well, and are key reasons why young people do not complete high school and/or run away from home. According to the National Longitudinal Survey of Children and Youth (NLSCY), students who reported bullying behaviours "sometimes" or "often" scored significantly lower in math and reading scores than those who reported no bullying behaviour (Totten and Quigley, 2003).

Non-abusive workplaces can provide opportunities for literacy. Since the mid-eighties when literacy was declared a national priority, a growing number of workplace literacy programs have been provided. The Conference Board of Canada found that at least one-third of employers had problems in their workforces attributable to low-literacy and basic skills (Darville, 1992). There is increasing attention being paid to healthy school environments, as the "workplace" for approximately one fifth of the population. Improving school environments has proven to be important for improving student health and achievement (WHO, 2003).

**Culture**
Literacy is also linked to culture. Francophones, Aboriginal peoples, and immigrants tend to have lower literacy scores in Canada (Statistics Canada, 1991). For the Francophone community, differences tend to disappear among the younger generations. In the U.S., racial and ethnic minority populations, including Aboriginals and Spanish-speakers, are more likely than others

to have lower literacy scores (Kirsch et al., 1993). Literacy studies have drawn attention to the importance of first language acquisition and support for improvement in one of Canada's official languages. Aboriginal literacy practitioners have found Native language studies to be an important precursor or complement to literacy studies in English or French. The reasons for this can only be speculated about but are likely related to the influence of culture, social connectedness, and support networks on health and well-being, and the impact of health on learning. Social exclusion is thought to be a primary barrier to well-being and learning. Conceivably then, when one feels more grounded in one's own culture, language and traditions, literacy will improve.

## Gender

In less developed countries, women tend to have lower levels of literacy than men (Weiss, 2001). One of the strongest predictors of life-expectancy among developing countries is adult literacy, particularly the disparity between male and female adult literacy, which explains much of the variation in health achievement among these countries after accounting for per capita GDP. For example, among the 125 developing countries with per capita GDP less than $10,000, the difference between male and female literacy accounts for 40% of the variation in life-expectancy after factoring out the effect of per capita GDP. (Daniels et al., 2000).

Literacy rates for Canadian adult men and women are comparable, but lower literacy is more prevalent among immigrant women than men (Boyd, 1991). Nearly one third (32%) of foreign-born women have extreme difficulty dealing with printed material or can use printed words only for limited purposes compared to over one-fifth (24%) of foreign-born men and approximately one-tenth of Canadian-born women and men (Boyd, 1991). Although most recent surveys of adult literacy show comparable literacy rates for men and women (Statistics Canada, 1996; Calamai, 1987), school age girls, at least in Ontario in grades 3, 6, and 10, consistently score higher than boys (Education Quality and Accountability Office, 2003). Girls performed significantly better than boys on reading tests in all countries in the 2000 PISA (Totten and Quigley, 2003). The average score for fifteen year old Canadian females was 32 points above that of the males. In Ontario, girls scored on average 548 and boys 418. Forty percent of Canadian girls reported reading at least 30 minutes a day for enjoyment compared to about 25% for boys. Still, both genders scored at level three on a scale of one to five "capable of solving reading tasks of moderate complexity such as locating multiple pieces of information, making links between different parts of a text, and relating it to familiar everyday knowledge" (Totten and Quigley, 2003). There is some evidence that such gaps have narrowed in adulthood as women in domestic roles may require fewer skills than men in workplaces, but it remains unclear whether such trends will continue as women play a larger role in the workplace and men take on more domestic responsibilities.

## Early life

Children of parents with reading problems are more likely to have reading problems themselves (Puchner, 1993). In the 2000 PISA, parental attitudes towards academic study were found to be a key variable: students with a home environment that stimulated learning did better than all students

Social Determinants of Health

across all countries. Students with parents who took them to a variety of cultural events and who discussed current affairs outperformed other students in all countries. As well, students who enjoyed reading, borrowed books from a library and had high career aspirations, did better than other students (Totten and Quigley, 2003). However, the impact of parents' education on literacy level is not as profound in Denmark, Finland, Norway, and Sweden as it is in Canada, Australia, Ireland, New Zealand, U.K., and U.S. (OECD and Statistics Canada, 2000). This suggests that the quality of education and life outside the family for children of the lowest SES play a strong role.

Recent research in brain development has drawn attention to findings that indicate highest capacity for learning in the early years. Studies show a "hard wiring" of the brain over time that affects capacity for future learning, lifelong attitudes, and problem-solving approaches (Mustard and McCain, 1999). Early child development programs, moreover, have proven capacity for breaking inter-generational cycles of disadvantage, and dramatically improving chances of high school graduation and workplace participation (Schweinhart et al., 1993). The critical period for learning a first language is thought to be between 0 and 3 years. Learning a second language becomes more difficult after 10 years of age (Begley, 1996).

Such findings have led to a relatively new trend in literacy programs—the recent proliferation of family literacy classes. These classes readily span the literacy and health arenas since health concerns and interventions during the early years are particularly frequent. Programs such as Rhymes that Bind, Books for Babies, and Health for Two have been developed in Canada, in part to apply new knowledge on healthy development of children from the attachment literature within the medical/ psychiatric field. Preliminary research indicates that retention is higher in family literacy than in traditional literacy programs; that the goal of supporting their children's learning is a powerful motivator for adults; and that embedding literacy in activities connected to daily life leads to greater sustainability (Shohet, 1997). There is also much to be learned from the intergenerational nature of many Aboriginal programs. Unfortunately, according to Dr. Eileen Antone, there is very little understanding of, or funding support for Aboriginal Adult Education programs that include intergenerational literacy participation and practices (Antone, 2003).

**Other factors**

A National Literacy and Health Research Program was launched in Canada in 2002. As a preliminary step, a conceptual diagram of the pathways linking literacy and health was developed and field tested in focus groups across the country. Based on feedback from the groups, the diagram was revised and presented in a summary paper on literacy and health research commissioned by the Canadian Institute for Health Research in 2003 (Rootman and Ronson, 2003).

In addition to the factors discussed above, factors of Aging and Personal Capacity were deemed important determinants of literacy, which in turn is a determinant of health. Other kinds of literacy were also thought to be important in relation to health. These include health literacy, media literacy, and cultural literacy. Finally, the conceptual diagram suggested five kinds of actions that can improve literacy: Health Communications, Capacity Development,

VANCOUVER - Roch Carrier, Canada's National Librarian and author of the beloved children's classic *The hockey sweater*, has declared October 27 to be National School Library Day in an effort to raise awareness about the erosion of school libraries across the country. Today teachers throughout British Columbia are echoing his call for a major reinvestment in libraries.

"As governments cut education budgets, school libraries are declining and librarians are struggling to maintain collections and meet students' needs," said Neil Worboys, president of the B.C. Teachers' Federation. "We've got to turn this trend around, because it has serious consequences for children's opportunities to learn."

Research shows that students who attend schools with well-funded, properly stocked libraries managed by qualified teacher-librarians have higher achievement, improved literacy, and greater success at the post-secondary level. For detailed information, see Dr. Ken Haycock's report *The crisis in Canada's school libraries: The case for reform and reinvestment,* online at www.peopleforeducation.com/librarycoalition/Report03.pdf.

Worboys noted that most Canadian students attain high levels of literacy, consistently performing near the top on international testing. "However, we must not allow the continued deterioration of our school libraries, especially as governments in the U.S., Europe and Asia are aggressively investing in school libraries and literacy programs," he said.

"Given all we know about the links between quality school libraries and high student achievement, it's disturbing to see the decline in B.C. school libraries," Worboys said. "In the past two years, 91 school libraries have closed altogether and many more are open only part-time. So many teacher-librarians have been cut due to funding shortfalls, we're afraid that they are practically becoming an endangered species in B.C. schools!"

"I encourage parents to inform themselves about the health of the library at your children's schools," Worboys said. "Is your library staffed by a qualified teacher-librarian? Does he or she have to work at more than one school? What about the condition of your library's collection: Are the classics there? Are the science books up-to-date? What about electronic resources? Is your library open throughout the day, every school day? If not, why not?"

Worboys urged parents, students and other concerned citizens to speak out for a strong school library. "The library is the heart of every school," he said. "It's the place where reluctant readers become avid ones, where children's imaginations can take them anywhere in the universe."

Source: Canada NewsWire, General News, Monday, October 27, 2003.

Community Development, Organizational Development, and Policy Development. In this chapter, policy development approaches to improve health through improving literacy will be discussed, and policy development will be looked to as a means of encouraging the other kinds of actions that can improve literacy.

# The role of policy in determining the level of literacy within jurisdictions

Policy plays a crucial role in affecting levels of literacy across countries around the world. Rootman (1991) summarizes the policy recommendations arising from the

LSUDA study. Among other things, the study authors recommend that governments: improve the educational system for young people; develop an adult education and training system; create policy and funding commitments to ensure adults have access to a variety of literacy and learning opportunities in their home communities; support public participation in the health care system; strengthen community health services; develop and co-ordinate public health policies in a variety of sectors; ensure information and materials provided by the government are written in plain language; provide incentives to organizations that attempt to make information more accessible to people with low literacy skills; encourage and fund projects aimed at increasing accessibility of information; and ensure attention be paid to literacy when health promotion strategies are developed (Rootman, 1991).

In this chapter, the following kinds of policy recommendations for the improvement of literacy will be discussed: (1) Research needs; (2) Need for a new definition of accountabilities and goals in our education system; and (3) Need for new mechanisms for inter-ministerial collaboration.

**Research needs**
More research needs to be done on the effectiveness of various kinds of actions to improve health though improving literacy. In particular, the following research needs have been identified by various studies as being of some priority: costs of health care delivery related to direct and indirect impacts of literacy (Health Canada, 2003; Rudd et al., 1999; American Medical Association, 1999); longitudinal studies of potential changes in health status following changes in literacy skills (Breen, 1997); effective communication approaches (including the

use of multi-media) for health providers (Health Canada, 2003; American Medical Association, 1999); evaluation of promising approaches and practices (e.g., Community Development and Participatory Education) addressing literacy, lifelong learning, and health issues (Health Canada, 2003; Canadian Public Health Association, 2003); the role of literacy and other factors in enabling people to feel more confident and empowered to take action regarding their own health (Health Canada, 2003); understanding the causal pathway of how literacy influences health (American Medical Association, 1999); and studying literacy and health within the unique circumstances of the Aboriginal and Francophone communities, and culturally diverse and challenged groups (Canadian Public Health Association, 2003).

In addition, more research needs to be done on the effectiveness of capacity development approaches such as education and training. Much research supports the need to design programs based on learners' interests and motivations. Mary Norton, Pat Campbell, Tammy Horne, Priscilla George, Eileen Antone, and Mary Breen are some of the Canadian literacy specialists who have written about literacy, health, and participatory education based on practical experience. Participatory approaches involve learners in issue selection and content development. Numerous examples of participatory development of health information were found in a recent assessment of Canadian research needs in literacy and health (Rootman et al., 2003). One example is a video and Discussion Guide called *A better you: The benefits of a healthy lifestyle* produced by the Dartmouth Literacy Network in Nova Scotia. Another example is Heart Health Nova Scotia's work on *Literacy and health promotion: Four case studies*. A third example is Canadian Public Health Association's *What the health! A literacy and health resource for youth*. The quality of these products suggests that it is well worthwhile to do more such participatory development and evaluation within literacy classes.

As noted above, Health Canada suggested that there is a need for evaluating a wider range of promising approaches and practices such as community development (Health Canada, 2003). A number of resources have recently been developed that can enhance literacy practitioners' skills and knowledge of effective community development approaches. Grass Roots Press' Adult Literacy Resources Catalogue for 2003 includes the following: Arnold, Burke, James, Martin and Thomas, *Educating for a change*; New England Literacy Resource Center's *Civic participation and community action sourcebook: A resource for adult educators*; Carmen Rodriguez's *Educating for change: Community-based/sudent-centred literacy programming with First Nations adults*; Pat Campbell and Barbara Burnaby's *Participatory practices in adult education* and *tools for community building: A planning workbook for northern Canadian community-based literacy*. At minimum, it would be worthwhile to evaluate the usefulness of these resources.

A better understanding of the unique situation of new Canadians interested in literacy programs is needed as well. We also need to better understand what are the effective messages and methods of delivery in terms of different ethnic groups (Canadian Public Health Association, 2003). Foreign born women and men with low literacy are less likely to be burdened by shame about low skills in English or French, but more likely to work long hours and be unable to participate in programs outside the workplace. A large percentage of foreign-born Canadians with low literacy skills participate in the workforce. Of all women in the workforce testing at the lowest levels of literacy, 52% are foreign born though they represent only 17% of the female workforce. Foreign born males represent 18% of the workforce and 34% of the men in the workforce who have low literacy levels 1 and 2 (Boyd, 1991).

## Need for new definitions of goals and accountabilities in our school system

One of the most pressing needs may be a better understanding of literacy testing itself on health and literacy levels of children and youth. This is important given that hundreds of thousands of Canadian students are being tested for literacy level every year and now, at least in Ontario, a passing mark on the grade 10 literacy test (or alternate assignment) is required for a high school graduation diploma. Also needed is a better understanding of means to identify academic and social goals of our education system. Many provinces have recently spent much time and effort developing new curricula for our schools with detailed lists of outcome criteria. Yet it is expected, for example, in Ontario, that such specific outcomes be achieved within 110 hours of class time. There is little leeway for students who may actually take much less or more time to meet academic goals. Yet, a certain amount of in-school hours is likely needed to make a difference in the socialization and citizenship skills of children and youth. In particular, a sense of school bonding or connectedness has been associated in the literature with a variety of indicators of academic success and well-being (DeWit et al., 2002).

More research needs to be done on creative ways of disentangling and/or combining academic, citizenship, and health goals of our education system. If we have met some kind of literacy threshold whereby increasing years of schooling beyond elementary school do not translate into decreasing numbers of people who are unable to read and write well enough to function in society through employment and other socially acceptable activities, it may be time to rethink how we fund and define education entirely.

One of the key recommendations of the first Ontario Public Health Association report is "the creation of a major shift in the education system to allow for lifelong learning. This would establish a drop-in drop-out philosophy allowing people to acquire the skills they need when they need them" (Perrin, 1989, p. 34). Peter Calamai's most recent publication on literacy is called *The three L's: Literacy and life-long learning* (Calamai, 2000). The Movement for Canadian Literacy, the hub of Canada's literacy network, has recently advocated for a National Literacy Action Agenda that is grounded in a life-long learning strategy. They suggest that such an agenda be a key part of the federal government's new Innovation Agenda supported by Industry Canada and Human Resources Development Canada. The Ontario Ministry of Education defines literacy education as:

> part of a process or cycle of lifelong learning, based on life experience, shared knowledge, and decision-making by learners supported by their instructors. Literacy education contributes to the development of self knowledge and critical thinking skills. In turn, this development empowers individuals and communities. (Parkland Regional College, 1998, p. 9)

The recent National Workshop on Literacy and Health Research supported this direction, in concluding that "studying the impact of literacy and life-long learning on health" was one of the top four priorities (Canadian Public Health Association, 2003). An agenda for life-long-learning may better address new understandings about multiple literacies and encourage learners previously held back by stigma. An agenda for life-long learning could begin to treat adults and teenagers on more similar terms and make high schools or community education centers welcoming and appealing to the young and old who are ready to learn. It would also go some way towards reducing the stigma of dropping out, and reducing the number of students who are not engaged in their school work, if alternatives such as extended co-op placements can be found for them.

### Need for new mechanisms for interministerial collaboration

This chapter, like the others in this book, highlights the degree to which health status is affected by areas of jurisdiction of government ministries other than health. Sectors such as education, social services, culture and immigration, justice, and social security are thought to have primary influence on health. Yet, when it comes to the health of individuals, too often, frontline people from every sector decide that the problem is within the jurisdiction of another sector. Fragmentation in our communities exacerbates problems with health for our children. For example: many schools are empty after school and on weekends while children and youth in the neighbourhood have no safe places to play and no constructive activities to do; many recreation centres now charge user fees which discourage participation of at-risk children and youth who are most in need of constructive outlets; children and youth who need special services are bounced from one provider to another with little communication between them, and over 40,000 remain on waiting lists in Ontario; and many schools do not have specialist teachers or access to professional support staff.

Clearly, a higher level of support for community collaboration between multiple sectors is needed. Nowhere is this more evident than within our school communities. Phyllis Benedict of the Ontario Teachers' Federation also supports better collaboration between Ministries. Healthy Schools were recognized as a direction to pursue at the "Realizing the Promise of Public Education" Forum held by the Federation in the Spring of 2003. In the most recent investigation of Ontario's school system, Dr. Mordechai Rozanski has recommended that "the government establish a Cabinet-level advisory council on integrated services for children and families, composed of representatives from the Ministries of Community, Family, and Children's Services, Education, Health and Long-Term Care, Public Safety and Security, and Tourism and Recreation, to meet on a regular basis to align the work and the funding mechanisms of the ministries that serve families, children, and youth." If such a step is taken, along with a deep look at the definition of literacy and the goals of our education system, the health and well-being of our population will undoubtedly be much better addressed.

## Conclusion

Much progress has been made in defining and measuring literacy and understanding the relationship between literacy and health, and in particular, the concept of literacy as a determinant of health. More needs to be done to refine our understanding of literacy and its impact on health, particularly in light of social trends. Some of the trends we are facing that make this kind of work so timely are that our ethnic and linguistic make-up is changing rapidly; the use of computers and new technologies is proliferating; there are greater literacy requirements today for functioning in our knowledge economy; and there are unprecedented stresses on our health care and education systems. Finally, we urgently need multi-sectoral collaboration to solve many kinds of problems. The field of health promotion has a history of experience in partnership building, and literacy and health research can be a guiding light for the kind of work and methods that are needed.

## Note

1.   For more information on the history, definition and measurement of literacy as a concept see the paper written by Rootman and Ronson (2003).

## Recommended readings

OPHA and Frontier College. (1989). *Literacy and health project phase one: Making the world healthier and safer for people who can't read*. Ontario Public Health Association and Frontier College, online at www.opha.on.ca/resources/literacy1summary.pdf.

This report describes the methods, findings and recommendations of the first phase of the Ontario Literacy and Health project sponsored by the Ontario Public Health Association and Frontier College.

Breen, M. (1993). *Partners in practice: The literacy and health project phase two.* OPHA and Frontier College.
This report summarizes the activities carried out during the second phase of the Ontario Literacy and Health Project and examines some of the questions which arose during the conduct of the project as well as recommendation for future work. It also contains descriptions of various literacy and health projects underway in Canada in 1993.

Shohet, L. (2002). *Health and literacy: Perspectives in 2002,* online at www.staff.vu.edu.au/alnarc/onlineforum/AL_pap_shohet.htm.
This paper discusses the links between literacy and health as they are currently represented in the discourse communities of the medical profession and of adult literacy. After comparing the positions taken by the medical field and the adult literacy field, and examining some selected government policies, the author outlines some directions for the future.

Rootman, I., Gordon-El-Bihbety, D., Frankish, J., Hemming, H., Kaszap, M., Langille, L., Quantz, D., and Ronson, B. (2003). *National literacy and health research program: Needs assessment and environmental scan,* online at www.nlhp.cpha.ca/clhrp/needs_e/needs_e.pdf.
This paper describes the methods and findings of a Canadian environmental scan, a needs assessment conducted during 2002 to identify gaps in knowledge in literacy and health research in Canada, current and proposed initiatives in literacy and health and opportunities for research.

Canadian Public Health Association. (2003). Literacy and Health Research Workshop: Setting Priorities in Canada, Final Report, online at www.nlhp.cpha.ca/clhrp/index_e.htm#workshop.
This document reports on the process, conclusions, and recommendations of a national workshop held in October 2002 to consider the implications of the above-noted environmental scan and needs assessment for literacy and health research and practice in Canada.

# Related websites

CPHA Literacy and Health Program—www.nlhp.cpha.ca
This website describes the National Literacy and Health Program and its associated services and projects including the National Literacy and Health Research Program.

National Adult Literacy Database—www.nald.ca
This website describes the National Adult Literacy Database, lists literacy organizations in Canada, presents information about what's new and events in the field, as well as awards and contacts. It also provides access to literacy discussion groups and to expert advice, newsletters, a literacy collection, full-text documents, a resource catalogue, links to internal resources and to data.

Harvard School of Public Health, Health Literacy Studies—www.hsph.harvard.edu/healthliteracy
This site contains introductions to health literacy, power point presentations, videos, literature reviews, annotated bibliographies, research reports, health education materials, guidelines on creating and evaluating written materials, curricula, highlights of talks and presentations, news items, insights, and links to related web sites.

# Part Three

———————●———————

# FOUNDATIONS OF
# LIFE-LONG HEALTH: FOOD AND SHELTER

CANADA IS THE SIGNATORY to a number of international agreements that guarantee the provision of basic needs such as food and shelter. Yet, one of the most shocking developments in Canada over the past 20 years has been the increasing incidence of food and housing insecurity. Canadian policy decisions related to the provision of adequate income and shelter have greatly weakened the state of these social determinants of health. In its most extreme but not particularly rare manifestation, these policy decisions have led to frightening levels of hunger and homelessness among Canadians. The explosive growth in the number of Canadians forced to rely upon food banks for food and temporary shelters for housing are the most obvious indicators of this situation. In its less extreme, but more pervasive forms, the effects of food and housing insecurity are associated with increasing numbers of Canadians being unable to acquire quality diets and spending disproportionate amounts of monetary resources on shelter. What is particularly disturbing about this image of Canadians being unable to meet the basic needs of food and shelter, is that this is occurring during a time when economic resources in Canada have never been at higher levels. This section details the extent of food and housing insecurity in Canada and the factors that have led to this situation. The health effects of the situation are reviewed and policy options to alleviate these crises are presented.

**Lynn McIntyre** provides a history of food insecurity in Canada. She then provides the latest available information on the incidence of food insecurity—including hunger—in Canada. She identifies who is most at risk for food insecurity and relates these factors to lack of available income resources. Factors leading to food insecurity are primarily financial; issues of financial management, and lack of nutritional knowledge of the food insecure are of minor importance. Nutritional implications are presented as are a number of policy options to address food insecurity in Canada that highlight the contribution and inter-relationship to food insecurity of other social determinants of health such as income, housing, and employment.

**Valerie Tarasuk** shows how food insecurity threatens healthy nutritional status, interferes with chronic disease management, and can lead to body weight problems. Food insecurity is related to the health of children, youth, adults, and the elderly. It increases the likelihood of emotional and health problems among the elderly, leads to poor academic and psychosocial development of younger children, and to depressive disorders among adolescents. Since health issues of food-insecure Canadians are similar to those associated with low income and other indicators of material deprivation, policy solutions require providing people—especially those out of work—with enough income to cover the costs of meeting basic needs.

**Michael Shapcott** outlines the scope of the housing crisis in Canada today and how it is a result of a number of policy decisions by the federal and provincial governments. Data is provided on the increasing number of housing insecure and homeless Canadians. The Aboriginal situation and the barriers faced by Canadian women to acquire adequate housing are especially problematic. Canada has gone from a leader in providing adequate housing to its citizens to one whose housing crisis has drawn critical and negative international attention. Latest developments in housing policy are outlined and policy solutions presented. The contrast between government statements and actions on housing issues is particularly interesting.

**Toba Bryant** details the health effects of homelessness and housing insecurity. Traditional epidemiological approaches to studying housing and health are limited and new ways of conceptualizing the relationship are required. Federal and provincial housing policies threaten health by increasing homelessness and increasing housing insecurity. The stresses associated with increasing housing insecurity also threaten health. Housing insecurity affects other social determinants of health by leaving fewer resources available for food, education, and recreation. Bryant provides a model of the policy change process that can be applied to provoke action on housing and other social determinants of health.

# Chapter Twelve

# FOOD INSECURITY

## Lynn McIntyre

## Introduction

Food used to be called a basic human need along with water, peace, shelter, education, and primary health care. It has also been called a prerequisite for health. Food security is a determinant of a lot of things—of life, health, dignity, civil society, progress, justice, and sustainable development. In this chapter, food security is considered as a determinant of health.

This chapter is organized to first present a conceptual framework of hunger and food insecurity in developed societies. It then outlines a brief social history of food insecurity in Canada, describes its current status, and offers several policy recommendations. While presenting a national picture of food insecurity, the specific situation of women and their children is explored is some detail.

## Understanding hunger and food insecurity

On World Food Day, October 16, 2000, The *Canadian Medical Association journal* published a paper, "Child hunger in Canada" (McIntyre et al., 2000). The story was featured that night on both the CTV and CBC National News and the next day in the highly respected newspaper *The Globe and Mail*. The following day, *The National Post*, an overtly "right wing" yet influential newspaper, wrote an editorial entitled "Junk food report." The editor wrote: "There is a big difference between hungry people in Canada and in the Third World, and it is preposterous and offensive to suggest otherwise as Lynn McIntyre ... has done."

That editorial has been an inspiration. Why is hunger so threatening to *The National Post* and its sympathetic readership? Unpacking the meaning of hunger is key to its understanding, and to understanding why we permit hunger and food insecurity to persist.

Food insecurity is the term used to describe hunger in developed countries. For a comparative discussion of hunger in developing countries, see Box 12.1. The generally accepted definition of food insecurity is "the inability to acquire or consume an adequate diet quality or sufficient quantity of food in socially acceptable ways, or the uncertainty that one will be able to do so." The experience of food insecurity is dynamic. It occurs at both the level of households and individuals. Household members may have different experiences of food insecurity and hunger due to intra-household food provisioning that favours the needs of one or more family members over those of others. Mothers, in particular, may experience more severe food insecurity than their children. The sequence of stages that define the experience for individuals reflects graded levels of severity, ranging from food anxiety to qualitative compromises in food selection and consumption to quantitative compromises in intake to the physical sensation of hunger. At its most severe stage, food insecurity is experienced as absolute food deprivation (i.e., individuals not eating at all). Only insufficient intake in this model is equated with classical hunger.

---

## Box 12.1: Comparing hunger in developing and developed countries

The United Nations Food and Agriculture Organization (FAO) report, *The state of food insecurity in the world* (2002), chronicled the 840 million people who were undernourished in 1998–2000, of whom 11 million or 1.3 percent lived in industrialized countries; the remaining 799 million resided in developing countries. Clearly there is difference in scale and severity of hunger in developed versus developing countries.

Malnutrition is synonymous with hunger in developing countries. Malnutrition is defined as the failure to achieve nutrient requirements which can impair physical and/or mental health. "Hidden Hunger" is the popular term used for developing country-acquired micronutrient deficiencies. Iron, iodine, and vitamin A deficiencies are quiet and unnoticed, although terribly health-damaging. Developing countries measure hunger through indicators of chronic energy deficiency; mild, moderate, and severe malnutrition; growth retardation; and serious key nutrient deficiencies at the population level. Sometimes absolute poverty and low per capita energy consumption are cited as indirect measures of hunger in the developing world.

In both developed and developing countries, hunger and food insecurity occur through a combination of individual through to international factors. In both contexts, nutritional adequacy is an essential, and arguably, the single most important determinant of health. Those with too little food, regardless of place, have too little because they are very poor or destitute; with adequate resources they could acquire food.

Hunger in developing and developed countries is starkly different in three ways: Hunger is lethal in developing countries. It is not obviously so in developed countries. In developing countries, food needs are a priority—they must be for both short-term and long-term survival. In developed countries the food budget is the most elastic, i.e., the most discretionary of all essential expenditures. Shelter needs come first. Thirdly, in developing countries we are seeing rapid increases in obesity and chronic disease associated with dietary preference change from even modest economic development, while at the same time gross malnutrition persists. In North America, those with obesity and chronic disease are often the poor, and often the hungry. In short, our hungry are often fat.

Social Determinants of Health

Validated instruments such as the Cornell-Radimer questionnaire, Community Childhood Hunger Identification Project questionnaire, and the Food Security Core Module directly measure the occurrence and severity of food insecurity. Food insecurity is also measured through smaller sets of indicator questions administered as part of both American and Canadian national surveys. Indirect measures of hunger and food insecurity include food bank use, adequacy of income, and homelessness.

The definition of hunger subscribed to is "the uneasy or painful sensation caused by a lack of food, the recurrent and involuntary lack of access to food" (Hamilton et al., 1997). This definition of hunger applies universally—and unfortunately, it is universally experienced. Canadian social work professor Graham Riches (1997) has argued that the hunger experience is socially constructed. One could argue that the hungry experience hunger universally—it is the lens of society that views the experience differently.

The Canadian debate on hunger has raised the issue of whether hunger is about absolute or relative poverty. Sarlo (1996), a conservative economist with the Fraser Institute argues that the poverty line is grossly inflated and that if we considered physical subsistence needs—only 2% rather than 19% of Canadian children would be deemed poor. Two percent does match the child hunger rate calculated from some national studies (McIntyre et al., 2000; McIntyre et al., 2001). In contrast, relative poverty relates to both material and social deprivation—a deprivation of resources required for a dignified participation in society.

Hunger, the "H" word conceptually has three elements: it is about suffering; it is about absolute poverty and the consequences of relative deprivation; and it is about political dismissal of a fundamental abrogation of human rights. Hungry children are illegal. Many international covenants have deemed that children have "an inalienable right to adequate nutritious food" (International Covenant on Economic, Social and Cultural Rights, 1966); and "the fundamental right of everyone to be free from hunger" (World Food Summit, Declaration of World Food Insecurity, 1995).

Individual food insecurity is linked with societal issues of food security and sustainable food production and distribution, topics that are beyond the scope of this chapter. However, it is important to recognize that globalized food systems, the international trade of food commodities, the agro-seed industry, agricultural policies that support or disadvantage local domestic producers, supply management of food staples by marketing boards, grocery distribution systems, processed food marketing and distribution, school food policies, and labour protections for agricultural workers are just some of the factors that make up a complex web of supra-individual factors that create or diminish conditions of individual and household food insecurity.

So why is it important that we understand that hunger does exist in Canada? Because to deny that among those with food insecurity in Canada are people who are truly hungry is to deny that we have gone too far.

## A brief social history of food insecurity of Canada

A very brief social history of food insecurity in Canada would read simply: poverty increased then it deepened. Food insecurity emerged then it increased in severity.

While poverty is a long-standing area of social study in Canada, food insecurity is relatively new. Canada has had its food problems before—decades of malnutrition before the First World War, drought and depression and charitable food delivery systems operating between the Great Wars, and a famine among the Inuit as late as 1950. But food insecurity, a child of the 1980s, was discovered when food banks emerged, and children's feeding programs in schools could be counted. Child poverty was on the map with the passage of the famous 1989 House of Commons resolution committing the government to the elimination of child poverty by the year 2000.

Globally Canada is a rich country, ranking first in the United Nations' Human Development Index between 1997 and 2000. Nonetheless, the nineties were marked by a fundamental restructuring of Canadian social programs. Global recession shifted federal spending priorities away from social union programs. Provincial deficit reduction or cost-control strategies concurrently reduced social expenditures in health, education, and community services. In Canada, the result was increased levels of food insecurity as one manifestation of growing poverty and inequity.

Over the past two decades, communities across the country have initiated a host of food programs in an effort to alleviate food insecurity locally. Responses to food insecurity in Canada have been community-based, *ad hoc*, and largely focused on the provision of free or subsidized food (e.g., food banks, targeted meal programs). Health promotion and community development initiatives have typically been smaller in scale and focused on either enhancing food shopping and preparation skills (e.g., community kitchens, targeted education programs) or on alternative methods of food acquisition (e.g., community gardens, farmers' markets, field-to-table programs, "good food" boxes). 1,800 new food banks opened between 1997 and 2002 (Wilson and Tsoa, 2002).

Food security is a central issue in the call for domestic action in Canada's Action Plan for Food Security. Food supplement and coupon programs for poor pregnant women and their children are run through federally-funded national networks. Children's feeding programs have been implemented throughout the country, representing a social movement predicated on Canadians' beliefs that virtually all poor children would go to school hungry without them. It is generally conceded that food banks are stop-gap measures, offering important immediate assistance but not yielding sustainable solutions. Similarly, the implications (positive, negative, or neutral) of other community-based strategies are not well understood but such programs have not been shown to significantly reduce food insecurity or improve nutritional status among vulnerable populations.

Since 1989, the date used for most comparisons, we have sadly counted the poor, poor children, hungry children, emergency food bank users, and now the homeless. Local, regional, and national food insecurity studies have been released with similar shameful results. We have launched and re-launched child poverty initiatives. This brief social history of food insecurity in Canada concludes that since 1989 we have failed to eliminate or even significantly reduce hunger and food insecurity despite a high level of public activity, awareness, and sympathy for those who do not have enough to eat. How can that be? Perhaps it lies in the numbers—they are alternately considered too low or too high.

Social Determinants of Health

# Current status of hunger and food insecurity in Canada

## Prevalence in Canada

The 1995 United States Current Population Study reported food insecurity in 17% of households with incomes less than 50% of the poverty level (Hamilton et al., 1997). U.S. child hunger rates calculated through the Community Childhood Hunger Identification Project revealed that 8% of children under the age of 12 experienced hunger (Wehler et al., 1996). While there is a growing body of literature on household food security in the United States, social, political, cultural, economic, and geographic differences between Canada and the U.S. make the simplistic extrapolation of U.S. findings to Canadian settings inappropriate. Literature on food insecurity in the United Kingdom, New Zealand, and Australia is sparse and reflects differing socio-economic conditions and social policy frameworks. Canadian prevalence estimates are needed to document the extent of food insecurity in this country and to develop effective responses.

Some insight into the scope of food insecurity in Canada is beginning to emerge from analyses of limited sets of indicator questions included in some recent population surveys. Child hunger is an extreme manifestation of household food insecurity. Further understanding of this problem has come from the 1994 and 1996 cycles of the National Longitudinal Survey of Children and Youth (NLSCY), in which 22,000 and 16,000 households were asked respectively, "Has your child ever experienced hunger because there was no food in the house or money to buy food? If yes, how often?"

In the study reporting on the 1994 survey, hunger occurred in 1.2% or 57,000 Canadian families with children under 11 years of age; 35.0% of whom reported that their child experienced hunger at least every few months (McIntyre et al., 2000). The adjusted rate for 1994 and 1996 comparisons was 1.3%. In 1996, 1.6% of the sample reported child hunger, representing 75,615 Canadian families of children under 13 years of age. In 1996, 37.5% of these families reported frequent hunger defined as hunger experienced at least every few months. Among these, hunger most often occurred regularly at the end of the month (McIntyre et al., 2001).

The 1998–1999 National Population Health Survey (NPHS) included three screening questions for food insecurity. Recent results revealed food insecurity among 10.2% of Canadian households representing 3 million people (Che and Chen, 2001). Additionally, the most severely food insecure, termed the food poor, represented 4.1% of households, and 4.9% or 338,000 children (Rainville and Brink, 2001).

In March 2002, the Canadian Association of Food Banks reported that its annual count of emergency food program users for the month was 747,665 or 2.4% of the total Canadian population—double the 1989 figure; 41% of the food bank users or 305,000 were children under the age of 18. While food bank use is not a specific marker of food insufficiency (about two-thirds of the hungry in the NLSCY did not seek food bank support), it is highly sensitive to the hunger state (i.e., few people who use a food bank are not truly hungry).

A recent study examined the food insecurity and hunger of 141 low-income lone mothers with children in Atlantic Canada over the past year and during the course of one month. Virtually every household experienced food insecurity over the past year (96.5%). This was reduced only modestly to 78% over the past four-week period. Maternal hunger was reported by 42% of mothers over the previous year and 23% over the month of the study. Child hunger was very similar to maternal hunger over the study period. Using the Food Security Core Module to assess food insecurity in women attending Metropolitan Toronto food banks, Tarasuk and Beaton (1999) found that 94% reported some degree of food insecurity, with 70% reporting quantitative compromises in food intake ("hunger") over the past year and 57% reporting such problems in the past 30 days. Both studies documented the problem of food insecurity among low-income women with children, and both identified variation in the severity of food insecurity. As with other studies, it is difficult to compare the prevalence of hunger and food insecurity without using comparable measures.

Every study of hunger and food insecurity in Canada uses slightly different measures and terms according to the food insecurity spectrum. There is food anxiety, food insufficiency, food poverty, compromised diet quality, and actual hunger.

We do not make a distinction in heart attack counts by percent cardiac muscle damage or in stroke counts by density of paralysis. Yet in food insecurity reporting, what exactly is being measured and how that translates into a palatable (pardon the pun) number, seems to matter a lot. National child hunger rates seem too low, and national population food insecurity rates seem too high to mobilize Canadians or their policy-makers into action.

**Best estimate of food insecurity in Canada**

A conservative estimate of the number of Canadians who are food insecure today would be the 7.8% or 2.3 million 1998/99 National Population Health Survey households that experienced at least a compromised diet; 10% of such households or 678,000 children were thus affected (Rainville and Brink, 2001; see Table 12.1).

**Risk factors for hunger and food insecurity in Canada**

The socio-demographic characteristics of hungry families are similar from study to

**Table 12.1: Numbers and proportions of Canadian population living in food-secure and food-insecure households, NPHS, 1998–1999**

| Category, n (%) numbers in thousands | Food Secure | Food Insecure | | | |
|---|---|---|---|---|---|
| | | Total | Anxious | Compromised diet | Food poor |
| Total Canadian population | 26,458 (89.8) | 3,015 (10.2) | 2,360 (8.0) | 2,290 (7.8) | 1,211 (4.1) |
| Adults | 20,470 (90.7) | 2,098 (9.3) | 1,655 (7.3) | 1,612 (7.2) | 873 (3.9) |
| Children (0–7) | 5,988 (86.6) | 924 (13.4) | 705 (10.2) | 678 (9.8) | 338 (4.9) |

Source: Adapted from Rainville, B., and Brink, S. (2001). *Food insecurity in Canada, 1998–1999*, Research paper R-01-2E, May. Ottawa: Applied Research Branch, Human Resources Development Canada.

Social Determinants of Health

study. Risk factors for hunger and food insecurity are also similar from one study to another—there are few surprises left among the descriptive and analytic studies of food insecurity and hunger in Canada. These misery surveys need not be reproduced again and again. Instead, intervention studies targeted at reducing the determinants of food insecurity are required.

1994 NLSCY families headed by lone mothers were eight times more likely to report that their children were hungry compared to other families. Children from families receiving welfare or social assistance income were 13 times more likely to experience hunger than non-welfare or social assistance income earners. 1996 NLSCY families with hungry children were six times more likely to be lone parent-led than other families with over half of such families reporting hunger. While 54% of all hungry families received their main income from employment in the 1996 survey, families whose incomes included social assistance had greater than an eight-fold risk for child hunger and half of such families reported hunger. The only ethnic group that was significantly associated with hunger was persons of Aboriginal descent who were four times more likely to report hunger than other respondents (this survey includes only off-reserve Aboriginal persons).

1996 NLSCY logistical regression models identified the following predictors of hunger in addition to low household income: there was a four-fold risk of hunger when the mother reported that her health was fair or poor. When the family was led by a single parent, the risk increased three-fold, and Aboriginal status increased the risk by 60%. We also found that a higher total number of siblings in the household independently increased the risk of hunger by 40%.

According to the 1998/99 NPHS, the odds of reporting food insecurity increased with declining income adequacy and reliance on social assistance; prevalence was greatest among lone mothers with children.

It is well-documented that low-income Canadians have poorer health than others, but it is unclear what role long-term food insecurity plays in observed health inequities. In the 1998–99 NPHS, food insecurity was associated with increased odds of poor/fair self-rated health, multiple chronic conditions, distress, and depression. The two NLSCY studies found that the primary caregivers in families reporting hunger themselves reported significantly poorer health status than non-hungry primary caregivers. Tarasuk (2001) found that women who reported more severe food insecurity were more likely to have long-standing health problems and activity restrictions and to describe their health as poor or fair when compared to women with less severe food insecurity. Tarasuk's accompanying chapter is this volume further discusses the relationship between food insecurity and health.

## Coping strategies

The national surveys asked hungry families how they coped when they had insufficient food. The NPHS analysis of all age groups found that among those reporting food insecurity, 22% sought food from charitable sources, almost half reduced the quality of their foods, and about a quarter skipped meals or ate less. Similar to the 1994 survey, among 1996 NLSCY respondents, 21.2% reported that they reduced the variety of foods usually eaten when the family had run out of food or money to buy food; 33.2% of hungry families reported that the parent skipped meals or ate less; and 4.9% reported that the child skipped meals or ate less. Thirty-five percent of respondents sought help from food banks, seeking help from relatives and friends was reported by 31% and 29% respectively.

Clearly food bank use grossly underestimates the number of hungry families but food bank visitors are distinct from other hungry families. From the 1996 NLSCY analysis, the independent predictors of food bank use were lone parenthood, higher number of siblings in the household, and income from social assistance. Tarasuk (2001) also found that food bank use was related to a higher number of children in the family. These families are the poorest, the most isolated, and among the hungriest. The Atlantic Canada study of lone mothers and their children asked the mothers about sources of free food. Less than 10% of mothers DID NOT receive free food and a startling 54% visited the food bank. Another 4 in 10 received food from relatives. Reflective of a rural population, some women had their own hunting licences to acquire food, and gardened. Again for such a complex social phenomenon, socio-demographic and behavioural results from one food insecurity study to another are remarkably similar.

## Nutritional implications

Food insecurity arises in the context of low income and financial insecurity. Low income has long been associated with increased likelihood of sub-optimal nutrient intake and decreased likelihood of food consumption patterns consistent with "healthy eating." Within low-income groups, food insecurity appears to impart additional risk of dietary inadequacy. Controlling for other social, cultural, and economic influences on dietary intake, Rose and Oliveira (1997a, b) found systematically lower nutrient intake levels among individuals in households characterized by food insecurity (indicated by a single question on household food

sufficiency) than those in food secure settings. A smaller study of 193 women with children in New York State found food insecurity to be associated with a significant decline in household food availability and fruit and vegetable consumption (Kendall et al., 1995). In Tarasuk's (2001) study of women with children using food banks, women in households characterized by more severe food insecurity also had systematically lower intakes of fruit and vegetables and meat and meat alternates than those in more food secure settings.

The Atlantic Canadian study of 141 women and children examined not only the food security status, but also the dietary intake of the mother and her children weekly for a month. Figure 12.1 depicts caloric intake of mothers and children over the month. At the first of the month, mothers' and children's intakes are quite close but mothers' consumption declines over time. Children have an increase during the third week of the month—what was called the T3 or second cheque of the month effect. This second cheque is often the Child Tax Credit or Goods and Services Tax refund. The same pattern was found for minerals and vitamins (Figure 12.2). Children's dietary intake was consistently better than their mothers, and generally exceeded adequacy levels in comparison with their mothers whose prevalence of inadequacy was high. The T3 effect reappeared for children (McIntyre et al., 2003).

If these results are generalizable to other vulnerable mothers, the implications are clear. In the Atlantic Canada study, mothers' dietary intakes were consistently poorer than their children's intakes. The difference in adequacy of intake between mothers and children widened from the beginning to the end of the month concurrent with the

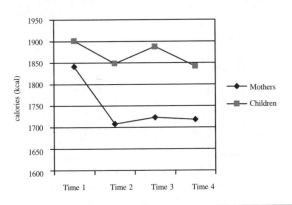

**Figure 12.1: Mean calorie intake of Atlantic Canada lone mothers and their children over one month**

Source: Reproduced from McIntyre, L., Glanville, N.T., Raine, K.D., Dayle, J.B., Anderson, B., and Battaglia, N. (2003). "Low-income lone mothers compromise their nutrition to feed their children," *Canadian Medical Association journal* 168, 686–691.

depletion of income resources. Dietary improvement occurred in children when a small amount of cash was infused into the home and in fact, except for a few nutrients, children attained dietary adequacy. The study is a demonstration of gender as a determinant of food insecurity as mothers compromise their own nutritional intake in order to preserve the adequacy of their children's diets.

Chronic food insecurity not only has implications for nutritional inadequacy and poor health but possibly also for altered body composition and prevalence of obesity. In Canada, obesity differs by gender and is associated more with low education than with low income. Che and Chen's (2001) analysis of the 1998–99 NPHS revealed, however, that people in food-insecure households had significantly higher odds of obesity (defined as body mass index or BMI ≥30) even when age, sex, and household income adequacy were taken into account. Cross-sectional comparisons suggest a curvilinear association between food insecurity and body mass index with overweight apparent among chronically food-insecure persons and thinness occurring most often with extremes of food insecurity (Olson, 1999).

Townsend and colleagues (2001) recently examined the relationship between BMI and food insecurity using the 1994–1996 U.S. Continuing Survey of Food Intakes by Individuals. They found that food insecurity was positively related to overweight in women, with mildly-food-insecure women 30% more likely than other women to be overweight (BMI >27.3). In particular, food insecurity was related to overweight over and above the effect of income, demographic, and lifestyle variables. They proposed a "food stamp cycle" hypothesis meaning that an injection of new food at the beginning of the month to a food-depleted household might lead to over-consumption. This area of inquiry is further expanded upon in Tarasuk's accompanying chapter.

## Figure 12.2: Selected dietary intakes of Atlantic Canada lone mothers and their children over one month

### Figure 12.2a: Vit A consumed by mothers and children over time as % RDA of median intake

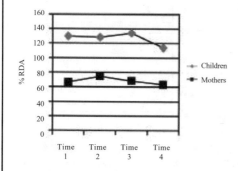

### Figure 12.2b: Calcium consumed by mothers and children over time a % adequate intake (AI) as mean intake

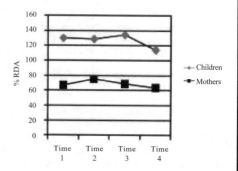

Source: Adapted from McIntyre, L., Glanville, N.T., Raine, K.D., Dayle, J.B., Anderson, B., and Battaglia, N. (2003). "Low-income lone mothers compromise their nutrition to feed their children," *Canadian Medical Association journal* 168, 686–691.

### Figure 12.2c: Zinc consumed by mothers and children over time as % RDA of median intake

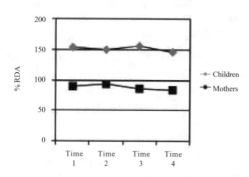

Source: Adapted from McIntyre, L., Glanville, N.T., Raine, K.D., Dayle, J.B., Anderson, B., and Battaglia, N. (2003). "Low-income lone mothers compromise their nutrition to feed their children," *Canadian Medical Association journal* 168, 686–691.

## Hunger dynamics

Another food insecurity descriptor is the dynamics of hungry households. While persistent hunger is a problem, hunger transitions are also worthy of study. There were 358 families in the NLSCY cohort for both 1994 and 1996 who ever reported hunger. Only 22.6% of them reported persistent hunger, i.e., hunger in both time periods.

Families with persistent hunger were remarkable for their lack of any meaningful change in circumstance. But that does not mean that these families were in some type

Social Determinants of Health

**Table 12.2: Risk factors among NLSCY families who report hunger in 1996 and no hunger in 1994**

| Risk factor | Odds ratio (95% confidence interval) |
| --- | --- |
| **Another mouth to feed** | |
| >1 new sibling in home | 5.75 (2.18–16.03) |
| Change in number of parents in household | 2.06 (1.02–4.21) |
| **Job loss** | |
| Father lost full-time work | 5.64 (1.15–26.57) |
| Mother unemployment status change | 2.57 (1.58–4.21) |
| **Health problems** | |
| Mother health status worse | 3.45 (1.27–8.52) |
| Child health status change | 2.25 (2.09–5.70) |

Source: Adapted from McIntyre, L., Walsh, G., and Connor, S.K. (2001). *A follow-up study of child hunger in Canada,* Working Paper W-01-1-2E. Applied Research Branch, Strategic Policy. Ottawa: Human Resources Development Canada, June.

of equilibrium. They reported the highest levels of family dysfunction (McIntyre et al., 2001).

There were many factors that could tip a family into the hunger state (Table 12.2). They are categorized as another mouth to feed (one or more siblings added to the household; change in number of parents in household); job loss (father lost full-time work; mother's unemployment status changed); and health problems (mother's health status worsened; child health status changed for either better or worse).

Getting out of hunger depended upon one change only—mother gets a full-time job, and the family's income rises accordingly (McIntyre et al., 2001).

Annual income changes were calculated for families by hunger state. Total family income needed to increase by $3,827 in order for a family to leave the hunger state but a loss of only $2,690 could tip a family into hunger indicating that these families are fragile already. These results related to change in hunger status underscore not only the fluidity of hungry families but their predictability.

## Conclusion

The data presented support the fact that hunger and food insecurity are real issues in Canada created by social policy that increases rather than reduces disparities. Policy recommendations required to address food insecurity and hunger are easy to name but they do require the political will to address them:

1.  **Real incomes must rise, whether from minimum wage or social assistance.**
    Food insecurity results from anything that limits household resources or the proportion of those resources available for food acquisition. Limited employment opportunities, low minimum wage scales and social assistance benefits, and increases

in non-discretionary non-food expenditures such as the cost of housing, utilities and child care all contribute to insufficient income to purchase food.

2.  **Healthy foods must be affordable, particularly the food staples such as milk.**

    Food must meet not only caloric needs but provide essential nutrients for optimal health. Community-based food assistance programs such as food banks do not support the achievement of healthy diets among recipients. These initiatives represent a poor policy alternative to the family purchase of healthy foods.

    Many developing countries monitor and support the price of food staples, e.g., tortilla flour in Mexico. Canada's marketing board policies protect the supply of staples and the incomes of producers but not the affordability of food staples for consumers. Fluid milk is one example. Despite its superior nutritional value, inadequate consumption of milk products is consistently observed in low-income populations. It may be time for Canada to adopt a food staples policy that supports opportunities for healthy eating among its most vulnerable citizens.

3.  **Because food needs give way to shelter needs in the poorest households, affordable housing is urgently required.**

4.  **In families with children, lack of affordable, quality daycare is often a significant barrier to employment.**

5.  **Some self-sufficiency demonstration projects have shown the promise of work-related supports, health and recreation provision, and other transition assistance. These types of employment support programs should be widely disseminated.**

    This grouping of recommendations speaks to the determinants of food insecurity and together, they are the subjects of wide policy debate. There is strong evidence supporting their contributions individually and collectively to poverty reduction and improved life quality.

6.  **There should be a monitoring system for hunger and food insecurity—not to survey misery but to determine progress, deterioration or shifts among those affected. In turn a food security policy lens must be applied to social policies to ensure that they reduce genuine hunger rather than exacerbate it.**

    The data presented for this paper have been assembled by individual effort and through the retrieval of disparate sources. Canada's Nutrition Plan of Action and other documents and lobbying efforts by non-governmental bodies call for a systematic monitoring of food insecurity with an eye to rapid policy translation.

Food security is perhaps the most precious of all determinants of health. If Canada is prepared to make the necessary investments, it can reap a food security dividend that enriches all of society with payoffs in health, social capital, sustainability of our physical and social environments, justice, and both cost savings and wealth creation.

# Recommended readings

Riches, G. (Ed.). (1997). *First World hunger, food security and welfare politics*. London: Macmillan.

This book provides the reader with comparative perspectives of hunger in the developed world; Australia, Canada, New Zealand, U.K. and U.S. Additionally emerging strategies are discussed in the fight against increasing hunger in developed countries.

Tarasuk, V. (2001). "A critical examination of community-based responses to household food insecurity in Canada," *Health education and behaviour* 28(4), 487–499.

Over the past two decades, household food insecurity has emerged as a significant social problem and serious public health concern in the "First World." This article reviews the recent emergence of hunger as a Canadian concern and the development of responses to this problem. The author provides a critical examination of the community development strategies that attempt to respond to food insecurity.

McIntyre, L., Glanville, N.T., Officer, S., Anderson, B., Raine, K.D., and Dayle, J.B. (2002). "Food insecurity of low-income lone mothers and their children in Atlantic Canada," *Canadian journal of public health* 93, 411–415.

This article examined the occurrence and predictors of hunger and food insecurity over the past year and month among low-income mother-led households in Atlantic Canada. The Cornell-Radimer Questionnaire to Estimate the Prevalence of Hunger and Food Insecurity was administered weekly for a month, with modifications, to 141 lone mothers taking part in a larger dietary intake study. Food insecurity over the past year occurred in 96.5% of households. Child hunger was similar to maternal hunger over the one-month study period (23%), however, it was lower than maternal hunger over the past year.

# Related websites

Centre for Studies in Food Security (CSFS) at Ryerson University—www.ryerson.ca/~foodsec/

The purpose of the CSFS is to facilitate research, community action, and professional practice to increase food security through focussing on the issues of health, income, and the evolution of food systems. The CSFS website provides links to the work of the Centre, publications, conferences, and affiliated organizations.

United Nations Food and Agriculture Organization—www.fao.org/docrep/005/y7352e/y7352e00.htm

The fourth edition of *The state of food insecurity in the world* presents the latest estimates of the number of chronically hungry people in the world and reports on global and national efforts to reduce that number by the year 2015. Detailed information is provided on the prevalence of undernourishment in developing countries and countries in transition and on food availability, dietary diversification, poverty, health, and child nutritional status.

Canadian Association of Food Banks (CAFB)—www.cafb-acba.ca/about_e.cfm

The CAFB represents food banks in every province. While providing member food banks with groceries for people in need day-to-day, they ultimately work toward a hunger-free Canada. This site provides information on CAFB, Public Education and Research, Finding a Member Food Bank and Supporters.

*HUNGERCOUNT 2003: "Something has to give": Food banks filling the policy gap in Canada.* Prepared by Lisa Orchard, Rob Penfold and Don Sage—www.cafb-acba.ca/pdfs/other_documents/HC2003_ENG.pdf

Initiated in 1989, *HungerCount* is the only national survey of emergency food programs in Canada. It has been conducted annually since 1997. The information the survey provides is invaluable, forming the basis for many CAFB activities throughout the year. *HungerCount* is a leading barometer of hunger, food insecurity, and poverty in Canada. Findings are used throughout the year by community-based organizations, government, researchers, media, and the corporate sector.

# Chapter Thirteen

———●———

# Health Implications
# of Food Insecurity

## Valerie Tarasuk

## Introduction

Household food insecurity has long been recognized as a public health problem in Canada.[1] It is also as serious a social problem (Riches, 2002; Riches, 1997), although this understanding of food insecurity has garnered less attention. The early research on household food insecurity in Canada and the United States was primarily qualitative in nature, focussed on eliciting an understanding of the everyday experiences of families with food access problems.[2] Qualitative research continues to importantly extend our understanding of food insecurity as social exclusion, as those affected are forced to adopt food consumption patterns and food acquisition strategies that fall outside social norms.[3] With the development of indicator questions and scales to measure food insecurity, quantitative research in this field has also burgeoned. Food insecurity questions have been included on several large population surveys in Canada and the U.S. in an effort to measure and monitor the problem. We are now faced with a plethora of studies examining associations between brief assessments of household food insecurity and dietary factors, health conditions, and various socio-demographic factors. The research highlights the conditions under which household food insecurity occurs and provides some insight into the possible health implications of food insecurity in Canada. Interpretation is limited, however, by the cross-sectional nature of the survey data, the brief indicators of food insecurity typically included, and the decontextualized nature of survey analyses.

This chapter begins with a review of the associations between food insecurity and nutrition. The evidence of relationships between food insecurity and various indicators of poor health is then critically examined, and these relationships are discussed within the context of other literature on social gradients in health. Finally, the policy implications of this research are discussed, with a particular focus on Canadian social policies as they appear to relate to local problems of food insecurity. A broader discussion of policy implications is presented by Lynn McIntyre elsewhere in this volume.

# Food insecurity and nutrition

## Indications of dietary compromise

Survey data from the 1998–99 National Population Health Survey (NPHS) indicated that 8% of Canadians reported qualitative and/or quantitative compromises in food intake in the previous 12 months because of a lack of money (Che and Chen, 2001). In the absence of dietary intake data, the nature and nutritional significance of these compromises can only be ascertained indirectly, through inferences from other literature. Although there have been some studies to investigate the relationship between household food insecurity and dietary intake among particularly vulnerable groups in our country (McIntyre et al., 2003; Tarasuk and Beaton, 1999; Tarasuk, 2001b), we have no empirical data from which to draw conclusions about the nature and magnitude of dietary compromises among food insecure versus food secure Canadians.

To date, Canadian studies of dietary intake in the context of food insecurity have been focussed primarily on low-income women with children, because of concerns about their particular vulnerability to food deprivation. Although small in scale, this research provides compelling evidence that self-assessments of household food security status are indeed indicative of the quantity and quality of food intakes among individuals (McIntyre et al., 2003; Tarasuk and Beaton, 1999; Tarasuk, 2001b). Further, the extent of dietary compromise, for adult women at least, appears to be a function of the severity of their household food insecurity. One study of women in families using food banks in Toronto found that those in households characterized by severe food insecurity (a determination based on the extent of food deprivation reported among adults and children over the period of study) reported significantly lower intakes of fruits and vegetables and meat and meat alternates (Tarasuk, 2001b) and lower intakes of energy, protein, carbohydrate, fat, vitamin A, vitamin C, folate, iron, magnesium, and zinc (Tarasuk and Beaton, 1999) than women in more secure settings. Most of these relationships remained statistically significant even after other economic, socio-cultural, and behavioural influences on diet had been taken into account, suggesting that the women's energy and nutrient intakes were independently related to their household food security status. Insofar as the results can be generalized, they suggest that the adequacy of dietary intakes among low-income groups is, in part, a function of their household food security.

Further indications that self-appraisals of household food insecurity are indicative of compromises in the nutritional quality of individuals' actual food intakes come from U.S. population surveys. Several U.S. studies have documented significantly lower intakes of energy and a number of nutrients among individuals in households characterized by food insufficiency[4] than those in food sufficient settings.[5] Multivariate modelling techniques were applied in two of these studies (Rose and Oliveira, 1997a; Rose and Oliveira, 1997b) to control for other social, cultural, and economic influences on dietary intake; results suggest that the observed differences in intake are specific to the state of household food sufficiency. Other measures of food insecurity have revealed similar associations with more conventional, nutritional assessments of dietary adequacy (Kendall et al., 1996).

In considering the nutritional implications of food insecurity, it is important to note that the distribution of resources within households affects the observed association between household measures of food insecurity and individuals' dietary intakes. Even when households are under no apparent economic constraints, foods and nutrients are not allocated in proportion to individual members' needs.[6] Disparities in intra-household food distribution appear to increase in the context of food insecurity. Poor women typically report that they deprive themselves of food in order to leave more for their children during periods of severe food shortages.[7] This behaviour is also suggested by studies reporting poorer quality dietary intakes among low-income women in comparison to their children.[8] It is further indicated by the absence of significant differences in the dietary intakes of preschool children, but the presence of significantly lower energy and nutrients intakes among other household members in food insufficient versus food sufficient households in the 1989–1991 Continuing Survey of Food Intakes of Individuals (a large U.S. nutrition survey) (Rose, 1999; Rose and Oliveira, 1997). These findings suggest that women's intakes may be particularly sensitive to deteriorations in household food security, but raise questions about expected correlations between household food insecurity and the dietary intakes of children and men.

**Implications for nutritional status**

Despite evidence of associations between household food insecurity and dietary intake, it is difficult to establish the impact of problems of food insecurity in Canada on individuals' nutritional status and long-term health. In the studies cited, food intake has been measured over only a few days at one point in time and the frequency, chronicity, and severity of experiences of food insecurity have generally not been assessed. Yet the consequences of food insecurity for individuals' nutritional health depend on the frequency, duration, and severity of the food insecurity. Episodic, short-lived perturbations in dietary intake may be inconsequential, but the chronic consumption of a diet low in essential nutrients can predispose individuals to compromises in nutritional status. Little is known about the extent to which this occurs. Dietary intake assessments are insufficient to draw conclusions about nutritional status, and very few studies of food insecurity have included clinical or biochemical measures of nutritional status.

Two recent U.S. studies in which biochemical measures of nutritional status were included highlight the complex relationship between indicators of food insecurity and nutritional status. In a U.S. population-based survey of elderly, disabled women, a measure of food insufficiency[9] was examined in relation to three biochemical indicators of nutritional status: hemoglobin, serum albumin, and total cholesterol (Klesges et al., 2001). Women who reported food insufficiency were three times more likely than food-sufficient women to have iron deficiency anemia. They also tended to have lower serum albumin and lower total cholesterol (measures that, in other studies, have been linked to increased risk of coronary heart disease and non-cardio-vascular diseases respectively among older persons), although these differences were not statistically significant. In contrast to these findings, an analysis of children's data from the U.S. National Health and Nutrition Examination Survey III revealed no association between iron deficiency and household food insufficiency among preschool and school-aged children, once other risk factors (i.e., socio-demographic and family characteristics, past health risk, health care risk, and environmental risk) were taken into account (Alaimo et al.,

2001c). This study did report a significantly increased risk of iron deficiency among children in low-income families, but no independent effect of food insufficiency could be detected.

## Barriers to "healthy eating"

Irrespective of whether the food insecurity experienced by Canadian households is of sufficient severity to impact the nutritional status of individuals, chronic food insecurity must limit the likelihood of "healthy eating." In affluent countries such as ours, problems of nutrient deficiency are generally thought to be rare. Attention is thus increasingly focussed on the identification and promotion of dietary practices that will reduce risk of heart disease and other diet-related conditions of public health significance. "Healthy eating" includes an emphasis on fruit and vegetable consumption, and the selection of whole grain breads and cereals, low-fat dairy products, and lean meats, fish, poultry, and meat alternatives (Health Canada, 1997). Yet a recent analysis of household food expenditure data in Canada indicates that the purchase of milk products and fruits and vegetables is constrained by low income (Kirkpatrick and Tarasuk, 2003). Further, many of the healthful dietary choices being currently advocated (e.g., specially formulated high-fibre or low-fat foods; margarines low in saturated or trans fatty acids; low-fat dairy products) represent increased food costs for low-income consumers (Travers et al., 1997). Household food insecurity can only exacerbate income-related constraints on food selection, making it even less likely that these households will be able to choose diets conducive to long-term health.

## Chronic disease management

Insofar as food insecurity is associated with dietary compromises, it can impede the management of chronic diseases in which nutrition is implicated. There is growing interest in diabetes in this regard because the consequences of even short-term food deprivation for individuals with diabetes can be profound and readily observable. Although many adults with diabetes report poor compliance to recommended dietary regimens, those on low incomes clearly face additional constraints. Food insecurity compounds problems of disease management for this group. One of the first published reports of this problem came when a 1997 study of food insecurity among a sample of adult patients at a U.S. urban county hospital revealed associations between hypoglycemia and hunger and food insecurity among diabetic patients, suggesting that food insecurity exacerbated the management of this condition (Nelson et al., 1998). In a more recent analysis of population data from the U.S. National Health and Nutrition Examination Survey III, adults with diabetes who were in food insufficient households reported significantly more physician encounters than those who were food sufficient (Nelson et al., 2001), again suggesting that they may experience poorer disease management. Both of these studies were cross-sectional in design, making it is impossible to draw causal inferences from the findings. Nonetheless, the results highlight a troubling association that merits further investigation.

The impact of food insecurity on the management of chronic conditions in which nutrition has been implicated is worrisome because people in food insecure settings appear more likely to report such conditions. A recent analysis of data from the 1996–1997 NPHS revealed significantly higher odds that individuals in food insufficient households would report heart disease, diabetes, high blood pressure, and food allergies compared to those in food sufficient households (Vozoris and Tarasuk, 2003). These associations persisted even after adjusting for age, sex, income adequacy, and education. Again, it is important to note that the observed associations are cross-sectional in nature, so it is impossible to infer causality. Regardless of why the associations exist, however, individuals in food insufficient households clearly face a serious obstacle to the effective management of chronic conditions through lifestyle modifications such as diet.

## Food insecurity and body weight

There has been considerable research into the relationship between food insecurity and body weight, driven in large measure by the quest to understand why both the prevalence of overweight and the prevalence of food insecurity are greatest among low-income groups in the U.S. Several studies have reported significant associations between cross-sectional measures of household food insecurity and overweight or obesity among adults.[10] One exploration of this question among a large sample of U.S. children found differences by age and race, with Non-Hispanic white girls, 8–16 year of age, in food insufficient households 3.5 times more likely to be overweight than girls in food sufficient settings, but younger girls (2–7 years of age) 1.6 times less likely to be overweight if they were in food insufficient households (Alaimo et al., 2001b). Such findings have spawned considerable speculation about possible mechanisms by which dietary choices or patterns of food intake characteristic of chronic food insecurity might predispose people to weight gain. The findings have also been interpreted by some to cast doubt on the legitimacy of individuals' claims that they have experienced food insecurity. The methodo-

logic limitations of this research are profound, however, and they merit much closer scrutiny before any conclusions about the relationship between food insecurity and overweight are drawn.

An examination of Canadian data highlights the difficulties in drawing meaningful conclusions about the relationship between food insecurity and body weight from cross-sectional survey data. Two analyses of measures of food insecurity in relation to body weight conducted using data from the National Population Health Survey have yielded opposite results. Working with data from the 1998–99 NPHS, Che and Chen (2001) reported that adults in food insecure households were 1.5 times more likely to be obese (i.e., body mass index (BMI) > 30) (Table 13.1). The determination of food insecurity in that cycle of NPHS was based on an affirmative response to one of three questions indicating worry about not having enough to eat, compromise in the quality or variety of foods eaten, and not having enough to eat. The regression model used to examine the odds of obesity in relation to food insecurity included age, sex, and income adequacy as covariates to control for the potentially confounding influences of these variables. Vozoris and Tarasuk (2003) subsequently examined this question using data from the 1997–98 NPHS (Table 13.2).

Because this cycle included a much larger sample than the 1998–99 cycle, they were able to stratify the analysis by gender and examine food insufficiency in relation to a broader range of BMI categories, while adjusting for age, education, and income adequacy. In contrast to Che and Chen, Vozoris and Tarasuk found no relation between household food insufficiency and body weight for women, and a significantly

**Table 13.1: Odds of obesity among individuals, by household food security status, as assessed in the 1998–99 National Population Health Survey[a]**

| Food security status | Odds ratio[b] (95th confidence interval) |
|---|---|
| Food secure | 1.0 |
| Food insecure | 3.2 (2.7, 3.8) |

a "Odds of obesity among individuals, by household food security status, as assessed in the 1998–99 National Population Health Survey," adapted from the article entitled "Food insecurity in Canadian households," published in the Statistics Canada publication *Health reports* (2000), Catalogue 82-003. 12(4), pp.11–22.
b Adjusted for age, sex, and household income.

**Table 13.2. Odds of women and men in food insufficient households having a body mass index (BMI) indicative of underweight, normal weight, overweight, obesity, or morbid obesity, as assessed in the 1996–97 National Population Health Survey.[a]**

| Body mass index classification | Odds ratio[b] (95th confidence interval) for women | Odds ratio[b] (95th confidence interval) for men |
|---|---|---|
| Underweight (BMI ≤ 19.0) | 1.0 (0.7, 1.5) | 1.6 (0.6, 3.9) |
| Normal weight (19.0 ≤ BMI ≤ 24.9) | 0.9 (0.7, 1.1) | 1.3 (0.9, 1.7) |
| Overweight (25.0 ≤ BMI ≤ 29.9) | 1.2 (0.9, 1.5) | 0.7 (0.5, 0.9) |
| Obesity (30.0 ≤ BMI ≤ 34.9) | 1.0 (0.8, 1.4) | 1.2 (0.8, 1.8) |
| Morbid obesity (BMI ≥35.0) | 1.0 (0.6, 1.6) | 1.3 (0.8, 2.2) |

a Adapted from Table 3 in Vozoris, N. and Tarasuk, V. (2003). "Household food insufficiency is association with poorer health," *Journal of nutrition* 133, 120–126. In all weight categories, the odds ratio for individuals in food sufficient households was 1.0.
b Adjusted for age group, education level, and household income adequacy.

*decreased* odds of overweight among men in food insufficient households (Vozoris and Tarasuk, 2003). In light of these findings, it is important not to assume that food insecurity is associated with overweight or obesity among Canadians, despite reports of this association in the U.S.

The contradictory results emerging from these two studies highlight the serious limitations of using population survey data to explore complex questions of etiology. The questions used to assess food insecurity on these cycles of the NPHS are crude, household-level measures. How well they indicate the experience of food insecurity for one randomly selected individual in the household (i.e., the person whose BMI is being considered in these analyses) is unknown, but the existing research suggests that experiences vary considerably among household members. Furthermore, although different indicators of household food insecurity were employed on the two cycles of NPHS, both assessed food insecurity over the past year; we have no idea how these indicators relate to household conditions in the more distant past. Nor do we have any data on individuals' weight histories, or whether they were in a state of weight gain or loss at the time of the survey. Depending on the severity, frequency, duration, and dietary manifestations of an individual's experience of food insecurity, it could conceivably predispose him or her to weight gain or weight loss. Cross-sectional comparisons of household-level indicators of food insecurity and BMIs based on self-reported heights and weights are unlikely to reveal such complex relationships.

## Implications for health

Individuals in households characterized by food insecurity appear to be more likely to suffer from poor health than those in more food secure situations. Several studies in Canada and elsewhere have documented significant relationships between indicators of household food insecurity and the likelihood of individuals reporting poor or fair self-rated health[11] and multiple chronic health conditions (Che and Chen, 2001; McIntyre et al., 2000; Vozoris and Tarasuk, 2003). In the 1994 National Longitudinal Survey of Children and Youth, for example, caregivers in families reporting child hunger were more likely to rate their health poorly and to report having at least one chronic health condition when compared to caregivers in families not reporting child hunger (McIntyre et al., 2000). In that study, the health of the children who experienced hunger was also reported to be worse than

the health of children who did not experience hunger (McIntyre et al., 2000). This finding is similar to that in an earlier U.S. study in which the severity of household food insecurity among low-income families was directly related to the number of child health problems they reported (Wehler et al., 1992). The relationship between food insecurity and poor health appears robust across the life cycle. In the U.S. study of elderly disabled women mentioned earlier, food insufficiency was associated with poorer physical performance among white women, and with more medical conditions among minority women (Klesges et al., 2001). Interestingly, financial variables were highly associated with the measure of food insufficiency in this study, but they were not found to mediate the observed relationships between food insufficiency and health.

Indicators of household food insecurity have also been linked to greater likelihood of emotional and mental health problems. Klesges et al. (2001) have documented higher levels of psychological depression among elderly disabled women reporting food insufficiency compared to women reporting no such problem. However, most of the research in this area has been with children. Research from the U.S. Community Childhood Hunger Identification Project (CCHIP) revealed that a variety of behavioural, emotional, and academic problems were more prevalent among children in food insecure versus food secure households (Kleinman et al., 1998; Murphy et al., 1998; Wehler et al., 1992). More recently, Alaimo and colleagues have examined associations within the U.S. National Health and Nutrition Examination Survey III and reported strong associations between household food insufficiency and poorer academic and psychosocial development among school-aged children (Alaimo

## Poorer people, poorer health
### The health of food bank recipients

Spring Food Drive, 2002
Daily Bread Food Bank

Each year since 1987, Daily Bread Food Bank has conducted a survey of more that 800 food bank households. The objective is to understand who needs to use a food bank, and why.

The annual survey covers a variety of issues. Periodically, surveys have questioned people about their perception of their own health.

With public health care on the public's mind at present, it is timely to look at the health of certain population groups beyond merely Medicare and hospitalization issues. For low-income people in general, nutrition is inadequate and health in general is poorer. This year's survey shows, too, that health has declined as incomes have declined.

### Nine years make a difference
The 2002 survey shows some dramatic declines in health among food recipients over time. In 1993 Toronto's Department of Health asked Daily Bread to gather information about the health status of food bank users. Food recipients were asked how they compared their health to others of the same age. We asked the same question again this year. The results are reported below—along with responses from the 2002 survey.

**Clearly food recipients are in poorer health now than then:**

|  | 1993 | 2002 |
|---|---|---|
| Rated health excellent | 17.2% | 11.8% |
| Rated health very good | 16.2% | 17.2% |
| Rated health good | 30.2% | 28.6% |
| Rated health fair | 19.0% | 25.4% |
| Rated health poor | 12.5% | 16.4% |

Furthermore, the health of food recipients is not only declining but is also considerably lower than that of the general population. 41.8% of food recipients rated their health as fair or poor. If one asks middle-income earners the same question, only 10% or 12% say their health is fair or poor.

With the after-rent incomes of food recipients at almost half what they were in 1993, there appears to be a relationship between significantly lower income and poorer health.

### Low-income equals poor health
There is ample and growing medical evidence that low-income people experience poorer health than those with more adequate means.

Dr. Dennis Raphael of the School of Health Policy and Management, York University, notes that "people with heart disease had almost a two times greater chance of living on low income than those Canadians without heart disease," and that "income differences

con't

con't

account for a 23.7% excess in premature dealths from cardiovascular disease among Canadians."[1]

Dr. Valerie Tarasuk of the University of Toronto's School of Nutrition has published on findings that the incomes of welfare recipients in Toronto are too low to buy nutritious food[2], and health suffers as a result.

**Inability to purchase needed food**
Food recipients were asked: "Are there foods which you think you should eat for your health, but cannot afford?"

> 45% couldn't afford meat, poultry, or fish
> 26% couldn't afford vegetables and fruits
> 5.4% couldn't afford milk and milk products

Their responses are hardly surprising: 57% of adults and 32% of children in food bank households report going hungry at least once a month because they cannot afford food —in spite of having used a food bank. Indeed, 26% report that they need more food than they can get from a food bank all the time, and 25% report they need more food most of the time. And 47% have had to borrow money from family or friends in the last month.

Food recipients are not asking for much, though: 41 % say an extra $100 a month would allow them to buy all the food they need for their health, and another 36.6% say that an extra $100 a month would buy some (but not all) the food they need for health.

**Access to health care**
Disturbingly, a quarter of those surveyed had been unable to get health care when then needed it. Of these

> 29% had a physical disability needing special care
> 5.7% had a mental disability needing special care
> 8% suffered from depression and needed special care

**Conclusion**
While we worry about the health care system, we must also worry about the causes of ill health—and poverty is a major cause. It is not enough just to fix Medicare—we must work to fix the inequality which is such a large determinant of good health. Doing so is an investment in health care—a healthier population means lower health care costs. In the long run, neglecting poverty will cost us all. Simple things would make a difference: giving people enough money to pay the rent so they don't go without food, allowing the poorest families to keep the federal child poverty money now clawed back by the province, helping the disabled get disability income instead of welfare.

Please help by giving food and volunteering. Please help us, too, to impress upon government officials that poverty is a health problem which must be addressed.

1 *Inequality is bad for our heart: Why low income and social exclusion are major causes of heart disease in Canada.* Toronto: North York Heart Health Network.
2 *The affordability of a nutritious diet for households on welfare in Toronto.* N. Vozoris, B. Davis and V. Tarasuk. *Canadian journal of public health,* 2002, p. 92.

Source: The Daily Bread Food Bank, 191 New Toronto Street, Toronto, M8V 2E7. Phone (416)203-0050 Fax (416)203-0049. email: info@dailybread.ca. website: www.dailybread.ca.

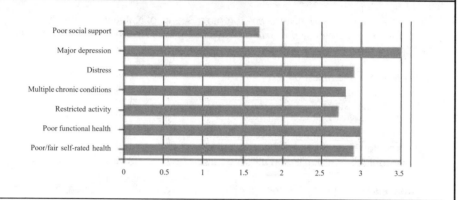

**Figure 13.1: Odds of individuals in food insufficient households reporting poor general, physical, mental, or social health and selected chronic conditions (1996–97 National Population Health Survey)**

Source: Vozoris, N. and Tarasuk, V. (2003). "Household food insufficiency is association with poorer health," *Journal of nutrition* 133, 120–126.

et al., 2001a), and depressive disorder and suicidal symptoms among adolescents (Alaimo et al., 2002).

When taken individually, each of the observed cross-sectional associations between an indicator of poor health and household food insecurity can give rise to speculation about possible mechanisms through which food insecurity influences health. It could be argued that household food insecurity predisposes individuals to poor health, but the reverse might also be true. However, a somewhat different picture emerges when food insecurity is considered in relation to multiple measures of poor health. In their analysis of data from the 1996–97 NPHS, Vozoris and Tarasuk (2003) found that individuals in households characterized by food insufficiency had significantly higher odds of reporting poor/ fair health, of having poor functional health, restricted activity, and multiple chronic

conditions, of suffering from major depression and distress, and of having poor social support (Figure 13.1). Given the broad spectrum of health indicators for which associations were observed, it seems unlikely that the effect of food insecurity on health is condition-specific.

The robustness of the association between indicators of household food insecurity and poor health is reminiscent of another particularly robust relationship—the relationship between income and health. In the general population, health tracks income across a wide variety of indicators. The observed associations between food insecurity and health may be an extension of the income-health gradient. Measures of household food insecurity are essentially measures of the dietary manifestations of acute financial insecurity. In this sense, food insecurity denotes a more extreme level of material deprivation than that identified by

Social Determinants of Health

conventional measures of low-income (Rose, 1999; Tarasuk, 2001b). As such, indicators of household food insecurity may be functioning as markers of the population subgroup who reside at the extreme end of the poverty-wealth spectrum. The extreme disadvantage associated with this social position is exemplified in the increased likelihood of poorer physical, mental, and social health among this group when compared even to others with low incomes.

## Policy implications

Since the 1980s, Canadian communities have struggled to find ways to respond effectively to concerns about problems of hunger and food insecurity in their midst. Most prominent among these responses have been food banks and children's feeding programs, but on a lesser scale, a variety of food-based "self-help" and community development programs have also been

---

### Food bank use up across the country

OTTAWA –The number of people who use a food bank in Canada is greater than the entire population of New Brunswick, says a new report on hunger.

A survey of food banks taken in March counted 777,869 people coming to a food bank at least once that month. That's an increase of more than five per cent over the previous year.

"It's a conservative estimate," said Matt Ferguson, who helped research the report for the Canadian Association of Food Banks (CAFB).

The survey was conducted in March, he said, because it is considered to be an "unexceptional" month for food bank use.

About 75 percent of the food banks and agencies responded to the survey, and not every food bank in Canada belongs to the association.

For comparison's sake, the population of New Brunswick, according to Statistics Canada's latest estimates, is 750,594.

"It's a national disgrace," said Charles Seiden, executive director of the CAFB.

The association conducts the same survey every year. This year, every province showed an increase except Manitoba.

Food bank use has more than doubled since 1989, according to CAFB.

Seiden said the federal government is not living up to its responsibilities to make sure everyone has enough to eat.

With a federal election expected next year, CAFB wants people to pressure politicians to put poverty and hunger on the federal government's agenda.

"We're committed to keep bringing the issue to the public's attention," he said.

Source: CBC News, www.cbc.ca/stories/2003/10/16/foodbanks031016.

---

initiated (Tarasuk, 2001a). Although it is beyond the scope of this paper to debate the effectiveness or strengths and weaknesses of these various responses, it is worth noting that problems of food insecurity do not appear to have diminished in the wake of these measures. The solution does not appear to reside in ad hoc, food-based community efforts.

The inclusion of food security indicator questions on population surveys in Canada has clearly delineated the socio-demographic factors associated with a vulnerability to household food insecurity in this country. Indeed this may be the most important contribution of measurement efforts to date. Analyses of NPHS data clearly indicate that the risk of food insecurity escalates as the adequacy of household income declines (Che and Chen, 2001; Vozoris and Tarasuk, 2003). Furthermore, income adequacy is by far the strongest predictor of household food insecurity in Canada (Che and Chen, 2001; Vozoris and Tarasuk, 2003). The findings are consistent with other research suggesting that problems of household food insecurity are primarily problems of financial insecurity (Gunderson and Gruber, 2001; Klesges et al., 2001; Tarasuk, 2001b), and not problems arising because of a lack of food preparation skills, poor budgeting skills, or the lack of motivation to prepare foods from scratch (McLaughlin et al., 2003; Travers, 1995).

Among low-income Canadians, those on welfare are particularly vulnerable to food insecurity (Che and Chen, 2001; McIntyre et al., 2000; Vozoris and Tarasuk, 2003). In the 1998–99 NPHS, 58% of households who were reliant on welfare, employment insurance or workers' compensation reported food insecurity (Che and Chen, 2001). Even when the influence of other socio-demographic factors on risk of food insecurity is taken into account (e.g., the increased risk of food insecurity associated with being in a single parent family), the odds of being food insecure is three times higher for households on welfare, employment insurance or workers' compensation (Che and Chen, 2001; Vozoris and Tarasuk, 2003). This finding reflects the impoverishment that has come to define welfare programs in Canada. Although welfare income levels are set by the provincial and territorial governments and these rates vary by household type, incomes rarely exceed two-thirds of the Statistics Canada Low-Income Cut-offs, and they are often much, much lower (National Council of Welfare, 2002). Income-expense comparisons indicate that, for many recipients, welfare incomes are insufficient to cover the costs of basic needs (Emes and Kreptul, 1999; Vozoris et al., 2002). Although welfare programs in Canada have never provided generous levels of income support, welfare incomes have declined over the past decade in most provinces and territories (National Council of Welfare, 2002).

## Conclusion

The compromises in dietary intake that are associated with household food insecurity appear to be one dimension of a more pervasive vulnerability to poor health that is experienced by people in states of severe material deprivation. With each new release of population health survey data by Statistics Canada, the failure of our social programs to protect low-income families from abject poverty is becoming clearer and clearer. If food insecurity is to be addressed, publicly funded income support programs like welfare must provide sufficient income to enable people to cover the costs of their most basic needs.

Social Determinants of Health

# Notes

1. See Campbell et al., 1988; Davis et al.,1991; Joint Steering Committee, 1996; The Canadian Dietetic Association, 1991.
2. See Campbell and Desjardins, 1989; Fitchen, 1988; Radimer et al., 1990; Radimer et al., 1992; Tarasuk and Maclean, 1990; Travers, 1995; Travers, 1996; Travers, 1997.
3. See Dowler and Leather, 2000; Hamelin et al., 2002; Lang, 1997; Leather, 1996.
4. "Food insufficiency" is an indicator of relatively severe household food insecurity. It is typically assessed by a single question in which respondents are asked how best to describe the food in their household over the past 12 months. Those who report that they sometimes or often did not have enough to eat are classed as "food insufficient."
5. See Cristofar and Basiotis, 1992; Kendall et al., 1996; Rose, 1999; Rose and Oliveira, 1997.
6. See Bull, 1991; Enns, 1987; Louk et al., 1999; Nelson, 1986.
7. See Badun et al., 1995; Campbell and Desjardins, 1989; Dowler and Calvert, 1995; Fitchen, 1988; McIntyre et al., 2002; National Council of Welfare, 1990; Tarasuk and Maclean, 1990.
8. See Cristofar and Basiotis, 1992; Dowler and Calvert, 1995; Lee, 1990; McIntyre et al., 2003.
9. In this study, food insufficiency was assessed through a single question, "How often does it happen that you (and your husband) do not have enough money to afford the kind of food you should have?"
10. See Basiotis and Lino, 2002; Olson, 1999; Sarlio-Lahteenkorva and Lahelma, 2001; Townsend et al., 2001.
11. See Alaimo et al., 2001c; Che and Chen, 2001; Cristofar and Basiotis, 1992; McIntyre et al., 2000; Radimer et al., 1997; Vozoris and Tarasuk, 2003.

# Recommended readings

Hamelin, A.M., Beaudry, M., and Habicht, J.-P. (2002). "Characterization of household food insecurity in Quebec: food and feelings," *Social science and medicine* 54: 119–132.

Drawing on data from in-depth interviews with a sample of 98 low-income households, Anne-Marie Hamelin and colleagues present a graphic portrait of the lived experience of food insecurity among Quebec families.

Riches, G. (2002). "Food banks and food security: welfare reform, human rights and social policy: Lessons from Canada?" *Social policy and administration* 36, 648–663.

Food banks remain the primary response to food insecurity in Canada. In this paper, Graham Riches critically examines the growth of food banking in Canada from three perspectives: the role of food banking in terms of advancing the human right to food, its effectiveness in achieving food security, and the extent to which food banking contributes to and/or counters the increasing emphasis by governments on welfare reform policies informed by a neoconservative ideology.

Tarasuk, V. (2001). "A critical examination of community-based responses to household food insecurity in Canada," *Health education and behavior* 28, 487–499.

This paper begins with a review of the recent emergence of food insecurity as a concern in Canada and the evolution of responses to this problem. The current application of community development strategies in response to food insecurity is then critically examined, drawing on insights from a qualitative study of community kitchens in southern Ontario.

# Related websites

The National Council of Welfare (NCW)—www.ncwcnbes.net/

The National Council of Welfare (NCW) is a citizens' advisory body to the Minister of Human Resources Development Canada on matters of concern to low-income Canadians. The NCW monitors the individual welfare programs that operate in the provinces and territories, producing regular reports on welfare incomes in relation to poverty lines and average incomes as well as policy analyses and public statements on policy developments of particular relevance to poverty and welfare in Canada. Their reports and statements can be viewed or downloaded from this website.

The Centre for Studies in Food Security, Ryerson University—www.ryerson.ca/~foodsec/

The Centre for Studies in Food Security at Ryerson University was established to "facilitate research, community action, and professional practice to increase food security through focusing on the issues of health, income, and the evolution of the food system (including attention to ecological sustainability and socio-cultural diversity)." The Centre's web site provides a broad spectrum of information about food security issues in Canada and internationally, including links to a wide variety of resources on this topic.

The Canadian Association of Food Banks (CAFB)—www.cafb_acba.ca/public_e.cfm

The Canadian Association of Food Banks (CAFB) conducts an annual survey of food bank use in Canada, as well as periodic surveys of public opinion on the problem of hunger in this country. As well, the CAFB occasionally releases position papers on policy issues of particular relevance to problems of food insecurity and hunger in Canada. These reports can be viewed and downloaded on their website.

Social Determinants of Health

# Chapter Fourteen

# HOUSING

## Michael Shapcott

## Introduction

Canada is, in global terms, a very rich country. There is plenty of money, and other resources, to ensure safe, good quality, affordable housing for all. However, about one-in-five Canadian households are unable to find affordable, acceptable homes. And about 250,000 people will experience homelessness every year.

The roots of this crisis lie in decisions by federal, provincial, and territorial governments to cut funding and programs for new social housing and cancel programs over the past two decades—which set the stage for the nation-wide housing crisis and homelessness disaster.

Canada's national government has been preaching "housing" globally, but back home has been setting in place policies that generated growing homelessness. At the same time that the federal housing minister was at Habitat II, the United Nations-sponsored global housing summit in Istanbul in 1996, to join with countries around the world in proclaiming the goal of "housing for all," the federal government announced plans to transfer responsibility for its housing programs to provincial and territorial governments. It had locked in place a plan for annual cuts to housing spending that will see national funding shrink to zero over the next three decades.

By the late 1990s, the federal government had signed housing transfer deals with the provinces and territories, abandoning a national role in affordable housing. Canada became one of the few countries in the world without a national housing strategy.

In 1998, the federal government "commercialized" Canada Mortgage and Housing Corporation (CMHC), shifting the mandate of the national housing agency away from its historic role of encouraging the development of a range of housing. CMHC now generates "profits" of hundreds of millions of dollars on its mortgage insurance program, but housing developers report that the high cost of the premiums is blocking development of new affordable units.

As governments abandoned their housing policies and programs, they believed or hoped that private markets would pick up the slack. After all, the majority of Canadians live in

"Whereas before the 1980s very few people went unhoused, and no one was born homeless, today many thousands of Canadians have no housing and are excluded from community networks and the mainstream patterns of day-to-day life ... Today, Canada has the most private-sector-dominated, market-based housing system of any Western nation (including the United States, where intervention on behalf of homeowners is extensive) and the smallest social housing sector of any major Western nation (except for the United States). Canada spends only about one percent of its budget on programs and subsidies for all the social housing ever built (about half a million units)."

—Dr. David Hulchanski, *Housing policies for tomorrow's cities*, Canadian Policy Research Network, 2002

homes that were built by the private sector, so why not turn over the entire housing sector to corporate development interests?

However, the private sector had already started to abandon affordable rental housing in the early 1970s, and that trend picked up in the 1990s. There is, quite simply, no money to be made in building housing for low, moderate, and middle-income households. With the potential for return on investments relatively low for new development in rental housing (versus, for instance, commercial properties or ownership developments), private money flowed out of the sector.

By the late 1990s, some smart operators had figured out a profitable niche in the rental market. Real estate investment trusts started buying up existing buildings with moderate rents. Taking advantage of lax rent regulation laws in most parts of the country, they drove up the rents and banked significant returns on investment. This was good for wealthy investors, but bad for tenants as rents rose and moderate-priced units were lost.

With no new government funding and a declining private role, Canada's rental housing sector has slipped from one crisis to another (CMHC, 2003):

- vacancy rates for affordable units are extremely low.

- rents are increasing well beyond the incomes of low-income households while tenant household incomes are stagnant or declining.
- the existing stock is aging and there are significant concerns about declining quality of the units, and
- existing rental units are being demolished or converted to more financially lucrative uses.

The rental housing crisis has triggered a big increase in homelessness, not just in big urban areas, but in small towns, and in remote, rural, and northern communities. The mayors of the country's biggest cities, gathering in Winnipeg in 1998, declared that homelessness is a "national disaster" and called on senior levels of government to restore funding for housing programs.

In the early 2000s, concerted political pressure convinced the federal government, and several provinces, to make commitments for new funding and programs. But those commitments have not translated into much net new housing.

The federal government in 2001 announced plans to invest $680 million over five years into new affordable housing, and topped that up with an additional $320 million in 2003. But, by November of 2003, the federal government had actually spent only $88 million—less than 9% of the $1 billion that was promised (Mahoney, 2003). And the bulk of that new spending has been offset by spending cuts at the provincial level, which means few real gains in terms of new units. Canada's nation-wide homelessness disaster is a manufactured crisis, triggered by the government and private sectors.

## A nation-wide housing crisis

Canada's national affordable housing crisis is hidden behind a picture of relative comfort.

Owner households in most parts of Canada have incomes that are, on average, about double the household income of renters (Hulchanski, 2001). Mortgage rates are relatively low, the supply of new and existing housing is generally good, and there are a number of government funding programs to assist homeowners (including direct subsidies and tax incentives).

All in all, conditions are good for homeowners. This relative prosperity obscures the housing crisis facing millions of low and moderate-income tenant households.

Canada's renter households have incomes, on average, half of the income of owners. While owner incomes have increased since the recession of the early 1990s, tenant household incomes have been stagnant. Some of the poorest households—including families living on social assistance (welfare)—have seen their income drop in real terms.

Low income makes it increasingly difficult for tenant households to move into ownership, especially in the biggest cities. But about one-third of Canadians are renters (a total of 4.8 million households—or about 13 million women, men and children) and for them, the affordable housing crisis and homelessness disaster is a devastating reality.

Median incomes for renter households are less than half those of owner households, and they have been falling since 1984. In a research bulletin for the University of Toronto's Centre for Urban and Community Studies, Dr. David Hulchanski analyzed this "tale of two Canadas" and concluded:

> The household income and wealth of renters is dramatically below that of owners, and the gap is growing. Renter households may find it increasingly difficult to move into home ownership. Government policies that focus on incentives for home ownership (such as tax-exempt savings plans or the Ontario government's waiver of land transfer taxes) do not address the housing needs of the vast majority of renter households. The federal government has not provided new social housing for low- and moderate-income renters since 1993.
>
> A comprehensive national housing policy, with complementary regional policies, must address the very low income and wealth of renters. Canada, more than most Western nations, relies on the private sector to provide housing. Renters must find adequate housing in housing markets in which prices are driven by the income and wealth levels of homeowners.
>
> Social policies and traditional income assistance programs (social assistance, unemployment, disability pensions, and so forth) must better address the growing income inequality between owners and renters.

Federal and provincial/ territorial housing policies must recognize that very few renters have incomes high enough to pay the rent levels required by unsubsidized new construction. Increased supply—the construction of new rental housing—is the only answer to low vacancy rates. Given the income and wealth profile of Canada's renters, only significant public-sector intervention will increase the supply of affordable rental housing.

In summary, there is a growing *social need* for affordable housing among renters. As the data from the Statistics Canada survey of financial security demonstrates, there is very limited *market demand*. The income and wealth levels of most renter households are much too low—and continuing to fall relative to homeowners.

(Hulchanski, 2001, p. 4)

Many tenant households cannot afford conventional rental units, or can't find them in the tight urban markets, and turn to the "non-conventional" or secondary rental market. These are condominiums (ownership housing bought by investors and rented to tenant households), illegal and substandard housing (basement apartments and other units that don't meet building and safety codes), and other rented units. But the secondary market is providing no relief for tenant households. Much of the housing is illegal and unregulated, and there are serious concerns about security of tenure for low-income tenants.

The housing crisis has grown so severe that even the big banks have started to notice. TD Economics, the research division of the

TD Bank Financial Group, released a major study on housing in June of 2003. TD noted in their introduction:

Housing is a necessity of life. Yet, after ten years of economic expansion, one in five households in Canada is still unable to afford acceptable shelter—a strikingly high number, especially in view of the country's ranking well atop the United Nations human-development survey. What's more, the lack of affordable housing is a problem confronting communities right across the nation—from large urban centres to smaller, less-populated areas. As such, it is steadily gaining recognition as one of Canada's most pressing public-policy issues ...

We are used to thinking of affordable housing as both a social and a health issue. This is not altogether surprising, given the fact that many social housing tenants receive their main source of income from government transfer payments. As well, in study after study, researchers have shown that a strong correlation exists between neighbourhoods with poor quality housing and lower health outcomes.

However, working to find solutions to the problem of affordable housing is also smart economic policy. An inadequate supply of housing can be a major impediment to business investment and growth, and can influence immigrants' choices of where to locate. Hence, implementing solutions to resolve this issue ties in well with the TD goal of raising Canada's living standards and overall quality of life. (TD Economics, 2003, p. i)

# Growing homelessness disaster

Nowhere is the housing crisis more visible than in the huge and growing number of homeless people living—and dying—on the streets of Canada. There are no reliable numbers on the number of homeless people in the country. Even figures for the number of people taking shelter in temporary hostels and other facilities for the homeless are not collected on a consistent basis. The National Housing and Homelessness Network released a comprehensive overview of homelessness in Canada in 2001 (NHHN, 2001). The following material is taken from the report *State of the crisis, 2001* (NHHS, 2001).

During the International Year of Shelter for the Homeless in 1987, the Canadian Council on Social Development estimated that 100,000 people would experience homelessness during that year.

By 1999, the Finance Committee of the Canadian House of Commons (the national legislature) had accepted an estimate that there were 250,000 people who would experience homelessness during that year.

A survey of eight Ontario communities in 1998 found that there were 1.5 million overnight stays in homeless shelters. Other studies suggest that the number of homeless people "sleeping rough," that is, outside of shelters, is often as high or higher than the number sleeping inside.

Toronto, the largest city in Canada, has the biggest number of homeless people and that number is staggering. Almost 32,000 people stayed in homeless shelters in that city in 2002, an increase of 21% from 1990.

In recent years, Toronto has reported that the biggest increase among the homeless is among children. About 6,200 children took shelter in Toronto in 1999, up 130% from the 2,700 in 1988. One-third of those children were under the age of four. The city's housing crisis is forcing people to stay longer in the emergency shelter system. More households are moving in and out of homelessness. The city is also reporting a growing number of seniors in city homeless shelters.

One measure of the serious state of the homelessness disaster in Toronto is the crowded shelters. Average occupancy in Toronto's homeless shelters has been over 90% for years. That means that every available bed is filled, and even the mattresses on the floor are mostly occupied. In the winters, hundreds of mats are placed on church basements to accommodate homeless people who cannot find room in the regular shelters.

Almost everywhere in the country, the numbers are up.

Muskoka, a rural area in central Ontario known as "cottage country" since it provides vacation homes to many people in southern Ontario, reported that in 1998 there were 219 admissions at Interval house, 38 emergency housing vouchers, and 43 motel rooms used by homeless people.

The main homeless shelter in London, Ontario, saw a 22% increase in homeless admissions from 4,319 people in 1995 to 5,269 in 1999.

The Peterborough (Ontario) Social Planning Council surveyed 206 homeless or near-homeless households (a total of 502 family members) in March 2000. They found:

- as many people were staying temporarily with friends or on the streets as in shelters.

- nine families (18 children) were homeless.
- one in four homeless were employed.
- two-thirds of homeless are not on waiting lists for social housing.
- among the near-homeless, 70% could not afford basic necessities such as food, clothing, personal hygiene products, telephone transportation or recreation, and
- the lack of affordable rents is the biggest barrier to finding housing.

Among those surveyed, the top solutions were more supply of affordable housing (77%) and better income (59%) through improved wages and social assistance programs.

Sudbury, a mid-sized city in northern Ontario, has the highest rental vacancy rate in the country. In theory, its rental market should provide plenty of vacant, lower-cost rental units as the market adjusts to meet demand. In fact, Subdury is trapped in the same homelessness cycle as other communities. An October 2000 study by the regional municipality found that during a seven-day period, 407 people were identified as homeless in the region. More than a quarter (28%) were children or adolescents. During that time, there were only 68 available beds in homeless shelters.

The study reported that the most frequent cause of homelessness in Sudbury was related to employment, followed by problems with social assistance (in particular, the inadequacy of social support payments), a lack of affordable housing, and domestic violence.

"Homelessness is one of the most pressing social issues affecting communities across the country today, and unfortunately, the Sudbury Region is no exception," said regional councillor Doug Craig.

In London, Ontario, a prosperous community in the province's south-western region, there are about 400 households per month using shelters—up by 13% from 1995. In nearby Windsor, the only hostel for the homeless had a licensed capacity for 90 beds in 1998, but it commonly sheltered 150 to 165. Hamilton, Ontario, has over 230 beds for homeless people and families escaping domestic violence. Shelter usage in Hamilton jumped by 35% between November 1998 and March 2000.

In Saint John, New Brunswick, a comprehensive review in early 2001 found that "the high rate of poverty in the city (27%) and the numbers of people who can't afford adequate housing (56% of unattached individuals and 18% of all families living in Saint John), along with the lack of affordable, adequate housing (low vacancy rates, long waiting lists, and the ghettoizing of subsidized housing)" were among the key factors in generating housing and homeless problems. "Those in highest needs are lone parent families and non-elderly singles," according to the study.

At last count in 2000, 1,300 people were homeless or used shelters in Calgary, Alberta, in the heart of Canada's booming oil patch. That's a 31% jump from 1998. The 1998 figure was up 61% from 1996. In addition, there are about 20,000 people a paycheque away from homelessness—they're just living right on the edge and if something disruptive happens to their lives, they can't make the rent.

A tour of the rest of the country shows:

- a 97% occupancy rate at shelters for the homeless in Edmonton, Alberta. Shelters for abused women were so full that they had to turn away 3,000 families in 1997. About 1,980 families used shelters in the city during 1998.

- shelters in Montreal, Quebec, offered space to about 12,660 people in 1996. Most of the centres report that they have reached a saturation point and often turn people away.
- Regina, Saskatchewan, in Canada's prairies, has a relatively small number of homeless people (there were only 60 beds in the city in 1998), but staff report a large increase in the number of "repeat" clients who use the shelters as "permanent" housing rather than temporary relief.
- the other major city in Saskatchewan, Saskatoon, reports that 68% of the people using its homeless shelters are First Nations people, even though they represent only 8% of the city's population. A total of 6,700 people stayed in shelters in 1998, with 28% of them children.
- St. John's, Newfoundland, on Canada's eastern coast, reports a major problem with "hidden" homeless; that is, people living in illegal and substandard housing.
- on Canada's west coast, there are about 300 to 400 people who sleep in homeless shelters every night, and another 300 to 600 people who "sleep rough" in Vancouver. City shelters are almost always full. From 1995 to 1998, the number of people sleeping on the floor in one shelter tripled from 3,887 to 10,758.

A study of hostels by the Toronto Disaster Relief Committee (TDRC) in the winter of 2000 provided a grim list of the conditions in the shelters. It documents overcrowding, poor food quality, lack of hygiene facilities, theft and violence, disease, and death both in the shelters and on the streets.

The study concludes that shelters in the rich city of Toronto fail to meet the emergency shelter standards set by the United Nations High Commissioner for Refugees (TDRC, 2000).

## First Nations people

First Nations people, the original inhabitants of Canada, make up a disproportionately large share of the number of those experiencing homelessness or living in substandard housing. Conditions on native reserves (often in rural, remote or northern locations) are desperate. Some First Nations people leave the appalling conditions on reserves for urban areas, only to see a large number join the ranks of homeless people.

"The single most critical issue currently facing the Assembly of First Nations, Department of Indian and Northern Affairs, and First Nation leadership is on-reserve housing," according to the Assembly of First Nations (AFN), one of the national groups representing First Nations people. The AFN estimates that almost one-third of the existing on-reserve housing stock requires major repair or replacement.

In cities and towns, First Nations people face poverty and discrimination. Aboriginal households are three times more likely to be living in poverty than non-Aboriginal households. Combined with the lack of rental vacancies and rising rents throughout Canada, it adds up to a major crisis.

In the 1970s and 1980s, the federal government set targets for urban Aboriginal housing projects. About 10,000 units were developed before the federal programs were cancelled in 1993, according to the National Aboriginal Housing Association.

A 1998 study using Statistics Canada data found that Aboriginal women experience higher levels of unemployment than other women, have lower average earnings, tend to have less formal education and have a shorter life expectancy than other women (NHHN, 2001).

## Women and children

About three million women live in poverty in Canada. Single women-led families are among the poorest in the country. "A significant proportion of Canadian women live on low incomes, on their own or with others. [Women] have serious housing difficulties and are suffering because of them," according to Reitsma-Street et al. (2001). "Most discouraging is the realization that the scope and depth of the housing concerns of women living on low incomes have not changed much, despite years of housing policies, laws, and programs by all levels of government, and despite successful strategies to assist people with moderate income to find and keep suitable accommodation" (Reitsma-Street et al., 2001, p. 2).

Canada's housing crisis and homelessness disaster also puts children at risk: "Lack of reasonably priced housing in and of itself poses risks to positive outcomes for children, primarily via the enabling condition of adequate income. Parents stressed by overcrowding, for example, may not parent as well as they might if conditions were more favourable. Similarly, neighbourhoods in which poor housing is the norm are also likely (not necessarily) neighbourhoods with few services, higher than average levels of violence and so on" (Cooper, 2001, p. 7).

## The private sector

As federal and provincial governments in Canada have cut funding for non-market housing in the past decade, they have expected the private sector to take the lead in developing new affordable housing.

This represents a big change from the first 40 years after the second world war, when Canada relied on a strong and successful social housing program to deliver more than 600,000 social housing units for low-income households.

The Ontario government established a Housing Supply Working Group in the late 1990s to advise on this strategy. They tried to put a positive spin on the lack of new affordable development. The government's own advisers noted that the only possibility for new private housing is at the upper end of the rental scale, then said: "even rental development at the high end increases affordability, because it adds to the overall stock, putting downward pressure on rents and freeing up more affordable units as higher income tenants move into the new supply" (OHSWG, 2001). In other words, they claimed that wealthy tenants would abandon existing units to move into the newly-built, even more expensive private housing, and then the vacancies would eventually trickle down to the lowest-income households.

The Ontario government called this "filtering" and it was been the cornerstone of provincial housing policy from 1995 to 2003. But there are three main barriers to "filtering" as a means of delivering new affordable housing:

- Even with massive public subsidies, low-income households still don't have enough money to pay the rents required by private developers to make a "reasonable" return on investment after covering the high costs of developing and managing housing.

- In most parts of the country, even if new high-end rental housing is created, the vacancies created down the rental spectrum by filtering will result in massive rent increases across the board due to lax or non-existent rent regulation laws.
- Recent trends in the rental market show increasing vacancies at the high end. The rental market is flooded with expensive rental units that are sitting empty. No investor would want to build even more units that would remain vacant.

The cost of building a new housing project, or acquiring and renovating an existing building, is high, especially in the big cities of Canada. A review of construction costs prepared by the Federation of Canadian Municipalities (FCM) in 2001 range from a low of $47,000 to acquire an existing building in Halifax (on Canada's east coast) to a high of $132,000 to construct a new building in Vancouver (on Canada's west coast).

While conventional lenders (such as banks or credit unions) will lend a portion of the costs, the amount of capital grant required ranges from $26,000 for the Halifax unit to a high of $93,000 per unit for a new housing project in downtown Toronto.

Without a large capital subsidy (including free or low-cost land, waiving of taxes and fees and outright grants), the rent for the new or renovated housing would be $1,300 or more per month, well beyond the affordable range. Even with a subsidy, rents would still be in the $600 or $700 range in

most major urban areas, which is not affordable to the lowest income households (FCM, 2002).

## The swinging pendulum

Canada has a record of success in delivering a national social housing program that funds affordable social housing units. From the late 1940s to 1993, the federal government (with some cost-sharing from the provinces) funded about 650,000 social housing units. The Ontario government, in Canada's most populous province, funded a social housing program from the mid-1980s to 1995.

Canadian Finance Minister Paul Martin rose in the House of Commons in the spring of 2001 to announce a record federal surplus of $15 billion. A massive amount of money, but he would not commit a single penny to new spending on housing. Instead, Minister Martin—who is now the Prime Minister of Canada—announced plans for what would grow into the biggest tax cut in the history of the country: $100 billion over five years.

The two reasons for the large surplus are:

- spending cuts over the past decade, including cuts to housing programs, and
- increased revenues in recent years from an upturn in the economy.

Canada's federal government began to cut housing spending with the election of the Conservative government of Brian Mulroney in 1984. By 1993, the federal government had cut almost $2 billion from housing programs and had cancelled development of new social housing.

In opposition during this time, the Liberal Party created a housing task force headed by two Members of Parliament, Paul Martin and Joe Fontana. In May of 1990, they issued a scathing indictment of the federal withdrawal from housing. The Liberals promised to restore funding for social housing, including new housing co-ops (Martin and Fontana, 1990).

In the fall of 1993, the Liberals were elected to the government of Canada, and have been the governing party since then. MP Martin was promoted to Finance Minister, the second most powerful position in the government next to the Prime Minister.

Although Minister Martin controlled the books, he refused to implement the recommendations of his own task force of three years earlier. Not only did Minister Martin fail to keep his promise to bring in a new national housing strategy, but in his 1996 budget, the Finance Minister announced plans for the federal government to abandon entirely its responsibility for social housing.

The federal government has signed housing transfer agreements with most of the provinces and territories. While the federal government will continue to fund existing housing projects after administration has been shifted to the provinces and territories, it has locked itself into a steady and growing decline in housing spending.

The federal government currently spends about $1.7 billion subsidizing the hundreds of thousands of social housing units built until the program was cancelled in 1993. Funding will start to decline by 2010, falling to about $800 million by 2024 and then to zero by 2036. The annual drop is fairly small, but the cumulative amount represents the complete withdrawal of all federal funding for housing over three decades (CHRA, 2003).

In addition to an overall budgetary surplus, the federal government is also running a large surplus with its national housing agency, the Canada Mortgage and Housing Corporation (CMHC). The agency sells commercial insurance services and it is a lucrative business, especially the return on investments of the assets. In 2002, CMHC had a gross income of $854 million, and paid $310 million in income taxes, for a net income that was returned to the government of $544 million (CMHC, 2002).

But not one penny of that surplus in the housing agency budget will go to desperately needed new housing.

In 1996, the federal housing minister was in Istanbul to commit her government to support the principles of the Habitat Agenda, with its goal of "housing for all." At home, the same minister was presiding over a rapidly deteriorating housing policy.

During the 1990s, the federal government has:

- cancelled all spending on desperately needed new social housing,
- cut spending from existing housing programs,
- transferred its responsibility for administration of housing programs to the provinces and territories,
- locked itself into a downward spiral of decreasing spending.

All this in a decade that ended with the first of a growing number of budgetary surpluses.

The shrinking federal role in housing has been bad, but the record of Canada's subnational governments (provinces and territories) has been terrible. In the six years from fiscal 1993 to fiscal 1999, the federal government cut about $17 million from its overall social housing spending of $1.9 billion. The provinces, over the same time period, cut $463 million from their combined

## Table 14.1: Spending on housing by Canada, provinces and territories

| | 1993–1994 ($ millions) | 1999–2000 ($ millions) | Dollar change | Percent change |
|---|---|---|---|---|
| Newfoundland | 18.1 | 8.0 | -10.1 | -55.8 |
| Prince Edward Island | 2.3 | 3.2 | +0.9 | +39.1 |
| Nova Scotia | 24.2 | 14.3 | -9.9 | -40.9 |
| New Brunswick | 32.7 | 31.8 | -0.9 | -2.8 |
| Quebec | 286.3 | 288.3 | +2 | +0.7 |
| Ontario | 1,140.9 | 837.1 | -303.8 | -26.6 |
| Manitoba | 46.6 | 43.2 | -3.4 | -7.3 |
| Saskatchewan | 43.1 | 40.5 | -2.6 | -6.0 |
| Alberta | 287.3 | 93.2 | -194.1 | -67.6 |
| British Columbia | 83.4 | 90.9 | +7.5 | +9.0 |
| NWT / Nunavut | 69.7 | 114.4 | +44.7 | +64.1 |
| Yukon | 4.9 | 11.1 | +6.2 | +126.5 |
| Total—provinces, territories | 2,039.5 | 1,576.0 | -463.5 | -22.7 |
| Canada (CMHC) | 1,944.9 | 1,927.9 | -17 | -0.9 |
| Total—all Canada | 3,984.4 | 3,503.9 | -480.5 | -12.1 |

Source: Canada Mortgage and Housing Corporation. (2002). *Opening doors: Annual report.*

spending, bringing the total in fiscal 1999 down to $1.6 billion (Carter, 2000).

The three territories and just three provinces spent more money on housing, but the seven other provinces slashed housing spending. Most of the cuts came from two of the richest provinces—the oil-producing province of Alberta and the manufacturing heartland of Ontario. Both made hundreds of millions of dollars in housing cuts, even though their revenues were booming.

Ontario has downloaded both the cost and the administration of provincial social housing programs to cash-strapped local authorities. Alberta cancelled its entire seniors' supportive housing program.

Under Canada's constitution, jurisdiction over property matters (which includes laws that guarantee security of tenure, rent regulation laws, anti-discrimination statutes and other issues related to rental housing) is assigned to the provinces.

Tenant households across the country face a patchwork of laws offering a diminishing amount of legal protection. Ontario started the decade with the strongest tenant protection laws in the country. The province had laws to protect rental housing from conversion to non-rental uses (to protect affordable housing), rent regulation laws to protect tenants from sharp practices by landlords, security of tenure and a package of anti-discrimination laws. Most of those laws have been gutted or cut entirely.

Canada's vanishing housing policies have attracted critical comments from two separate United Nations' committees in recent years. Both the U.N. Human Rights Committee and the U.N. Committee on Economic, Social and Cultural Rights have called on governments in Canada to take positive steps to correct violations of international commitments.

The federal government has taken several positive steps in recent years in response to growing political pressure from national and local advocacy groups, along with opinion polls that show housing is a key issue for a majority of Canadians.

In December of 1999, it announced a national homelessness strategy, including the Supporting Community Partnerships Initiative (SCPI)—$753 million over three years. Using SCPI and other funding, innovative projects have created transitional housing and services in several cities.

In November of 2001, the federal government signed the Affordable Housing Framework Agreement with every province and territory. The federal government agreed to provide $680 million over five years. Provinces and territories agreed to match the federal dollars. However:

- most provinces are not paying their matching share. For instance, the federal government is contributing $245 million in Ontario, but the province is only providing $20 million.
- the definition of "affordable" has been changed to "average market rents," so the new housing will be rented at existing market. However, as many as two-thirds of renters cannot afford average rents, which puts the housing out of the reach of those who need it the most.
- even if the framework agreement was fully funded, the total number of units would be well short of the amount required to meet the massive and growing need for affordable rental housing.

The combined impact from the withdrawal of the private sector in the 1970s, and the government in the 1990s, led to a serious and growing shortfall in the supply of affordable housing by the end of the 20th century. At the same time, the gap between rich and poor Canadians was growing more extreme, exacerbating the affordability crisis.

## One percent solution

In 1998, the Toronto Disaster Relief Committee launched a national campaign called the One Percent Solution. The campaign grew out of an observation by Dr. David Hulchanski, a leading Canadian housing scholar, who noted that in the early 1990s, the federal, provincial, territorial, and municipal governments spent about one percent of their overall budgets on housing. The TDRC figured that doubling that amount—or adding an additional one percent—would create an envelope to fund a comprehensive, national housing strategy (TDRC, 1998).

In its 2000 pre-budget submission to the House of Commons Standing Committee on Finance, the Toronto Disaster Relief Committee joined with the National Housing and Homelessness Network (NHHN) to renew the call for implementation of the One Percent Solution:

The enhanced funding envelope (combined with existing housing spending) would allow the federal government to adopt a comprehensive national housing strategy with these key elements:

- supply (increase the number of rental units).
- affordability (ensure the new units are affordable to the households that need the new housing the most).
- supports (programs for those that require special services).

- rehabilitation (funding to maintain housing to a proper standard).
- emergency relief (special support for people who are already homeless).

The first four are prevention strategies, aimed at ensuring that everyone has access to good quality, affordable housing. The fifth is relief, aimed at providing a basic level of comfort for those who are on the streets and also assistance to help them secure permanent homes. Details of programs aimed at these five elements need to be developed in consultation with public, private and non-profit experts. New programs would have to be targeted to make sure that the housing and services meet the needs of low and moderate-income households (NHHN pre-budget submission, 2002).

The NHHN and its housing partners on the national stage—the Federation of Canadian Municipalities, Co-operative Housing Federation of Canada and the Canadian Housing and Renewal Association—has been successful in convincing the federal government to commit a limited amount of new funding for affordable housing.

But the latest national housing report card from the NHHN, released in November of 2003, noted that the federal government has failed to turn that commitment into real housing, largely because it is relying on federal-provincial cost-sharing (NHHN, 2003). Most provinces and territories appear to be unable or unwilling to match the federal dollars, which means that the hard-won federal commitment has not translated into desperately-needed new homes in most parts of the country.

Of the $1 billion over five years in spending promises made by the federal government, only $88 million had actually been spent on new housing by November of 2003—less than 9% of the total (Mahoney, 2003). The original amount was modest to begin with, and the actual amount that has been delivered has been only a fraction of that. And, even worse, many provinces continue to make housing cuts, which means that housing gains from the new federal money are offset by continuing losses of provincial funding.

---

**Box 14.2**

"The federal government has abandoned its responsibilities with regards to housing problems ... The housing crisis is growing at an alarming rate and the government sits there and does nothing; it refuses to apply the urgent measures that are required to reverse this deteriorating situation ... The federal government's role would be that of a partner working with other levels of government, and private and public housing groups. But leadership must come from one source; and a national vision requires some national direction. Homelessness is only the most visible manifestation of Canada's housing crisis. Though homelessness affects a relatively small percentage of Canadians, it is a reality which is symptomatic of a broader crisis in the supply of affordable housing ... The Task Force was told that though affordable housing is in desperately short supply across the country, the major contributing factor to the current crisis is poverty." Paul Martin, MP, and Joe Fontana, MP, *Finding room: National Liberal Task Force on Housing*, 1990.

---

**Table 14.2: Federal affordable housing program spending, 2001 to 2003**

| Province | Allocation ($m) | Recorded spending ($m) |
|---|---|---|
| Newfoundland and Labrador | $15.14 | 0 |
| Prince Edward Island | $2.75 | 0 |
| Nova Scotia | $18.63 | $0.07 |
| New Brunswick | $14.98 | 0 |
| Quebec | $161.65 | $43.72 |
| Ontario | $244.71 | $1.20 |
| Manitoba | $25.39 | $0.48 |
| Saskatchewan | $22.93 | $0.94 |
| Alberta | $67.12 | $8.50 |
| British Columbia | $88.70 | $26.70 |
| Northwest Territories | $7.54 | $1.89 |
| Yukon Territory | $5.50 | 0 |
| Nunavut | $4.96 | $4.96 |
| Total | $680.00 | $88.48 |

Source: Mahoney, Hon. S, Secretary of State with Responsibility for Canada Mortgage and Housing Corporation. *Letter to National Housing and Homelessness Network with update on spending commitments under the affordable housing program*, December 5, 2003.

The network and other advocates have continued to press the federal government to follow through on its commitments, plus add new spending to create a funding envelope that is large enough to meet the scale of the national need.

# Conclusion

The devastating reality of the nation-wide housing crisis concerns Canadians, even though two-thirds are comfortably housed by global standards. Numerous opinion polls starting in the late 1990s show growing public concern for housing and homelessness issues, and support for increased government funding for solutions. This polling, combined with effective political advocacy, is creating a powerful political dynamic.

The housing history of Canada over the past 100 years shows a cycle of rising concerns, which are eventually met by limited government responses.

The outbreak of disease in Toronto's slums in the early 1900s led to the development of the country's first affordable housing projects (Spruce Court and Bain Co-op—two townhouse developments built in 1913 that continue to provide good quality homes even today).

The appalling conditions in many communities in 1930s led to large-scale development of government-managed public housing starting in the late 1940s.

Concerns about conditions in the public housing projects, along with a more general housing crisis in the late 1960s, led to the national co-op and non-profit housing program of 1973 (which generated hundreds of thousands units until the program was cancelled in 1993).

The affordable housing crisis and homelessness disaster of the late 1990s has led to an emerging patchwork of responses from senior levels of government starting in 2001.

Housing advocates are trying to break this pattern with the One Percent Solution—a permanent, fully-funded comprehensive national housing strategy.

A manufactured response, they argue, is the only solution to a manufactured housing crisis and homelessness disaster.

## Recommended readings

Layton, J. (2000). *Homelessness: The making and unmaking of a crisis*. Toronto: Penguin.
 Jack Layton has been a leader in Toronto and nationally in the struggle for more affordable housing. His book provides a lively overview of the crisis and solutions.

Sewell, J. (1994). *Houses and homes: Housing for Canadians*. Toronto: James Lorimer.
 John Sewell, a former Toronto mayor, has also been both a leading advocate and actively involved in the management of social housing.

Hulchanski, J.D. and Shapcott, M. (2004). *Finding room: Policy options for a Canadian rental housing strategy*. Toronto: Centre for Urban and Community Studies, University of Toronto Press, forthcoming.
 A collection of current research and advocacy on key elements of the affordable housing crisis.

Carver, H. (1948). *Houses for Canadians: A study of housing problems in the Toronto area*. Toronto: University of Toronto Press.
 A classic in Canadian housing literature, especially chapter 6—the "ultimate housing problem," which is available online at www.urbancenter.utoronto.ca/pdfs/policyarchives/1948HumphreyCarver.pdf.

Rose, Albert (1958). *Regent Park*. Toronto: University of Toronto Press.
 Another classic of Canadian housing literature, which includes a detailed outline of housing initiatives at the local and national levels from the 1930s to the 1950s.

## Related websites

Housing Again—www.housingagain.web.net/
 A site maintained by housing advocates that includes an excellent on-line library with hundreds of articles on housing and related issues.

Centre for Urban and Community Studies—www.urbancentre.utoronto.ca/
 The University of Toronto research centre publishes policy-relevant research on local, national, and international housing and urban issues.

Toronto Disaster Relief Committee—www.tdrc.net/
 A local housing and homelessness advocacy group with an excellent resources section with material from the TDRC, Housing and Homelessness Network in Ontario, and the National Housing and Homelessness Network.

# Chapter Fifteen

———●———

# HOUSING AND HEALTH

### Toba Bryant

## Introduction

The *Ottawa Charter for Health Promotion* recognizes shelter as a basic prerequisite for health (World Health Organization, 1986). Yet, Canadian political leaders and the housing policies they offer are failing to meet the housing needs of many Canadians. As documented in Federal NDP leader Jack Layton's book on homelessness, the number of Canadians who sleep in the streets, use temporary shelters, or spend more than 30% or 50% of their income on housing is increasing at alarming levels (Layton, 2000). These developments have clear implications for the health of Canadians.

The first objective of this chapter is to provide the available evidence on how housing issues affect health. The first and most obvious question to be considered is *What is the effect of homelessness on health?* The second question is *What is the effect of poor housing conditions on health?* The third question is *How does spending an excessive amount of income on housing influence the quality of other social determinants of health?* Tying all of these questions together is the concept of housing insecurity and its effects on health.

The second objective of this chapter is to consider why health researchers and policy-makers have neglected housing as a health issue. Given the existence of a housing crisis, it would be expected that housing and health would be well-developed areas of Canadian research and policy concern. This does not appear to be the case. There is housing and health research in Canada, but much of it is carried out within rather limited models that examine how physical aspects of dwellings affect health. The role housing plays in relation to other social determinants of health is rarely considered. New ways of thinking about, and researching, how housing and health are related are presented.

The third objective of this chapter is to consider how policymakers can be influenced to address housing and health issues. There are policy options than can improve housing, thereby improving health. To see successful implementation of these options requires understanding how policy-makers use different forms of evidence to develop housing policies to support health.

## The housing crisis in Canada

A key issue in Canada, particularly in urban areas, is the lack of affordable private rental accommodation and the inability of the private rental market to produce affordable units. Rental housing affordability emerged as a major issue in the 1980s and remained largely unaddressed through the 1990s. Many analysts attribute the growing number of homeless and housing insecure in Canada to reduced state provision of social housing.

Indeed, Canada has the most private-sector-dominated, market-based system of any western nation. It also has the smallest social housing sector of any western nation with the exception of the U.S. A history of Canadian housing policy to the present is available (Hulchanski, 2002).

Other contributing factors to the crisis are continuing high levels of unemployment and lack of affordable rental accommodation. The result is increasing numbers of families and individuals with insecure housing. Growing numbers of Canadians are underhoused, living in motels, dependent on the shelter system or living on the street (Layton, 2000). Three aspects of the housing crisis have implications for health: homelessness, the experience of poor living conditions, and the effects of housing insecurity on other social determinants of health.

---

**Box 15.1: Women and housing in Canada: Barriers to equality**

Women and children are the fastest growing group using shelters. The increasing number of women in shelters is only a small fraction of women across Canada experiencing housing crises and homelessness in diverse ways—living with the threat of violence because there are no other housing options; sacrificing other necessities such as food, clothing, and medical needs to pay rent or to make mortgage payments or moving into overcrowded accommodation with family or friends.

The homelessness crisis facing women is also a poverty crisis and cannot be understood merely in relation to scarcity of appropriate housing. It is important to consider the interconnections between housing programs, subsidy eligibility and allocation, income security, access to credit, security of tenure, transportation, and service needs.

The withdrawal of federal funding for new social housing, culminating in the 1993 freeze in federal contributions to social housing and the cancellation of funding for any new social housing (except for on-reserve Aboriginal housing), had a particularly adverse effect on women, who are most likely to be in need of housing subsidies.

In most provinces and territories, the National Child Benefit Supplement is clawed back from social assistance recipients by agreement with the federal government. Despite the fact that women on social assistance may be most in need of this benefit and most unable to pay for housing and related expenses, they are excluded from the federal government's only initiative to address child (family) poverty.

Changes that have been put in place to Employment Insurance eligibility have placed many women at increased risk of eviction when dealing with loss of a job, pregnancy or disability. This is an area of direct federal responsibility for protecting the needs of women for income and housing security.

Source: *Women and housing in Canada: Barriers to equality.* (2002). Ottawa: Women's Program, Centre for Equality Rights in Accommodation. Online at www.equalityrights.org/docs/barriers_exec_summary.doc

---

## Homelessness

Shelter use is up across Canada. As of 2000, Layton (2000) reports that on an average night, shelter use was approximately 300 people in Vancouver, 1,200 in Calgary, 460 in Ottawa, and 4,000 in Toronto. In 1998, it was estimated that the number of homeless people in Canada on any given night is in the order of the tens of thousands (Hwang, 2001). And since then there have been increases in every city in Canada. Wherever more recent data is available, sharp increases are apparent (City of Calgary, 2002).

## Increased incidence of poor living conditions

CMHC created the term "core need" to track the number of households unable to afford suitable, adequate, rental accommodation in their community. Core housing need exists when one or more of the following issues is present (Layton, 2000):

- Affordability—tenants pay more than 30% of their gross income on their housing.
- Suitability—tenants live in overcrowded conditions, whereby household size exceeds recommended actual space.
- Adequacy—tenants' homes lack full bathroom facilities, or require significant repairs.

Recent data from CMHC indicates that over 1.7 million Canadian tenant households are in core need situations. These individuals had average incomes of $14,600 and are paying out, on average, 47% of income on rent. This leaves only $645 a month for other expenses such as food, health products, education, transportation, and other living costs.

## Weakening of other social determinants of health as a result of housing insecurity

In 1996, 43% of Canadian tenant households spent more than 30%, and 21% of Canadian households spent more than 50% of their income on rent. By 2000, the situation improved slightly with 40% spending more than 30% of gross income on rent (Statistics Canada, 2004). Tenants paying more than 50% of incomes on rent are in a revenue/expense structure that makes losing their housing a real possibility (Layton, 2000). Such conditions have both direct material effects on health and increase stress and insecurity, another established determinant of health (Brunner and Marmot, 1999).

## Housing and health

A recent review of the housing and health literature concluded that research has focused on, and identified findings in, four key areas (Dunn, 2000). Homeless people experience poor health status and have limited access to health care. Problematic dimensions of dwellings are associated with adverse physical and mental health outcomes. Stresses linked with unaffordable and/or inadequate housing can affect health status. Unhealthy individuals are disadvantaged in the housing market and are directed into substandard housing conditions.

The focus here is on three variants of these issues: the health effects of homelessness, how poor housing conditions influence health, and how spending excessive amounts of available income on housing influences health. The experience of homelessness and poor housing conditions are placed into a broader context of how individuals in Canada systematically differ in their access to economic and social resources. Poor housing is just one indicator of potential disadvantage in Canadian society.

The link between one's housing situation and health seems obvious (see Box 15.2). Homelessness, inadequate, and insecure housing have effects on health and well-being. While most of those who are homeless appear to be men, most of those living in poor housing conditions or insecure situations are women with children.

## Homelessness and health

It would hardly seem necessary to argue the case that housing—and homelessness in particular—are health issues, yet surprisingly few Canadian studies have considered it as such. In the U.K.—where the housing and health research tradition is more established—numerous studies have shown strikingly high incidences of physical and mental health problems among homeless people as compared to the general population. Among 1,280 homeless people in the U.K. who used hostels, bed and breakfast accommodation, day centres, and soup runs, numerous problems were more common than among the general population (Bines, 1994). Table 15.1 shows these data as comparisons with a representative sample of U.K. residents whose death rates are calculated as standardized—taking into account age and gender—morbidity ratios with a value of 100. All rates were higher than the general population with those sleeping on the street having the highest likelihood of experiencing these afflictions.

Many other studies find much greater incidence of a variety of conditions and ailments among the homeless population (see Hwang, 2001). These include greater incidence of mental illness, HIV infection, and physical violence (Dunn, 2000). A Toronto survey of homeless people found much higher risk than the general population for chronic respiratory diseases, arthritis or rheumatism, hypertension, asthma, epilepsy, and diabetes (Ambrosio et al., 1992). Tuberculosis is more common among the homeless in the U.K. (Ramsden et al., 1988) and Canada (Hwang, 2001).

Homeless people are at greater risk of premature death (Shaw et al., 1999). In the U.S., being without housing shortens life expectancy by 20 years. The average age of death of homeless people in Boston is 47 years and in Georgia, 46 years. In the U.K., it is 42 years. In Toronto, homeless people die at a younger age than the general population. Between 1979 and 1990, 71%

---

**Box 15.2: *Three evils of inadequate housing***

A pamphlet published in 1944 quotes the Chief Medical Officer at the then new Ministry of Health in United Kingdom at the time on the three "evils" of inadequate housing: "There is *diminished personal cleanliness and physique* leading to debility, fatigue, unfitness, and reduced powers of resistance. A second result of bad housing is that the *sickness rates* are relatively high, particularly for infectious, contagious, and respiratory diseases. Thirdly, the general *death-rates* are higher and the expectation of life is lower. The evidence is overwhelming, and it comes from all parts of the world—the worse people are housed the higher will be the death rate."
—J.N. Morris, *Health, No. 6: Handbooks for discussion Groups.* London: Association for Education in Citizenship. Reprinted in M. Shaw, "Health and housing: A lasting relationship," *Journal of epidemiology and community health* 55(2001), p. 291.

---

Social Determinants of Health

## Table 15.1: Standardized morbidity ratios[1] for reported health problems for hostel users and rough sleepers (Bines, 1994)

| Health problem | Hostels and B and Bs | Sleeping rough day centres | Soup runs |
|---|---|---|---|
| Musculoskeletal problems | 153 | 185 | 221 |
| Wounds, skin ulcers or other skin complaints | 105 | 189 | 298 |
| Chronic chest or other breathing problems | 183 | 259 | 365 |
| Fits or loss of consciousness | 651 | 2109 | 1892 |
| Frequent headaches | 264 | 338 | 365 |

[1] SMRs for the general population are 100.

Source: Bines, W. (1994). *The health of single homeless people*. York: Centre for Housing Policy, University of York.

of homeless people who died were less than 70 years old as compared to 38% in the general population (Kushner, 1998). A study of 9,000 men who used shelters in 1995 showed young homeless men in Toronto were eight times more likely to die than men of the same age in the general population (Hwang, 2000). Keyes and Kennedy found UK homeless people to be 34 times more likely to commit suicide while Grenier reported a 35 times greater risk of suicide among the homeless (Shaw et al., 1999).

It is sometimes argued that these health outcomes cannot be clearly attributed to being homeless as their presence may precede the experience of homelessness. It is clear that "while some health conditions may precede homelessness, it certainly is the case that the daily conditions of homelessness, both material and psychosocial, compound existing health problems, cause additional problems, (such as problems with feet and respiratory illness), and make access to healthcare more problematic" (Shaw et al., 1999, p. 232).

# Poor housing conditions and health

An extensive review of the health effects of housing conditions categorized findings as being either definitive, strong, possible, or weak (Hwang et al., 1999). *Definitive* findings were seen for health effects associated with the presence of lead, asbestos, poor heating systems, and lack of smoke detectors. *Strong/definitive* findings were seen for presence of radon, house dust mites, cockroaches, and cold and heat. *Strong* findings were seen for environmental tobacco smoke. *Possible* findings were seen for dampness and mould, high rise structures, overcrowding and high density, poor ventilation, and poor housing satisfaction. This review used a narrow set of criteria for isolating the effects of these factors independent of the presence of other factors, an issue discussed in following sections.

Many studies have investigated the effect of poor housing conditions such as inadequate heating and dampness on health. A U.K. survey of older people reported 25%

were not using as much heat as they would have liked because of cost (Savage, 1988). Studies have confirmed that dampness in homes contributes to, and exacerbates, respiratory illness. Strachan (1988) found children living in homes with damp and mould in Edinburgh had increased risk of developing wheezing and chesty coughs. Another study found higher levels of several symptoms for both child and adults in damp and mouldy houses as compared to those living in dry dwellings (Platt et al., 1989).

It is difficult to separate the effects of any single variable or sets of variables upon health, as indicators of disadvantage—poverty, poor housing, preexisting illness—frequently cluster together. One study was able to do this. In *Home sweet home: The impact of poor housing on health*, Marsh and colleagues (1999) used a lifespan approach to examine the link between housing and health. The study was based on an analysis of longitudinal data that examined the link between housing and health among more than 13,000 citizens. Housing conditions played a significant and independent role in health outcomes.

Greater housing deprivation shows a dose-response relationship—the worse the conditions, the greater the health effects—to severe/moderate ill health at age 33. Those who experienced overcrowded housing conditions in childhood to age 11 had higher likelihood of infectious disease as adults. In adulthood, overcrowding was also linked to increased likelihood of respiratory disease. Living in poor housing in the past and in the present make independent contributions to the likelihood of poor health.

Another study of childhood housing conditions and later mortality showed poorer housing conditions to be generally associated with increased adult mortality in selected

areas in the U.K. (Dedman et al., 2001). Statistically significant associations were found between lack of private indoor tapped water supply and increased mortality from coronary heart disease, and between poor ventilation and overall mortality.

## The effects of excessive spending on shelter on other social determinants of health

When spending on housing becomes excessive there is less money available for other needs. A Canada Mortgage and Housing Corporation survey compared welfare incomes with rental costs in Toronto (CMHC, 2001). The average monthly gross welfare income in 2001 for a single adult with one child aged 1 to 12 years was $957. For two adults with two children, it was $1,178. At the same time, rent for an average 1-bedroom apartment was $866 and for a 2-bedroom apartment was $1,027. This left less than $100 a month to cover food and other expenses. Clearly, having little after-rent income makes it difficult to cover other important expenses such as food, thereby contributing directly to food insecurity as well as housing insecurity, malnutrition, and consequent poor health. Excessive spending on housing reduces amounts to be spent on other social determinants of health.

This situation was clearly described in a recent report on the impacts of housing insecurity upon children's health (Watt, 2003). Thirty percent of Canadian families who rent have affordability—less money than needed for other expenses—problems. Fifty-eight percent of lone-parent—usually female-led—families who rent have affordability issues and if the parent of these lone-parent families is under 30 years of age, the figure rises to 76%. The striking rise in

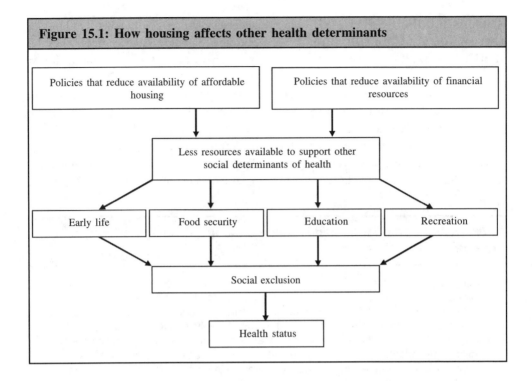

Figure 15.1: How housing affects other health determinants

| Policies that reduce availability of affordable housing | Policies that reduce availability of financial resources |

Less resources available to support other social determinants of health

| Early life | Food security | Education | Recreation |

Social exclusion

Health status

food bank use in Canada is also being attributed to continuing housing inadequacy and its impacts upon available monetary resources among the working and non-working poor (Daily Bread Food Bank, 2002). Figure 15.1 shows how housing insecurity and housing inadequacy impacts upon other social determinants of health.

Little housing research places the experience of homelessness or insecure housing into this broader context (Bryant, 2003). There is little research that considers how insecure housing and related health effects are integral to issues related to inequalities in material resources that exist among the population. Another way of putting this is to ask the question *How does the experience of poor housing reflect the general experience of being materially deprived within a society?* This places the issue of the clustering of disadvantage among

individuals into focus and how poor housing is part of a common pathway to poor health together with other indicators of economic and social disadvantage (Dunn, 1998; Hwang et al., 1999; Shaw et al., 1999).

There are significant health inequalities across the entire socio-economic spectrum in Canada. These inequalities are related to differences in access to material resources necessary for health including housing. Housing research has tended to focus narrowly on the concrete aspects of housing such as homelessness and material aspects of housing poverty (Dunn, 2000). There is a need for research that recognizes that housing is both part of and contributor to the social gradient in health by which Canadians of different income levels differ in health status. The goal is to understand the sources of disadvantage that manifests itself across the socio-economic spectrum.

## Reasons for the neglect and narrow focus of housing and health research

Despite such calls for an expanded analysis of housing and health issues, such research is uncommon in Canada. One reason may be the difficulties such research presents for those trained in traditional epidemiological methods. Epidemiological models attempt to understand the relationships between housing and health, but existent models may be insufficient to capture the complexity of these relationships. Epidemiologists argue it is necessary to isolate specific causes of an outcome such as poor health status. In the case of housing and health, this can be difficult if not impossible as housing disadvantage is associated with numerous other indicators of disadvantage (Box 15.3).

---

**Box 15.3: Traditional epidemiological model of housing effects on health**

Epidemiology is the study of the distribution and determinants of diseases and injuries in human populations. Epidemiologists frequently aim to identify the unique causal effects of single variables upon health outcomes through various analytical procedures. Identifying unique health effects of housing does not easily lend itself to such a model. Living in disadvantaged housing circumstances is associated with other indicators of disadvantage. Indeed, Shaw et al. argue that: "health inequalities are produced by the clustering of disadvantage—in opportunity, material circumstances, and behaviours related to health across people's lives" (1999, p. 65).

Epidemiologists therefore have tended to focus on aspects of housing and health that can be isolated for measurement such as the presence of mould and the development of respiratory infections in children, or overcrowding and its impact on mental health. But its models attempt to identify the effects of these factors independent of the contextual variables associated with disadvantage in general. Many problems are associated with this methodology.

Many studies have investigated the relationship between housing and health and have pointed to the confounding factors that make such research difficult. People in poor housing suffer many deprivations rendering it difficult to assess any one risk factor. In addition, the direction of cause and effect is often unclear. People with pre-existing ill health tend to live in substandard housing because of their low income. All of these factors contribute to methodological difficulties in designing and conducting appropriate research. Figure 15.2 is an example of a traditional epidemiological model that could be deployed to examine the relationship between housing and health.

Figure 15.2: Traditional epidemiological model

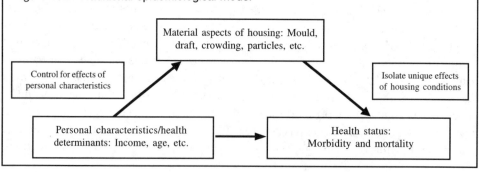

---

The model in Figure 15.2 identifies the material conditions of housing such as mould and draft as the area of interest. Studies attempt to control for the effects of personal characteristics of research participants. It then separates the unique effects of housing conditions from other potential variables that may influence health. To confirm such associations and identify causal relationships between variables, experiments or controlled trials would generally be carried out. Such activities are usually not possible for investigating housing and health.

The relationships investigated in such models do not explain how people end up in poor housing and the effects of housing on the other determinants of health. Attempts to identify the unique effect of poor housing are unable to measure or capture the complexity and interaction among the social determinants of health. *Some of these problems occur as a result of the rigid criteria of bio-medical research, particularly in establishing causal mechanisms, which contradicts the more ethnographic nature of research on the social causes of illness* (Wilkinson, 1999, p. 3). These models also focus on individuals instead of considering the effects of various policies and programs

on groups within society. They rarely consider the effects of income on both housing quality and health. They may end up blaming individuals for their poor housing conditions instead of addressing larger structural issues—such as housing policy—that may contribute to their housing circumstances.

Income affects the type of housing people have. If people have low income, they are likely to live in poor housing. High income increases choices for housing and influences general living conditions. Income and housing insecurity also create stress.

## An expanded model of the housing and health relationship

There is overwhelming evidence that social and environmental conditions determine the presence of health-damaging stress (Brunner and Marmot, 1999). Especially important conditions are the availability of adequate housing and income. Lack of monetary resources is frequently related to public policy decisions that reduce the availability of both affordable housing and monetary resources. Figure 15.3 shows how these factors come together to influence health.

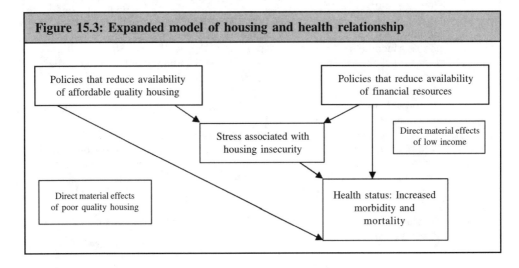

Figure 15.3: Expanded model of housing and health relationship

Policies that reduce availability of affordable quality housing

Policies that reduce availability of financial resources

Stress associated with housing insecurity

Direct material effects of low income

Direct material effects of poor quality housing

Health status: Increased morbidity and mortality

Researchers in Britain are leaders in investigations of how material deprivation creates health-damaging stress (Davey Smith, 2003). In fact, Brunner and Marmot (1999) report that social and psychological circumstances can "seriously damage" health in the long term. Chronic anxiety, insecurity, low self-esteem, social isolation, and lack of control over home and work weakens mental and physical health. The human body has evolved to react to emergencies. This reaction triggers a whole range of stress hormones that affect the cardiovascular and immune systems.

The ability to respond to a crisis is highly adaptive and can save life in the short term. However, if the biological stress reaction system is triggered too often and for too long, as it is for people living in poor or insecure housing and on low income, it results in considerable health damage. This includes depression, vulnerability to infection, diabetes, high blood pressure, and build up of cholesterol in blood vessel walls, with the related risks of heart attack and stroke. Individuals who are materially disadvantaged and experience income, housing, and food insecurity experience greater stress with associated increased risk of morbidity and premature death.

## Towards the future: Understanding the complexities of the housing and health relationship

There are many innovative models for examining the relationship between housing

---

**Box 15.4:** *Housing as a socio-economic determinant of population health: A research framework*

Canadian geographer James Dunn and others identified knowledge gaps in the understanding of the housing and health relationship (Dunn et al., 2002). Dunn argues that, *"Housing, as a central locus of everyday life patterns, is likely to be a crucial component in the ways in which socio-economic factors shape health"* (p. iii). The framework identifies three dimensions of housing relevant to health.

1) "Material dimensions" refer to the physical integrity of the home such as the state of repair; physical, biological, and chemical exposures in the home, and housing costs. Housing costs are critical because they are one of the largest monthly expenditures most people face. When housing costs eat up most of people's income, it affects other aspects of their lives.
2) "Meaningful dimensions" refer to sense of belonging and control in the home. Home is also an expression of social status—prestige, status, pride, and identity—all of which are enhanced by home ownership. These dimensions also provide for the expression of self-identity, and signify permanence, stability, and continuity in everyday life.
3) "Spatial dimensions" refer to a home and its immediate environment. For example, the proximity of a home to services, schools, public recreation, health services, and employment. This also includes systematic exposure to health hazards—toxins in the environment, asbestos insulation, etc. This dimension introduces the need for understanding geographic aspects of neighbourhoods and the kind of housing that is found within them. These concepts should stimulate new ways of Canadian thinking about and studying the role that housing plays in health.

Social Determinants of Health

and health. Box 15.4 provides one example. Interrelationships among housing and other determinants of health must be considered as should policy decisions that affect the presence of material resources such as income and affordable housing. Ethnographic studies of people's housing experiences could document the meaning that housing provides to people and how these affect health. Finally geographic studies are necessary to consider the spatial dimensions of housing and how these interact with other health determinants to influence health.

## Introducing the policy dimension into housing and health studies

As shown earlier in Figures 15.1 and 15.3, the availability and cost of housing have direct material effects on health. But the availability of both affordable housing and other economic resources are directly influenced by policy decisions made by governments. Both types of policy decisions contribute to housing insecurity, increased stress, morbidity and mortality, and increased incidence of social exclusion, illness, and disease.

Housing advocacy groups have brought forward solutions to the housing crisis, in particular to increase the availability of affordable housing and eradicate homelessness. The Toronto Disaster Relief Committee (TDRC) developed the One Percent Solution to end the housing crisis (TDRC, 1999). The TDRC argues that if all governments increased their spending on housing by 1% of overall spending, the homelessness crisis could be eliminated in five years. The One Percent Solution calls for three actions by government:

1) Annual funding for housing of $2 billion federally, and another $2 billion among provinces and territories;

2) Restoring and renewing national, provincial and territorial programs to resolve the housing crisis and homelessness disaster;

3) Extending the federal homelessness strategy with immediate funding for new and expanded shelter and services across the country.

Diverse policy strategies must be explored to address the housing crisis. Layton (2000) outlines several strategies developed as part of a Federation of Canadian Municipalities task force. A healthy housing sector should have four components: rental housing; ownership housing; social housing with mixed incomes; and support for people with special needs to enable them to live independently. The National Affordable Housing Strategy should consist of the following:

1) *Flexible Capital Grant Program for Housing*: a locally designed and administered program of initiatives financed by a federal or joint federal/provincial/territorial capital fund;

2) *A Private Rental Program* to stimulate private rental production;

3) *An Investment Pool of Money* to create Affordable Housing by attracting new funding for the development, acquisition or rehabilitation of affordable housing; and

4) *Provincially Administered Income Supplement Programs* to assist tenants who cannot afford private market rents. The program would complement capital grants to reach those most in need.

## Recent policy developments

The health reform reports of Romanow (2002), Kirby (2002), and Mazankowski (2002) all acknowledge the economic burden of illness and the role of social determinants in population health. Kirby recommends assessing federal policies and programs on their impact on the health status of Canadians.

In 2001, the federal and provincial governments signed housing agreements that commit them to building more social housing units. On the first anniversary of the signing of that agreement in November, 2002, the National Housing and Homelessness Network (NHHN) reported that, outside of Quebec, less than 200 new housing units have been built since the housing agreement was signed in November, 2001 (NHHN, 2002). Over half of the provincial governments have yet to fulfil their commitments to build more social housing units. Quebec and the three territories have taken action to match the federal commitment of $680 million over five years. The Network expressed concern that the definition of "affordable housing" has been undermined in the bilateral housing agreements. This weakening of the term will make the rents of many new units unaffordable.

Indeed, Canadians see little governmental activity to address these social determinants of health besides policy proclamations on housing and the other social determinants. Governments are not seriously addressing social and health inequalities and the role housing policy plays in widening these inequalities.

## Understanding the policy change process

An understanding of how these developments came about would help to identify some means of influencing new policy approaches toward housing. The policy framework presented in the next section can be used to consider how policymakers use evidence to inform their housing decisions regarding housing and other related public policy.

This framework was devised to guide case studies on housing policy and health policy changes in Ontario since 1995 (see Figure 15.4). It incorporates elements of different forms of knowledge, the means by which this knowledge can be applied, and those who are likely to apply such knowledge. This framework can serve as a template for analyzing the policy change process on a case by case basis. It also provides insights into a government's general approach to policy change over time. Fuller presentations of the model and its applications are available (Bryant, 2002; Bryant 2003; Bryant, in press).

Government policy is affected by civil society actors such as professional policy analysts (PPA) and citizen activists (CA). PPAs are university-based academics and policy analysts associated with think-tanks such as the Caledon Institute or the Canadian Policy Research Networks. CAs are usually volunteers. Different ways of knowing about a social issue refers to the different types of knowledge. Traditional or instrumental knowledge is derived from scientific or social science studies. Interactive knowledge is knowledge developed through dialogue. It can be local knowledge that residents have about their community such as its history and customs. Critical knowledge raises questions about social justice and begins to address how social structures influence the distribution of power and resources, questioning the organization of society and challenging the distribution of wealth and political power.

Different ways of using knowledge about a social issue are reflected in the

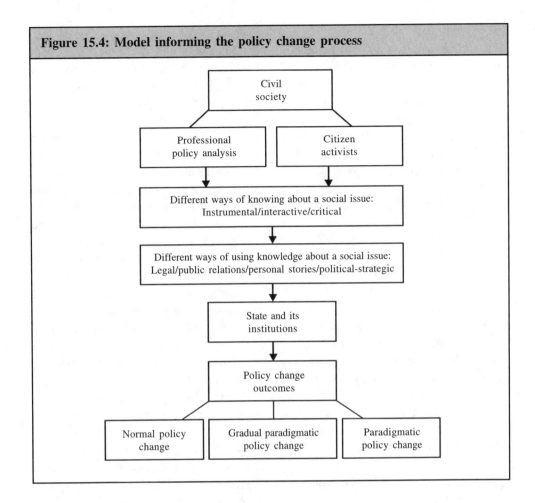

different strategies devised to present knowledge. Four strategies can be used to influence government policy and each of these strategies may be necessary to influence policy change in the housing area:

- Legal Approach refers to the use of legal knowledge, argumentation, and judicial rulings to convey knowledge about a social issue.
- Public Relations is marketing knowledge in order to target a message to a specific audience.
- Personal stories are the use of anecdotal evidence or the stories of individuals to illustrate the effects

of specific policies and programs or of a public issue.

- Political-Strategic is knowledge of how to use the political system to achieve particular policy change goals and objectives.

Finally, the last segment of the model identifies three different patterns of policy change. Routine or normal policy change is a change in policy instruments or policy settings such as a change in rental increases allowed (Howlett and Ramesh, 1995). In normal policy change, the overall policy goals and objectives remain the same. In contrast, paradigmatic policy change is a radical shift in the overall goals and objectives of a policy area, such as a shift from rent regulation such as rent control to vacancy decontrol or other methods of rent deregulation. Gradual policy change can be a series of routine policy changes over time that, taken together, signify paradigmatic policy change (Coleman et al., 1997). The framework attempts to address the following questions relevant to the consideration of housing policy and health in Canada:

- Who is trying to influence policy change?
- What type of knowledge can be used to communicate concerns and issues?
- How can this knowledge be used to influence policy change?
- How receptive is the government to these messages and to the messengers?
- What dynamics affect the receptivity of government to the messengers and the perspectives they present?
- What is the likelihood of achieving policy change?

In the case of Canadian housing policy, political ideologies of governments are significant barriers to progressive housing policy change. Housing policy appears to be especially sensitive to political ideology. Since federal and many provincial governments now have a strong pro-privatization and marketization agenda, housing is vulnerable to this agenda since it can be privatized and the public perceives it as a market issue (Bryant, in press).

Also important is the extent to which governments subscribe to neo-liberal approaches that see the market economy as the best allocator of resources and wealth (Coburn, 2000). This view is consistent with the Mulroney and Chretien government policies and the provincial governments of Alberta, British Columbia, and Quebec. The ideology of individualism espoused by Canadian governments and most western nations is strongly associated with notions of "deservingness." Jenkins (1982) argues that individualism can be defined as "a way of looking at the world which explains and interprets events and circumstances mainly in terms of the decisions, actions and attitudes of the individuals involved" (p. 88). In other words, this ideology pathologizes individuals with social problems. This is relevant in the case of people living under conditions of poor or no housing.

The notion of collective responsibility for social responsibility to vulnerable populations is no longer part of the political discourse. Although some consider neo-liberalism to be extreme and therefore temporary, the development of social policy that addresses the housing crisis and other social policy issues has yet to be seen. To date, only municipal governments have taken a strong stand to address housing and homelessness in Canada (see Sandeman et al., 2002; City of Calgary, 2002).

Also influencing housing policy is public perceptions of housing. Housing is an expense that most people are expected to cover themselves. Many low-income Canadians will be life-long tenants. These populations are particularly vulnerable to policy changes in housing and to policies that affect other social determinants of health. They also tend to have poorer health than the general population and homeowners in particular. The current political environment is not receptive to their concerns and impedes action on the social determinants of health such as housing from which these groups would benefit.

# Conclusion

In spite of the ample evidence on the relationship between housing and health, government actions at times are at odds with a social determinants approach to health. Governments are not seriously addressing health inequalities and the role housing policy plays in widening these inequalities. Political strategies are needed to highlight how these health inequalities threaten the health of all Canadians.

To illustrate the difficulties to be surmounted, in 1990, Paul Martin co-authored a Liberal Opposition task force on housing. The report agreed with the need for a strong federal role in housing:

> The federal role in housing must not be a residual one. The connection between housing and other aspects of both social economic policy means that the federal government must take a lead role ... Our market housing system has not responded adequately to all of society's needs ... The Task Force believes that all Canadians have the right to decent housing, in decent surroundings, at affordable prices. (Martin and Fontana, 1990)

After becoming Minister of Finance and well placed to take action on the housing crisis, Martin chose not to implement the task force's recommendations. Whether he will do so as Prime Minister remains to be seen.

# Recommended readings

Marsh, A., Gordon, D., Pantazis, C. and Heslop, P. (1999). *Home sweet home? The impact of poor housing on health*. Bristol: Policy Press.

This study looks in detail at the impact poor housing has on health using data from the National Child Development Study. It provides important information on how housing influences health.

Hwang, S., Fuller-Thomson, E., Hulchanksi, D., Bryant, T., Habib, Y. and Regoeczi, W. (1999). *Housing and population health: A review of the literature*. Ottawa: Canada Mortgage and Housing Corporation.

This report takes a traditional epidemiological approach towards identifying the health effects of housing conditions.

Watt, J. (2003). *Adequate and affordable housing: A child health issue*. Ottawa: Child and Youth Health Network for Eastern Ontario.

This very current report reviews the literature on housing and health with particular emphasis on the effects of housing insecurity on children. Online at www.child-youth-health.net/book%20english%20 revised.pdf.

Golden, A. (1999). *Taking responsibility for homelessness: An action plan for Toronto*. Toronto: City of Toronto. Online at www.city.toronto.on.ca/pdf/homeless_action.pdf.

An exhaustive report on the antecedents and solutions for the homelessness crisis in Canada's largest city.

Canadian Council on Social Development. (2003). *Selected annotated bibliography: Literature addressing the structural and systemic factors contributing to homelessness in Canada*. Online at www21.hrdc-drhc.gc.ca/research/projects/projectslist1_e.asp

The bibliography done for the Federal National Homelessness Initiative contains numerous articles related to health.

## Related websites

Housing and Health Website—www.cme.ucalgary.ca/housingandhealth/

This website was established as part of a Canadian Institute of Population Health research project on housing and health. It contains reports and links to related websites.

BC Homelessness and Health Research Network—www.bchhrn.ihpr.ubc.ca/

The purpose of the Network is to mobilize stakeholders and to develop a collaborative, multidisciplinary program of research around homelessness and health. Funded by the Canadian Institutes of Health Research, the work is initially based out of the Institute of Health Promotion Research at the University of British Columbia.

Toronto Disaster Relief Committee—www.tdrc.net/

The Toronto Disaster Relief Committee is a diverse group of individuals that have declared homelessness to be a national disaster and that Canada must end homelessness by implementing a fully-funded National Housing Program through the One Percent Solution.

The Centre for Urban and Community Studies—www.urbancenter.utoronto.ca/

The Centre promotes and disseminates multidisciplinary research and policy analysis on urban issues in Canada and around the world.

Social Determinants of Health

# Part Four

―――――――●―――――――

# SOCIAL EXCLUSION

T HE ISSUES RAISED in this volume, low income, unstable and poor quality employment, low levels of education and literacy, and food and housing insecurity, are clearly linked to each other. They are linked in that members of a society experiencing one form of deprivation usually experience other forms of deprivation. The issues are also linked in that governmental policy directions contribute to this linking of health-threatening conditions. In this section, the concept of social exclusion is explored as a means of understanding how this clustering comes about and why economic and social conditions in Canada appear to be under threat. Social exclusion is about the societal processes that systematically lead to groups being denied the opportunity to participate in commonly accepted activities of societal membership. It is an integrative concept that provides insights into how and why these groups experience material deprivation and how political, economic, and social conditions contribute to these conditions. In Canada, social exclusion is especially likely among Aboriginals, new Canadians, racialized groups, and women. The incidence of social exclusion has implications not only for the health of populations but also for the smooth functioning of societies. Increases in social exclusion threaten Canadian society and its institutions.

**Grace-Edward Galabuzi** provides an overview of social exclusion as both process and outcome. Social exclusion has four aspects: exclusion from legal processes, acquiring social goods, social production, and economic activities. He carefully outlines the components of social exclusion and the political, economic, and social forces that are driving this process in Canada. Social exclusion is a threat to individual, community, and population health, as well as to social cohesion and economic prosperity. The origins of social exclusion are primarily structural and complicated by racism and discrimination within Canadian society. Galabuzi provides evidence of how social exclusion is especially prevalent among new Canadians and racialized groups making them subject to all the types of material deprivation described in this volume.

**Ronald Labonte** reflects on how the concept of social exclusion—which is primarily focused on how society excludes peoples—has surfaced in Canada as an emphasis upon social inclusion. While few would dispute the need to include marginalized people from participation in Canadian life, a focus upon inclusion runs the risk of denying the sources of exclusion and placing blame for exclusion upon individuals. Labonte asks whether a society that has sytematically excluded people can be expected to include those it has excluded. Social exclusion has material and economic underpinnings. And some benefit from exclusion: when racialized workers receive lower wages, employers reap rewards. Researchers, community workers, and policy-makers can use the concept of social inclusion to advantage, but should maintain a critical eye on the political, economic, and social forces that continue to promote exclusion in Canadian society.

**Chandrakant P. Shah** provides a systematic examination of the health issues facing a particularly socially excluded group, Canada's Aboriginal peoples. Aboriginal peoples show significantly greater incidence of a range of afflictions and premature death from a variety of causes. These issues result from the poor state of any number of social determinants of health and reflect a history of social exclusion from Canadian society. Carefully reviewing what is known about the sources of ill health among Aboriginal Canadians, Shah concludes that improvement in Aboriginal health requires a greater sensitivity to Aboriginal culture, Aboriginal control of health service and other aspects of local government, increased opportunities for the success of Aboriginal peoples in various healthcare professions, and improvement in the socio-economic status of Aboriginal Canadians.

# Chapter Sixteen

———————●———————

# SOCIAL EXCLUSION

### Grace-Edward Galabuzi

Perhaps health is not so much a personal matter but the aftertaste of a society's other activities, the residue of all its policies. (Fernando, 1991, p. 2)

## Introduction

Poor social and economic conditions and inequalities in access to resources and services affect an individual's or group's health and well being. Groups experiencing some form of social exclusion tend to sustain higher health risks and lower health status. According to Health Canada, in Canada such groups include: Aboriginal Peoples, immigrants and refugees, racialized groups, people with disabilities, single parents, children and youth in disadvantaged circumstances, women, the elderly and unpaid caregivers, gays, lesbians, bisexuals, and transgendered people (CIHR, 2002). Poverty is a key cause and product of social exclusion. Its impacts on health status are now well established (Wilkinson, 1996; Wilkinson and Marmot 1998; Kawachi et al., 1999; Ross et al., 2000; Raphael, 1999, 2001). Racial and gender differences in health status tend to reflect differences in social and economic conditions (Wilkinson 1996). The "racialization of poverty" compounds inequalities in material conditions in socially excluded communities.[1] Such documented characteristics of racialized poverty as labour market segregation and low occupation status, high and frequent unemployment status, substandard housing combined with violent or distressed neighbourhoods, homelessness, poor working conditions, extended hours of work or multiple jobs, experience with everyday forms of racism and sexism, lead to unequal health service utilization, and differential health status. Recent research shows that the actual experience of inequality, the impact of relative deprivation and the stress associated with dealing with social exclusion tend to have pronounced psychological effects and to negatively impact health status (Wilkinson, 1996; Kawachi and Kennedy, 2002).

Canadian and international research has begun to confirm the links between the minority status of ethnic, immigrant and racialized groups and low health status (Adams, 1995; Anderson, 1995, 2000; Bolaria and Bolaria, 1994; Shaw et al., 1999; Hyman, 2001; Wilkinson and Marmot, 1998). It is now generally agreed that adverse socio-economic conditions in early life lead to increased health risks in adulthood. According to Health Canada, children whose health status is most at risk tend to live in low-income families, single families, or among racialized group populations, including immigrant and refugee families and Aboriginal families (CIHR, 2002). Racialized community members, recent immigrants and refugee women, men and their children, experience the psycho-social stress of discrimination and racism which contribute to such health problems as hypertension, mental health, and behavioural problems such as substance abuse. Vulnerability to compromised health is now documented even among recent immigrants, who have historically enjoyed higher health status because of the stringent health selection process; research shows a loss of ground over time under conditions of social exclusion (Hyman, 2001; Noh et al., 1999). Recent research also shows that the experience of racism and discrimination puts racialized group members and immigrants at higher risk of mental health problems (Beiser, 1988; OACW, 1990; Dossa, 1999; Noh et al., 1999). Research in women's health suggests similar impacts from gender discrimination (Agnew, 2002; Adams, 1995; Janzen, 1998). Canadian health research and the health system as a whole have not always appreciated the multiple influences on the health status of the affected groups imposed by these various dimensions of social exclusion. At a time when Canada's population growth and stability are increasingly dependant on immigration, with racialized group members now forming 13.5% of the population and growing (Census, 2001) and immigrants now 18.4% and projected to account for 25% of the population by 2015, these issues represent an important area of health policy and research.[2]

## Social exclusion

Social exclusion is used to broadly describe both the structures and the dynamic processes of inequality among groups in society which, over time, structure access to critical resources that determine the quality of membership in society and ultimately produce and reproduce a complex of unequal outcomes (Room, 1995; Byrne, 1999; Guildford, 2000; Duffy, 1997; Shaw et al., 1999; Littlewood, 1999; Madanipour et al., 1998). Social exclusion is both process and outcome. While it has its roots in European social democratic discourse, it has been increasingly embraced by mainstream policy makers concerned about the emergence of marginal subgroups who may pose a threat to social cohesion in industrial societies. In industrialized societies, social exclusion is a by-product of a form of unbridled accumulation whose processes commodify social relations and intensify inequality along racial and gender lines (Byrne, 1999; Madanipour et al., 1998).

White (1998) has referred to four aspects of social exclusion. First, social exclusion from civil society through legal sanction or other institutional mechanisms as often experienced by status and non-status migrants. This conception may include substantive disconnection from civil society and political participation because of material and social isolation, created through systemic forms of discrimination based on race, ethnicity, gender, disability, sexual orientation, and religion. In the post-September 11 era, racial profiling and new notions of national security seem to have exacerbated the experience of this form of social exclusion. Second, social exclusion refers to the failure to provide for the needs of particular groups—the society's denial of (or exclusion from) social goods to particular groups such as accommodation for persons with disability, income security, housing for the homeless, language services, and sanctions to deter discrimination. Third is exclusion from social production, a denial of opportunity to contribute to or participate actively in society's social and cultural activities. And fourth, is economic exclusion from social consumption—unequal access to normal forms of livelihood and economy.

Social exclusion can be experienced by individuals and communities, communities of common bond, and geographical communities. The characteristics of social exclusion tend to occur in multiple dimensions and are often mutually reinforcing. Groups living in low income areas are also likely to experience inequality in access to employment, substandard housing, insecurity, stigmatization, institutional breakdown, social service deficits, spatial isolation, disconnection from civil society, discrimination, and higher health risks. The resulting phenomenon is what some have referred to as one of an underclass culture (Wilson, 1987).

## Social exclusion in the late twentieth and early twenty-first century

Processes of social exclusion intensified in the late twentieth century. The intensification of social exclusion can be traced to the restructuring of the global and national economies which emphasized deregulation and re-regulation of markets, the decline of the welfare state, the commodification of public goods, demographic changes owing to increased global migrations, changes in work arrangements towards flexible deployment, and intensification of labour through longer hours, work fragmentation, multiple jobs, and increasing non-standard forms of work. These developments have intensified exploitation in workplaces, but also urban spatial segregation processes including the gendered and racialized spatial concentrations of poverty, among others. The emergence of a neo-liberal globalized political economic order has redefined the nature of the state, and redrawn the boundaries of citizenship as part of a process that seeks to institutionalize market regulation of social relations in societies around the world (Jenson and Papillon, 2000; Gill, 1995). Under this neo-liberal order, the social exclusion concept represents a critique of both the commodification of public goods such as health care services, social services, education and the like, brought about by the dismantling of the welfare state, and the market conditioned response to the resulting marginalization, euphemistically characterized simply as the failure of the individual to utilize their opportunities in the marketplace (Del Castillo, 1994). However, this atomisation of social exclusion is contested. For instance, Yepez Del Castillo has noted that "the many varieties of exclusion, the fears of social explosions to which it gives rise, the dangers of social disruption; the complexity of the mechanisms that cause it, the extreme difficulty of finding solutions, have made it the major social issue of our time" (Del Costillo, 1994, p. 614).

In this policy environment, the social exclusion concept seeks to shift the focus back to the structural inequalities that determine the intensity and extent of marginalization in society. It represents a shift of the burden of social inequality from the individual back to society, defining it as a social relation and allowing for the reassertion of welfare state-type social rights based on the concept of social protection as the responsibility of society and not the individual. It is in that respect that the policy discourse of social inclusion in response to marginalization has began to emerge. Yet, a caution is warranted because there is not necessarily a linear relationship between social exclusion—which seeks to unravel the structures and processes of mar- ginalization—and the more liberal conception of social inclusion, as presently constituted in policy discourse, which promises equal opportunity for all without a commitment to dismantling the historical structures of exclusion (Saloojee, 2002).

## Social exclusion in the Canadian context

In the Canadian context, social exclusion defines the inability of certain subgroups to participate fully in Canadian life due to structural inequalities in access to social, economic, political, and cultural resources arising out of the often intersecting experiences of oppression as it relates to race, class, gender, disability, sexual orientation, immigrant status, and the like. Along with the socio-economic and political inequalities, social exclusion is also characterized by processes of group or individual isolation within and from such key Canadian societal institutions as the school system, the criminal justice system and the health care system, as well as spatial isolation or neigbourhood segregation. These engender experiences of social and economic vulnerability, powerlessness, voicelessness, a lack of recognition and sense of belonging, limited options, diminished life chances, despair, opting out, suicidal tendencies and, increasingly, community or neighbourhood violence. Aside from numerous health

implications, the emergence of the institutional breakdown and normlessness characterized by such phenomena and the turn to an informal economy and community violence represents a threat to social cohesion and economic prosperity.

In Canada, the discourse on social exclusion has tended to focus on Canadians living on low incomes. Guildford's (2000) work on social exclusion and health in Canada is ground breaking but limited because of the focus on the generic low income experiences of social exclusion. Here, we suggest the need to interrogate the multiple dimensions of the phenomena as well as identify the subgroup dimension of the victims of social exclusion, precisely because of the extent to which their experiences are differentiated by the nature of the oppressions they suffer. Social exclusion is an expression of unequal relations of power among groups in society which then determine unequal access to economic, social, political, and cultural resources. The assertion of certain forms of economic, political, social, and cultural privilege, or the normalization of certain ethnocultural norms by some groups occurs at the expense of, and ultimately, marginalization of others. This is especially true in a market regulated society where the impetus for state intervention to reduce the reproduction of inequality is minimal as is increasingly the case under the neo-liberal regime. Social exclusion takes on a time and spatial dimension. In different societies, there are particular groups that are at higher risk of experiencing social exclusion depending on the historical social relations in the societies. In Canada, four groups have been identified as being in that category of special risk: women, new immigrants, racialized group members, and Aboriginal peoples (CIHR, 2002). The focus in this chapter is on the experiences of racialized group members and immigrants.

## Social exclusion, racialized groups, and recent immigrants

"The name Chinatown continues to express the deeply embedded white desire for us to one day return from whence we came." (Pon, 2000, p. 230)

Canada welcomed an annual average of close to 200,000 new immigrants and refugees over the 1990s. Immigration accounted for more than 50% of the net population growth and 70% of the growth in the labour force over the first half of the 1990s (1991–96), and it is expected to account for virtually all of the net growth in the Canadian labour force by the year 2011 (HRDC, 2002). According to the 2001 census, immigrants made up 18.4% of Canada's population, projected to rise to 25% by 2015. Since the shift from a European centred immigration policy in the 1960s, there has been a significant change in the source countries, with over 75% of new immigrants in the 1980s and 1990s coming from the so-called Third world or Global south—the majority of them falling into the category of racialized immigrants.

Racialized groups and recent immigrants encounter processes of marginalization in many spheres of life. The racialization of poverty, in particular, represents two increasingly prevalent intersecting experiences of marginalization faced by Aboriginal peoples, and non-Aboriginal women and men from racialized groups (hereafter referred to as racialized peoples) and immigrant groups. Not only are these groups the subject of these processes of marginalization, they have received very limited treatment in the research on the social determinants of health. The preponderance

of the experiences the chapter explores are those of the non-Aboriginal racialized populations whose experiences with racial and gender inequality, disproportionate low income status, unemployment and underemployment, low occupation status, low standard housing, intensified workplace exploitation, disproportionate residence in neighbourhoods with social deficits etc., render them disproportionately vulnerable to low health status. The persistence of the racial and gender discriminatory structures, income and employment inequality, economic and social segregation, and political and cultural marginalization means that increasingly, a disproportionate number of racialized group members exist within a reality of exclusion from mainstream Canadian society (Galabuzi, 2001).

## Dimensions of social exclusion: The racialization of poverty

The racialized community is divided into Canadian-born members (roughly 33%) and immigrants (about 67%). During the last census period (1996–2001), the growth rate of racialized groups far outpaced that of other Canadians. While the Canadian population grew by 3.9% between 1996–2001, the corresponding rate for racialized groups was 24.6%. Over the same period, the racialized component of the labour force grew by 28.7% for males and 32.3% for females compared to 5.5% and 9% respectively for the Canadian population. Over much of the 1990s, over 75% of Canada's newcomers were members of the racialized group communities. But with that shift has come a noticeable lag in social economic performance among members of the groups. These patterns seem to be holding both during and after the recession years of the late 1980s and early 1990s.

## Box 16.1: The impact of racialization

- A double digit racialized income gap as high as 30% in 1998
- Two to three times higher than average unemployment rates
- Deepening levels of poverty
- Differential access to housing leading to neighbourhood racial segregation
- Disproportionate contact with the criminal justice system (criminalization of youth)
- Higher health risks

These developments have had numerous adverse social impacts, leading to differential life chances for racialized group members.

A most significant development is the one described as the racialization of poverty. The racialization of poverty refers to the emergence of structural features that pre-determine the disproportionate incidence of poverty among racialized group members. What explains these trends are structural changes in the Canadian economy that conspire with historical forms of racial discrimination in the Canadian labour market to create a process of social and economic marginalization. The result is a dispropor-tionate vulnerability to poverty among racialized group communities. Racialized groups are also disproportionately highly immigrant communities and suffer from the impact of the immigration effect. However, current trends indicate that the economic inequality between immigrants and native-born Canadians is becoming greater and more permanent. That was not always the case. In fact, immigrants tended to outperform native born Canadians because of their high educational levels and age advantage.

The racialization of poverty is directly linked to the process of the deepening oppression and social exclusion of racialized and immigrant communities on one hand and the entrenchment of privileged access to economic opportunity for a small but powerful section of the majority population on the other. The concentration of economic, social, and political power that has emerged as the market has become more prominent in social regulation in Canada explains the growing gap between rich and poor as well as the racialization of that gap (Yalnyzian, 1998; Kunz et al., 2001; Galabuzi, 2001; Lee, 2000; Dibbs et al., 1995; Jackson, 2001). Racialized community members and Aboriginal peoples are twice as likely to be poor than other Canadians because of the intensified social and economic exploitation of the racialized and Aboriginal communities whose members have to endure historical racial and gender inequalities accentuated by the restructuring of the Canadian economy and more recently racial profiling. In the midst of the socio-economic crisis that has resulted, the different levels of government have responded by retreating from anti-racism programs and policies that would have removed the barriers to economic equity. The resulting powerlessness and loss of voice has compounded the groups' inability to put issues of social inequality and, particularly, the racialization of poverty on the political agenda.

Social Determinants of Health

## Racialized group members are twice as likely as other Canadians to live in poverty

In 1995, 35.6% members of racialized groups lived under the low income cut off (poverty line) compared with 17.6% in the general Canadian population. The numbers that year were comparable in urban areas— 38% for racialized groups and 20% for the rest of the population, a rate twice as high (Lee, 2000). In 1996, while racialized groups members accounted for 21.6% of the urban population, they accounted for 33% of the urban poor. That same year, 36.8% of women and 35% of men in racialized communities were low-income earners, compared to 19.2% of other women and 16% of other men. In 1995, the rate for children under six living in low income families is an astounding 45 percent—almost twice the overall figure of 26% for all children living in Canada. In Canada's urban centers, in 1996, while racialized groups members account for 21.6% of the population, they account for 33% of the urban poor. The improvements in the economy have not dented the double digit gap in poverty rates. Family poverty rates were similar—in 1998, the rate for racialized groups was 19% and 10.4% for other Canadian families (Lee, 2000; Jackson, 2001).

Some of the highest increases in low income rates in Canada have occurred among recent immigrants. Low-income rates among successive groups of immigrants almost doubled between 1980 and 1995, peaking at 47% before easing up in the late 1990s. In 1980, 24.6% of immigrants who had arrived during the previous five-year period lived below the poverty line. By 1990, the low-income rate among recent immigrants had increased to 31.3%. It rose further to 47.0% in 1995 but fell back somewhat to 35.8% in 2000. In 1998, the annual wages of racialized immigrants were up to one-third less those of other Canadians, partly explaining why the poverty rate for racialized immigrants arriving after 1986 ranged between 36% and 50% (Jackson, 2001). This was happening at a time when average poverty rates have been generally falling in the Canadian population. Studies show that former waves of immigrants were subject to a short term "immigration factor" which over time—not longer than 10 years for the unskilled and as low as 2 years for the skilled—they were able to overcome and either catch up to their Canadian born counterparts or even surpass them in their performance in the economy. Their employment participation rates were as high or higher than the Canadian-born, and their wages and salaries rose gradually to the level of the Canadian-born.

However, recent research indicates persistent and growing difficulties in the labour market integration of immigrants, especially recent immigrants. Rates of unemployment and underemployment are increasing for individual immigrants, as are rates of poverty for immigrant families (Galabuzi, 2001; Ornstein, 2000; Pendakur, 2000; Reitz, 1998, 2001; Shields, 2002). So the traditional trajectory that saw immigrants catch up with other Canadians over time seems to have been reversed in the case of racialized immigrants. Of course the irony is that over that period of time, the level of education, usually an indicator of economic success, has been growing.

Recent Statistics Canada analysis shows that male recent immigrant full time employment earnings fell 7% between 1980 and 2000 (Kazimapur and Hou, 2003). This compares with a rise of 7% for the Canadian born cohort. Among university educated the drop was deeper (13%). For female recent

## Table 16.1: Unequal access to full employment (Unemployment rate in %)

|  | 1981 | 1991 | 2001 |
|---|---|---|---|
| Total labour force | 5.9 | 9.6 | 6.7 |
| Canadian born | 6.3 | 9.4 | 6.4 |
| All immigrants | 4.5 | 10.4 | 7.9 |
| Recent Immigrants | 6.0 | 15.6 | 12.1 |

Source: "Unequal access to full employment (%)," adapted from the Statistics Canada publication *The changing profile of Canada's labour force, 2001 census* (Analysis series, 2001 Census), Catalogue 96F0030, February 11, 2003.

## Table 16.2: Labour force participation (Employment rate in %)

|  | 1981 | 1991 | 2001 |
|---|---|---|---|
| Total labour force | 75.5 | 78.2 | 80.3 |
| Canadian born | 74.6 | 78.7 | 81.8 |
| All immigrants | 79.3 | 77.2 | 75.6 |
| Recent Immigrants | 75.7 | 68.6 | 65.8 |

Source: "Labour force participation (%)," adapted from the Statistics Canada publication "The changing profile of Canada's labour force, 2001 Census (Analysis series, 2001 Census)," Catalogue 96F0030, February 11, 2003.

immigrants full time employment earnings rose but by less than other female full time employees. More alarming are the low income implications of these trends. While low income rates among recent immigrants with less than high school graduation increased by 24% from 1980 to 2000, low income rates increased by 50% among high school graduates and a whopping 66% among university educated immigrants!

Recent immigrants' rates of employment declined markedly between 1986 and 1996. The result is that Canada's immigrants exhibit a higher incidence of poverty and greater dependence on social assistance than their predecessors, in spite of the fact that the percentage of university graduates is higher in all categories of immigrants including family class and refugees as well as economic immigrants than for the Canadian-born (CIC, 2002).

The Ornstein report (2000) revealed that high rates are concentrated among certain groups such as Latin Americans, African Blacks and Caribbeans, and Arabs and West Asians—with rates at 40% and higher in 1996, or roughly three times the Toronto rate. This research is confirmed by accounts in the popular press, which reveal a dramatic increase in the use of food banks by highly-educated newcomers (Quinn, 2002).

A significant factor in these trends is the under-utilization of immigrant skills within the Canadian labour market. Reitz (2001) has looked at the quantitative significance of this issue using a human-capital earnings analysis which identified immigrant earnings deficits as arising from three possible sources: lower immigrant skill quality, or under-utilization of immigrant skills, or pay inequities for immigrants doing the same work as native-born Canadians.

Social Determinants of Health

He concluded that in 1996 dollars, the total annual immigrant earnings deficit from all three sources in Canada was $15.0 billion, of which $2.4 billion was related to skill under-utilization, and $12.6 billion was related to pay inequity. He observed as well that employers give little credence to foreign education and none to foreign work experience, that discrimination specific to country of origin or visible minority status is mainly related to pay equity rather than skills utilization, and that the economic impact of visible minority status and immigrant status is very similar for both men and women. In addition Reitz noted that race appears to be a more reliable predictor of how foreign education will be evaluated in Canada than the specific location of the origin of the immigrant from outside Europe.

## Economic exclusion in the labour market

The third category of the relative surplus population, the stagnant, forms a part of the active labour army, but with extremely irregular employment ... hence it furnishes to capital an inexhaustible reservoir of disposable labour-power. Its conditions of life sink below that of the average normal level of the working class; This makes it at once the broad basis of the special branches of capitalist exploitation ... it is characterized by a maximum of working hours, and a minimum of wages ... But it forms at the same time a self-reproducing and self-perpetuating element of the working class, taking a proportionally greater part in the general increase of that class than the other elements. (Marx, 1977, p. 602)

The neo-liberal restructuring of Canada's economy and labour market towards flexibility has increasingly stratified labour markets along racial lines, with the disproportionate representation of racialized group members in low income sectors and low end occupations, and under-representation in high income sectors and occupations. These patterns emerge out of a context of racial inequality in access to work and in employment income, and the growing predominance of precarious forms of work in many of the sectors racialized group members are disproportionately represented in. They point to racially unequal incidence of low income and racially defined neighbourhood segregation. It is these broader processes that explain the emergence of the phenomenon of the racialization of poverty whose dimensions can primarily be identified by such indicators as disproportionate levels of low income and racialized spatial concentration of poverty in key neighbourhoods.

Economic social exclusion takes the form of labour market segregation, unequal access to employment, employment discrimination, and disproportionate vulnerability to unemployment and underemployment. These are both characteristics and causes of social exclusion. Attachment to the labour market is essential to both livelihood and to the production of identity in society. It determines both the ability to meet material needs but also a sense of belonging, dignity and self-esteem, all of which have implications for health status. Labour market related social exclusion has direct implications for health status not just because of the impact on income inequality, but also because of the extent to which working conditions, mobility in workplaces, fairness in the distribution of opportunities, and utilization of acquired skills all have a direct bearing on the levels of stress that are generated in workplaces.

The Canadian economy and labour market are increasingly stratified along racial lines, as evidenced by the disproportionate representation of racialized group members in low income sectors and low end occupations, and under-representation in high income sectors and occupations. These patterns emerge out of a context of neo-liberal restructuring of the economy conditioned by global competition and demands for flexible deployment of labour, persistent racial inequality in access to employment, and the growing predominance of precarious forms of work in many of the sectors in which racialized group members are disproportionately represented. Labour market research shows this racial stratification as observable in the disproportionate participation of racialized groups in industries increasingly dominated by non-standard forms of work such as textiles, clothing, hospitality and retailing, and an over-representation of racialized group members in low income jobs and low end occupations. On the other hand, they are under-represented in such high income sectors as the public service, automobile making and metal working, which also happen to be highly unionized.

The fastest growing form of work in Canada is precarious work, also referred to as contingent work or non-standard work—contract, temporary, part-time, and shift work with no job security, poor and often unsafe working conditions, intensive labour, excessive hours, low wages, and no benefits. In the early 1990s, it grew by 58%, compared to 18% for full time employment

(Vosko, 2000; de Wolf, 2000). Racialized workers are disproportionately represented in this form of work, as a consequence of their vulnerability to the restructuring in the economy (Galabuzi, 2001).

Most of this work is low-skilled and low paying and the working conditions are often unsafe. Such non-regulated service occupations as newspaper carriers, pizza deliverers, janitors and cleaners, dish washers, and parking lot attendants are dominated by racialized group members and recent immigrants who work in conditions with little or no protection—conditions similar to low end work in the hospitality and health care sectors, light manufacturing assembly plants and textile and home-based garment work. Many employees are "self-employed" or sub-contracted on exploitative contracts by temporary employment agencies, with some assigning work based on racist stereotypes.

Racialized women are particularly over-represented in another form of self-employment—unregulated piecemeal homework. Gendered racism and neo-liberal restructuring have conditioned the emergence of what some have called Canada's sweatshops, especially in the garment and clothing industry (Yanz, et al., 1999; Vosko, 2000). The intensity of the experience of exploitation imposes stressors especially on racialized and immigrant women who continue to carry a disproportionate bulk of house work, to go with the sub-contract wage work, and many of whom are single parents.

Because of the intensified exploitation characterized by demands for longer working hours and low pay, and/or multiple part-time jobs, the intensity of work under a deregulated labour market becomes a major source of stress and related health conditions. In the case of immigrants and racialized group members, the failure to convert their educational attainment and experience, whether internationally or domestically acquired, due to the structures of racial and gender inequality or barriers in employment relating to immigrant status, has been identified increasingly as a major stress generator.

## Social exclusion and racialized neighbourhood selection

*Space is a key function of social exclusion.*

The fact that people live in certain places can either sustain or intensify social exclusion. (Hutchinson, 2000, p. 167)

The racialization of poverty has also had a major impact on neighbourhood selection and access to adequate housing for new immigrants and racialized groups. In Canada's urban centres, the spatial concentration of poverty or residential segregation is intensifying along racial lines. Immigrants in Toronto and Montreal are more likely than non-immigrants to live in neighbourhoods with high rates of poverty as Table 16.3 below shows. Social exclusion is increasingly manifest in urban centres where racialized groups are concentrated through the emergence of racial enclaves and

a growing set of racially segregated neighbourhoods. In what is becoming a segregated housing market, racialized groups are relegated to substandard, marginal and often overpriced housing. These growing neighbourhood inequalities act as social determinants of health and well-being, with limited access to social services, increased contact with the criminal justice system, and social disintegration, and violence engendering higher health risks.

Recent studies by Hou and Balakrishnan (1998), Kazemipur and Halli (2000), Eric Fong (2000), and Ley and Smith (1997) suggest that these areas show characteristics of 'ghettoization' or spatial concentration of poverty, concentrating in urban cores, tightly clustered, with limited exposure to majority communities. Increasingly these geographical areas represent racialized enclaves subject to the distresses of low income communities.

A racialized spatial concentration of poverty means that racialized group members live in neighbourhoods that are heavily concentrated and "hypersegregated" from the rest of society and often with disintegrating institutions and increasingly dealing with social deficits such as inadequate access to counseling services, life skills training, child care, recreation, and health care services (Kazemipur and Halli, 1997, 2000; Lo et al., 2000).

**Table 16.3: Toronto-area racialized enclaves and experience of high poverty rates**

|  | University degree | Unemployment | Low income | Single parent |
|---|---|---|---|---|
| Chinese | 21.2% | 11.2% | 28.4% | 11.7% |
| South Asian | 11.8% | 13.1% | 28.3% | 17.6% |
| Black | 8.7% | 18.3% | 48.5% | 33.7% |

Source: "Toronto Area racialized enclaves and experience of high poverty rates," adapted from the Statistics Canada publication *Visible minority neighbourhood enclaves and labour market outcomes of immigrants* (Analytical Studies Branch research paper series), Catalogue 11F0019, July 2003.

Young immigrants living in low income areas often struggle with alienation from their parents and community of origin, and from the broader society. The social services they need to cope with dislocation are lacking, the housing on offer is often sub-standard, or if it is public housing it is largely poorly maintained because of cutbacks. They face crises of unemployment, despair, and violence. They are disproportionate targets of contact with the criminal justice system.

Finally, a word about homelessness and the recent immigrant and racialized groups. Homelessness is said to be proliferating among racialized group members because of the incidence of low income and the housing crises in many urban areas (Lee, 2000; Peel, 2000). Homelessness is an extreme form of social exclusion that suggests a complexity of causes and factors. Increasingly, recent immigrants and racialized people are more likely to be homeless in Canada's urban centres than they were ten years ago. It compounds other sources of stresses in their lives. Homelessness has been associated with early mortality, health factors such as substance abuse, mental illness, infectious diseases, and difficulty accessing health services. The complex interactions among these factors, homelessness and access to health services have not received enough study and represent a key gap in both the anti-racism and social determinants of health discourses.

## Racialization, social exclusion and health

The importance of power relations, social identity, social status, and control over life circumstances for health status follows from the evidence upon which the population health perspective is based. This evidence can be usefully grouped into three broad categories: social inequalities in health within and between societies; social support and health; and workplace characteristics and health. (Dunn and Dyck, 1998, p. 2)

If today's immigrants have higher rates of illness than the native-born, the increased risk probably results from an interaction between personal vulnerability and resettlement stress, as well as lack of services, rather than from diseases they bring with them to Canada. (Health Canada, 1998, p. 1)

There is no doubt that universal access to health care is now a core Canadian value, espoused broadly by all segments of the political elite as defining Canadian society. But beyond the policy articulation of universality of coverage, other determinants such as income, gender, race, immigrant status, and geography increasingly define the translation of the concept of universality as unequally differentiated. A review of the limited available literature indicates that the processes of social exclusion we have discussed above affect the health status of racialized and recent immigrant communities. The extent of exclusion is expressed through the gap between the promise of universal access to health care and the reality of unequal access to health service utilization, or inequalities in health status arising out of the inequalities in the social determinants of health. It is the gap between the promise of citizenship and the reality of exclusion that represents the extent of social exclusion and the unequal impact on the well-being of members of racialized groups and immigrants in Canada. While there is limited empirical research to draw on, there is significant anecdotal evidence to make the case.

It follows though that given the landscape of exclusion we have painted above, a perspective based on a synthesis of a diverse public health and social scientific literature, which suggests that the most important antecedents of human health status are not medical care inputs and health behaviours (smoking, diet, exercise, etc.), but rather social and economic character-istics of individuals and populations, would suggest significant convergence between social exclusion and health status (Evans et al., 1994; Frank, 1995; Hayes and Dunn, 1998). For racialized groups and recent immigrants, power relations, identity and status issues, and life chances are influential on the processes of immigration and integration (Dunn and Dyck, 1998).

However, one of the more significant studies of immigrants and health by Dunn and Dyck (1998) using the "social determinants of health" approach and based on a review of NPHS data perspective found no obvious, consistent pattern of association between socio-economic characteristics and immigration characteristics on the one hand, and health status on the other (Dunn and Dyck, 1998). Hyman (2001) has observed, neither did it find evidence to the contrary.

## Racialization and health status

It is now generally agreed that racism is a primary source of stress and hypertension in racialized group communities. Everyday forms of racism, often compounded by sexism and xenophobia, and the related conditions of underemployment, non-recognition of prior accreditation, low standard housing, residence in low income neighbourhoods with significant social deficits, violence against women and other forms of domestic and neighbourhood violence, and targeted policing and disproportionate criminalization and incarceration define an existence of those on the margins of society, an existence of social exclusion from the full participation in the social, economic, cultural, and political affairs of Canadian society. They are also important socio-economic and psycho-social determinants of health. While empirical research is under-developed, there is significant qualitative evidence, collected from group members, service providers, and some qualitative community based research to suggest that these act as determinants of health status for socially marginalized groups such as racialized women, youth and men, immigrants and Aboriginal peoples (Agnew, 2002; Tharoa and Massaquoi, 2001). These conditions contribute to and mediate the experience of inequality into powerlessness, hopelessness, and despair contributing to the emotional and physical impact on health of the members of the groups. These conditions in turn negatively impact attempts by affected individuals, groups, and communities to achieve full citizenship because of their inability to claim social and political rights enjoyed by other Canadians—including the right to physical and mental well-being of residents (Canada Health Act, 1984).

While there is limited literature in the Canadian context, research done internationally shows the connection between race and health more clearly. Research in the United States shows the connection between racism and health status (Randall, 1993). Wilkinson has investigated the processes of racialization, which result in the social and economic marginalization of certain social groups and shown that "racial" differences in health status can largely be accounted for by differences in individuals' social and economic circumstances (Wilkinson, 1996; Anderson, 1987, 1991).

Institutionalized racism in the health care system characterized by language barriers, lack of cultural sensitivity, absence of cultural competencies, barriers to access to health service utilization and inadequate funding for community health services has been identified as impacting the health status of racialized group members. Mainstream health care institutions are Eurocentric, imposing European and white cultural norms as standard and universal and, by extension, their cultural hegemony imposes a burden on racialized and immigrant communities. Insights from the critical race discourses help us understand that the cumulative burden of the subtle, ordinary, persistent everyday forms of racism, compounded by experiences of marginalization also determine health status. The psychological pressures of daily resisting these and other forms of oppression add up to a complex of factors that undermine the health status of racialized and immigrant group members. They are compounded by low occupation, housing and neighbourhood status, high unemployment, and high levels of poverty. Racist stereotypes by health practitioners also tend to impact health status.

## Social exclusion, stress, and mental health

Many racialized group members and immigrants with mental health issues and mental illnesses identify racism as a critical issue in their lives. The magnitude of the association between racism and poverty and mental health status was said by low income racialized group community members surveyed to be similar to other commonly studied stressful life events such as death of a loved one, divorce or job loss (Healing Journey, 1999).

Racism is a stress generator as are family separation through immigration, the intensification of work, devaluation of one's worth through decredentialism, and the very experience of inequality and injustice. Stress in turn is a major cause of a variety of health problems. It has been observed that one of the reasons the health status of immigrants declines is because of the the experiences of discrimination and racism (Hyman, 2001). State imposed barriers to family reunification through immigration policy that discourages reunification in favour of independent class immigration leads to extended periods of family separation. Family separation, and failure to effect reunification robs family members of their support network but also engenders separation anxiety, thoughts of suicide, lack of sufficient support mechanisms and even death.

Racism and discrimination based on immigrant status intensify processes of marginalization and social exclusion, compounding the experiences of poverty and its impacts on mental health status. The everyday darts that arise from put downs and diminishing self-esteem tend to undermine the mental health of racialized group members.

The stigma of mental illness often bars members from seeking treatment, some being afraid that such a stigma would compound their marginalization. The Canadian Task Force on Mental Health Issues Affecting Immigrants identified a mental health gap between immigrants and the Canadian-born population based on the socio-economic status of immigrants. Concluding that this was a determinant of mental health, it called for increased access to mental health services for immigrants, more appropriate culturally sensitive and language specific services to help close the gap (Beiser, 1988).

The serious gap in the research on the mental health of immigrants can be significantly closed by using a framework that recognizes the impact of racism and immigrant status on the process of social exclusion and social determination of health. Beiser et al. (1993) identify the persistence of the gap in health care utilization between immigrants and native born Canadians, its impact on the mental health status of immigrants, and the need for research to better understand the phenomenon.

## Skill deployment: Internationally trained

Many skilled immigrants are experiencing mounting barriers to making full use of the skills and talents in both the economic sphere and in public life. Increasingly they are dealing with frustration at the barriers they face. Such a strong sense of inequality and injustice has implications for their mental health (Beiser, 1988). Moreover, as the Anderson et al. (1993) study on chronic illness shows, for immigrant women living on meagre incomes and sustaining a marginal status in the labour market, the daily struggles of this meagre existence and the desire to hold on to their low paying jobs tend to take precedence over disclosing chronic illness to ensure its active management with the support of health professionals. Along with such livelihood considerations, they often face the daunting prospect of navigating the mainstream health care system, with its barriers to access, lack of culturally appropriate services, and inability of health care professionals to understand the choices that those living in poverty and at the margins have to make to survive.

Research shows that immigrant youth sometimes find the stresses of integration on top of the challenges of adolescence overwhelming. Their feelings of isolation and alienation are linked to perceptions of cultural differences and experiences of discrimination and racism. While these are often complicated by intergenerational issues, support from friends, family and institutions is key to overcoming the challenges—in essence it presents them with a recreated community in response to the exclusion they face in mainstream institutions like the school system (Kilbride, 2000).

## Conclusion: The dearth of research on health and race

I have suggested that social exclusion describes both the structures and the dynamic processes of inequality among groups in society which, over time, structure access to critical resources that determine the quality of membership in society and ultimately produce and reproduce a complex of unequal outcomes. Social exclusion speaks of both the process of becoming and the outcome of being socially excluded. It has received the attention of policy-makers concerned about the impact of marginal subgroups on social cohesion and has provided them with the social inclusion framework for responding to this phenomenon. However, its use in health policy and health research is limited although the social determinant of health approach seems to share its philosophical orientation. Its potential is especially suggestive when dealing with the complexity of issues faced by racialized and immigrant communities and their impact on health status, an area where there is limited research. Racialized groups and immigrant groups are disproportionately impacted by labour market segregation, unemployment and income inequality, poverty, poor neighbourhood selection, to go with experiences of discrimination based on race, gender, and immigrant status. The multidimensional approach of social exclusion as a framework for understanding the multiplicity of non-behavourial influences on health status may provide a more adequate basis for assessing the health status of not just racialized and immigrant communities but other socially excluded groups like women, persons with disability, gays and lesbians, bisexual and transgendered, and even the "generic" poor.

## Notes

1. The racialization of poverty here refers to the disproportionate and persistent incidence of low income among racialized groups in Canada.
2. There has been a significant change in the source countries, with over 75% of new immigrants in the 1980s and 1990s coming from the Global South. Most immigrants end up in urban centres—75% in Toronto, Vancouver, and Montreal.

## Recommended readings

Galabuzi, G. (2001). *Canada's creeping economic apartheid: The economic segregation and social marginisation of racialised groups*. Toronto: CSJ Foundation for Research and Education. Online at www.socialjustice.org.
    This report calls attention to the growing racialization of the gap between the rich and poor, which is proceeding with minimal public and policy attention, despite the dire implications for Canadian society. It challenges some common myths about the economic performance of Canada's racialized communities and shows how historical patterns of differential treatment and occupational segregation in the labour market, and discriminatory governmental and institutional policies and practices, have led to the reproduction of racial inequality in other areas of Canadian life.

Percy-Smith, J. (Ed.). (2000). *Policy responses to social exclusion: Towards inclusion?* Open University Press.
    A definitive U.K. analysis of social exclusion, its processes and causes. It contains numerous chapters concerned with presenting possible policy solutions to this emerging problem.

Guildford, J. (2000). *Making the case for economic and social inclusion*. Ottawa: Health Canada.
    Groundbreaking work in Canada that brought the concept of social exclusion to Canada.

Omidvar, R. and Richmond, T. (2003). *Immigrant settlement and social inclusion in Canada*. Toronto: Laidlaw Foundation. Online at www.laidlawfdn.org/programmes/children/richmond.pdf.
    This report is part of the Laidlaw Foundation Initiative on Social Inclusion.

Ornstein, M. (2002). *Ethno-racial inequality in Toronto: Analysis of the 1996 census*. Toronto: Institute for Social Research. Online at ceris.metropolis.net/Virtual%20Library/Demographics/ornstein1.pdf
    A careful analysis of the growing gap in income among people of different races in Toronto, Canada's largest city.

# Related websites

Social and Economic Inclusion in Atlantic Canada—www.acewh.dal.ca/inclusion-preface.htm

The "Inclusion Project" is a partnership project facilitated by the Maritime Centre of Excellence for Women's Health (MCEWH) and funded by the Population and Public Health Branch of Health Canada, Atlantic Region Office. The Project considers the problem of poverty and the shift in thinking away from a concentration of child poverty and towards an analysis of social and economic exclusion of women and their children.

The Centre for Analysis of Social Exclusion (CASE)—sticerd.lse.ac.uk/case/

CASE is an ESRC Research Centre, core-funded by the Economic and Social Research Council since October 1997. CASE is a multidisciplinary research centre located within the Suntory and Toyota International Centres for Economic and Related Disciplines (STICERD) at the London School of Economics and Political Science.

Laidlaw Foundation—www.laidlawfdn.org

Building inclusive cities and communities is the new focus of the Children's Agenda Program of the Laidlaw Foundation. The foundation has commissioned twelve working papers that have contributed to understanding social inclusion and pointed to the importance of cities and communities as places where inclusion and exclusion are first experienced by children and families.

The Townsend Centre for International Poverty Research—www.bris.ac.uk/poverty/

The Centre was launched on 1st July 1999 at the University of Bristol. It is dedicated to multidisciplinary research on poverty in both the industrialised and developing world.

Social Exclusion Unit—www.socialexclusionunit.gov.uk/

Social exclusion is a shorthand term for what can happen when people or areas suffer from a combination of linked problems such as unemployment, poor skills, low incomes, poor housing, high crime environments, bad health, and family breakdown. The Social Exclusion Unit was set up by the U.K. Prime Minister to help improve Government action to reduce social exclusion by producing "joined-up solutions to joined-up problems." It provides an example of how a government is defining the problem and attempting to resolve it.

# Chapter Seventeen

———⬤———

# SOCIAL INCLUSION/EXCLUSION AND HEALTH: DANCING THE DIALECTIC

## Ronald Labonte

## Introduction

The last decade has seen many of the "community" concepts in health (community empowerment, community capacity) replaced by "social" concepts (social capital, social cohesion). The continuous re-labelling of roughly similar phenomena may be a necessary stratagem to attract attention to the economic and power inequalities that arise from undisciplined markets. "Social" concepts also have an advantage over "community" ones by directing that attention to higher orders of political systems. The latest construct being wielded by health practitioners, researchers, and policy-makers is the twinned concepts of social inclusion and social exclusion. These represent sophistication over social capital and social cohesion. Like their predecessors, however, there are risks in their adoption without a critical examination of the premises that underpin them. For example, how can one "include" people and groups into structured systems that have systematically "excluded" them in the first place? The cautions expressed in this article do not dissuade use of the concepts. Their utility, however, particularly at a time when not only inequalities, but also their rate of growth, is increasing, requires careful questioning. This chapter, then, poses two basic questions:

1. How does the social inclusion/exclusion concept advance our understanding of the social determinants of health, in the broadest, deepest sense?
2. How can its uncritical use lead us to a focus on socially excluded groups rather than socially excluding structures and practices?

The chapter answers these questions indirectly by, first, exploring briefly the "community" and "social" concepts that preceded social inclusion/exclusion and then examining the "embedded contradiction" in the social inclusion/exclusion concept. It then discusses who is socially excluded, and why; and frames this in the context of two competing social justice norms, "equality of opportunity" and "equality of outcome." The chapter concludes with a reflection on the global aspects of social inclusion/exclusion, and the implications this new concept has for practitioners, researchers and policy-makers.

## From society to community to society once more

Thirty years ago, bristling with newly employed activists from the social movements of the 1960s and the 1970s (the New Left movement, the environment movement, the women's movement, the civil rights movement), many rich world governments rediscovered community. From processes—community participation, community development—to attributes—community competence, community capacity—to services—community health, community education—it seemed that all we had to was drop the adjective of *gemeinschaft* ("community") in front of the noun of our particular preoccupation and the impersonal structures of *gesellschaft* ("society") disappeared. Of course, we quickly learned it was more complex than this. We confronted the vagaries of power in our workplaces, which supported communities when they weren't threatening to established rules and authority; in our assumptions, which often imposed a romantic localism on poorer people who simply wanted some of the same networked privileges we enjoyed; in communities themselves, which were far from the loving, homogenous, always wise and self-knowing entities we contrasted against our own organizational hierarchies.[1] More fundamentally, we bumped against the lesson best expressed in the 1989 *Worldwatch Institute report*: small may be beautiful, but it may also be insignificant (Durning, 1989). Decisions conditioning and constraining the possibilities of local empowerment were drifting further and higher away from the purview of, and accountability to, the places where, as health promoters like to express, "people live, work and play."

In the 1990s, our glance widened to broader social phenomena with a new, appropriately social lexicon. Community competence and capacity gave way to social capital. Community participation and development yielded to social inclusion. Social cohesion became the unstated aim of diminishing state programs and services to patch back together communities unravelling with digitized, marketized, and globalized inequalities. Even as a "new" population health research—concerned not with reproductive health in the narrow sense, but with the social production of health in the broadest sense—broached a new government slogan:

> WARNING: Inequalities may be bad for your health. Avoid excessive greed, intolerance, and poor parents.[2]

Neo-liberal economic assumptions continued their global domination, cementing their gospel of liberalization, privatization, de-regulation, and welfare minimalism in the policies of the International Financial Institutions (the World Bank and the International Monetary Fund) and the rules of the World Trade Organization. It is in this brave, new, "history-ending world" (as conservative analysts quickly dubbed life after the fall of the Berlin Wall and the demise of the communist "other") that we need to consider whether the twinned concepts of social inclusion/social exclusion help or hinder our development of actions that will shrink the preventable differences in health, well-being and quality of life that still demarcate and segregate our communities and nations.

## An advance on social cohesion and social capital

The twinned concept of social inclusion/exclusion is more helpful than its other "social" cousins: social cohesion and social capital. Social cohesion resides more in the realm of moral philosophy than in the grit of human relations. It is a counterfactual ideal, and perhaps even a dangerous one if we ever forget its essential idealism and let it become the driver for how we approach social change. Here it is useful to consider the school of thought known as "conflict sociology," which holds on the basis of a few thousand years of cumulative empirical evidence, that societies have always been a tenuous arrangement of fluid groupings in some degree of conflict with one another—for resources, for authority, for legitimacy; in a word, for power. Where there is no conflict, Ralf Dahrendorf once offered, there is suppression (Dahrendorf, 1959). This does not mean that we should espouse or tolerate civil or any other form of war. But it does challenge us to accept some degree of social conflict as healthy, albeit in discomforting ways. We need to retain a healthy scepticism of concepts that direct us towards a wishful desire for social harmony, however important that desire is as an ideal. Such concepts can blunt the sharp edges of mobilized criticism that has always been one of the necessary fuels for social reform.

Social capital fares little better. For one, no one can settle on a definition of what it is or what it does, apart from a melange of psychosocial variables of differing interest to different researchers—trust, reciprocity, participation, social network density. More

fundamentally, individuals and organizations with quite different visions of how societies should govern themselves can become social capital bedfellows, though perhaps with a quite different understanding of what are "means" and what are "ends." To the World Bank, social capital is the means to the end of economic growth, the necessary social glue that allows unfettered markets to work the magic of their invisible hands (Labonte, 1999). Its absence, it is conjectured, explains why liberalized market reforms (with a few Asian exceptions) have had a dismal record of delivering on their promises in Africa, Latin America and the so-called Transition Economies. To others, economic growth is the sometimes-necessary means to the end of building social capital. ("Sometimes-necessary" because many of today's rich countries could benefit more by *developing* their economies to be more equitable and sustainable, rather than simply growing them to become larger.) Economic growth provides a sufficiency of wealth required by states for universal programs and resource redistribution that, in turn, are essential to what Nobel economist, Amartya Sen, describes as the foundations for the capabilities that allow people "to live a life they have reason to value" (Sen, 2000). To its credit, social capital builds a linguistic bridge between those in the market and those in civil society. To its detriment, and I borrow here from how a disgruntled environmentalist once lamented the concept of sustainable development, *they* got the noun, which defines, while we got the *adjective*, which merely modifies.[3]

## Social inclusion/exclusion: The embedded contradiction

Social inclusion/exclusion is more interesting and dynamic than either social cohesion or social capital, for it is poised on the very contradiction evinced by all of these terms: How does one go about including individuals and groups into a set of structured social relationships that were responsible for excluding them in the first place? Or, put another way, and in deference to Michel Foucault's brilliant essays on the positive practices of power, the seductive ways in which people internalize their own powerlessness and become their own prison guards, to what extent do efforts at social inclusion *accommodate* people to relative powerlessness rather than challenge the hierarchies that create it (Foucault, 1979, 1980)? To what degree might we consider wilful social exclusion by groups an important moment of conflict, an empowered act of resistance to socio-economic systems that, by their logic and rules, continue to replicate and heighten the material hierarchies of inequality?

I pose these questions because many who embrace the concept of social inclusion emphasize how it goes beyond simply matters of income or material inequalities and their state-enforced redistribution (Barata, 2000), or even of securing basic human rights (Bach, 2002). Rights and redistribution, it is argued, are necessary but not sufficient conditions for people "to be accepted and to participate fully within our families, our communities, and our society," as one definition of social inclusion defines

---

### Box 17.1: Resistance is not futile

Many years ago I was involved in community organizing activities with single mothers receiving social assistance. Many of these women had low self-esteem. A principal reason for this was that the dominant discourse of welfare recipients was as non-autonomous, wholly dependent and publicly accountable individuals who were, effectively, public property, objects of the state. These women had internalized their lesser eligibility; they had become lesser persons. The women complained bitterly, for example, of the "spouse in the house" regulation, and of welfare workers who would call them up at all hours or drop by for surprise visits to make sure they weren't "cheating." The "spouse in the house" regulation required single mothers on family benefits allowance to remain single, which in some instances was interpreted to mean not having lovers stay in their apartment or house.

Some recipients claimed that they were careful to lower the toilet seat prior to welfare worker visits in order to avoid suspicion that they may be seeing a male lover, or to trade in their double for a single bed. This is an evocative example of what Foucault described as the *modus operandi* of the "positive practice" of power: the gaze of authority that judges what it sees and, in so judging, controls the choices of those who are gazed upon. The only form of struggle against this form of power, to Foucault, was resistance to the gaze, a concealment of one's life from those with authority over the gaze and the world of judgements it creates, a deliberate act of *social exclusion*, at least from those forms of social regulation that nominally claim to promote social inclusion. Two British researchers, studying the response of poor single parents to home visitors (a hybrid public health nurse and social worker), similarly found that many of these women deliberately hid certain messy rooms, or cupboards, or ill children from the gaze of the home visitors (Bloor and McIntosh, 1990). The authors interpreted these "laconics" or acts of concealment as a rudimentary form of empowering resistance to the hegemonic power-over induced by welfare state policies and the roles they created for both welfare recipients and home visitors.

the territory (Guildford, 2000, p. 1). There is little to disagree with in these sentiments. But are there not also risks in pursuing policies and programs that assume *a priori* that income redistribution and human rights are solidly in place, when most of the evidence for much of the world is that they are not?

## Who are the excluded, and why?

Consider, first, the list of the excluded in need of greater inclusion: women, racial minorities, the poor and the sick, those with disabilities, children and youth, especially if they face developmental challenges or disadvantaged circumstances. Like members of our previously designated "high risk groups" for health problems, our attention turns to anyone who is not a white, middle-aged and minimally middle-incomed male. Conceptually, social exclusion is an improvement over its predecessor; it defines disadvantage as an outcome of social processes, rather than as a group trait. But in attempting to take us away from a narrow focus on material or income inequality, the concept can falter on an even subtler victim blaming. People are no longer at fault for their disadvantage. But their disadvantage is seen to lie in their *exclusion*, rather than in *excluding structures* predicated on inequality. Let me explain.

Striding alongside social inclusion's references to acceptance by and participation in family, community and society, is social exclusion's complaint that people "do not have the opportunity for full participation in the economic and social benefits of society" (Guildford, 2000, p. 1). People are excluded from these benefits, we are told, because they are poor. But people are poor because they lack these benefits. They lack these benefits because capital and state structures

allow wealth to accumulate unequally, and powerful others benefit directly and immediately from this. People are excluded from these benefits, we are also told, because they are women. But women for the past two centuries have been cast economically as a source of cheap and surplus wage labour, and of free reproductive labour. Powerful others benefit directly and immediately from women's relative exclusion from economic and social benefits. This has changed tremendously in the world's wealthier nations over the past half century. But the identical script, directed by the same cast of scriptwriters, is now being enacted globally.

People are excluded from these benefits, we are finally told, because they are black, or yellow, or red, or at least "not white." But contemporary racism, though its roots may be obscured in historic competition over resources, is firmly planted in contemporary capitalism. As Brazilian writer Eduardo Galeano thirty years ago showed in his brilliant essay, *Open veins of Latin America* (1973), only the wealth of the exploited colonies—their resources, their peoples, their enslavement—allowed Western capitalism to depose feudalism. As British novelist, Barry Unsworth, recounts vividly in his Booker-winning novel, *A sacred hunger* (1993), African slavery was the fuel of both England's early capitalist wealth, and American colonial wealth. Slavery collapsed when it was no longer economically efficient, not without a bloody civil war but not because of it. Its undertow remains. Internationally, ethnic conflicts from the tribalism of Africa to the cleansings in the Balkans have powerful roots in the economic structures and political systems that allow wealth to accumulate unequally and powerful others to benefit directly and immediately from this.

This is not to say that the complexities of gender and race exclusion can be reduced to a simple stock of class and materialism. Patriarchal practices and racial exclusions predate feudal societies, much less capitalism. But every example of contemporary social exclusion based on gendered or racialized difference will also have a material and class-based component, with some people deriving benefit from it. When a recent Canadian study tells us that, all other things being equal, workers of colour earn 16% less than white workers, this is not only racism. This is also economic advantage to employers (*Globe and Mail*, November 29, 2002, p. B2).

Uncritical use of social inclusion can blind us to the use, abuse and distribution of power. Power has non-zero sum elements—the win/win empowerment of trusting, respectful relationships. So, too, does social inclusion. But power has distinctly non-zero sum aspects—the win/lose of dominance, exploitation, and hegemony. This is manifest in social inclusion's obverse of exclusion. We should not let the warmth of our inclusive ideal smother our anger over exclusivity's unfairness. Anger is often the magnet of mobilization; mobilization is often the tool for social transformation that shifts power relations in ways that allow societies to become more inclusive.

In one sense, we can be generous about concepts, especially new and contested ones such as social inclusion/exclusion. Provided people define carefully what they mean when they use these terms, there is no problem. But people rarely do. More importantly, there is a lesson in the metaphor of a frog in a pot of water. If you throw a frog into a pot of boiling water, it immediately jumps out. It is not that stupid. If you throw it into a pot of cold water and then turn on the heat, it swims about contently as the water slowly

rises to a boil and then, suddenly, it dies. It is not that smart. So it can be with certain concepts. Like cold water, we immerse ourselves in them, only to find after a time, and quite suddenly, we arrive at a place we did not originally want to be, colonized by a set of assumptions we did not initially assume. Social inclusion could be one of these concepts, unless we maintain a very keen eye on the background temperature and who is in control of the gauge.

## And just what are we including them in?

This problematic of who benefits most by an emphasis on inclusion, rather than a critique of exclusion, becomes more apparent when we examine the different ways its advocates define its end. The first major policy shift based on the concept was in France, in 1988.

As with many of the economically advanced countries, France was faced with high unemployment, particularly amongst its traditional semi-skilled manufacturing workers. This was due to capitalism's transformation to a digital economy and its liberalized ability to locate more labour intensive production in low-wage countries. Fearing a loss in social cohesion, the centre-right government adopted a *revenue minimum d'insertion*, a guaranteed minimum income, but only if people "inserted" themselves into economic or civil life through training and work programs with the private sector, government and voluntary associations (Guildford, 2000). A slightly more nuanced form of "workfare" programs, this was not the first time France attempted a project of social reintegration necessitated by fundamental shifts in capitalist production. A century earlier, rural farmers and craft persons, economically marginalized by another great shift in capitalism, the development of factory production, drank more and killed themselves quite regularly. This led French sociologist, Emile Durkheim, to coin the concept of *anomie*, a loss of personal meaning that arises with deep tears in the social fabric that normally binds people together. His policy recommendation: creation of "corporative organizations"—community betterment groups—whose purpose would be to change how people thought of themselves, essentially transforming their social identities to conform with how the economy had changed (Taylor and Ashworth, 1987). This is a gloss of Durkheim's sociological thought, but it makes my point: that social inclusion or social integration tends to adapt people to the needs of markets, rather than regulate markets to the needs of people.

We see this even more sharply in the U.K., where social inclusion has been truncated to labour market attachment (Lister, 2000). If you have a job, you're OK and more likely to display socially inclusive and nicely cohesive attitudes and behaviours. If you don't, you're more likely to be poor, a drain on social welfare and prone to "anti-social" drug abuse, hooliganism and crime. This isn't to minimize the importance of work to peoples' lives. Work satisfies far

---

**Box 17.2: Social inclusion the "A-way"**

Persons with mental health disabilities often face social exclusion. In the mid-1980s, many psychiatric institutions began closing their wards and releasing psychiatric "consumer/survivors," as they began calling themselves, into communities, often without adequate support services. Key problems faced by many of these people were adequate income, social support, and something to do.

A-Way Express, a Toronto community economic development program for psychiatric consumer/survivors founded in 1987 by two agencies, offers a good example of both the possibility and the problematic of promoting health using a social inclusion approach.[4] A-Way Express is a courier service operating in Metropolitan Toronto run by people who have had some treatment for mental health difficulties. Couriers utilize public transit, especially the subway system, as their main source of transportation. All of its couriers work for welfare top-up. None of them are employed full-time, most working three 5-hour shifts a week. Several professional staff manage, co-ordinate, and train couriers for the service. A-Way Express is proud of its ability to integrate economic development activities with support services for psychiatric consumer/survivors. Income, a sense of meaningful social contribution, social support, and self-confidence are all part of the health promoting, social inclusion "package" that A-Way, and many other consumer/survivor industries, are able to offer. Employment generally provides one sense of community to people. In enterprises such as A-Way, this sense of community is heightened due to the integrated participation of employees in the formation and implementation of the policies of the organization. But the "social inclusion" offered by such community economic development projects is not primarily about strengthening participants' labour market attachment, or making them wholly independent of state-funded support programs. Indeed, such projects are unlikely to become fully self-sufficient in the short, or even medium, term, owing partly to the historic social exclusion of many of the people for whom they create part-time employment. The economic dimension of social inclusion is merely one facet of a more holistic approach they are taking to the successful social integration of persons with long-term psychiatric histories.

---

more dimensions of our being than simply the monthly wage packet. Rather than neighbourhoods, workplaces are where people form many of their enduring friendships. (See Box 17.2.) But we also know the bleaker side of work: its physical hazards, its psycho-social threats and, subsequent to today's liberalized capital and episodic encounters with a crisis of over-production, its increasing non-standard form in which regular hours, living wages, extended benefits and longer-term security are being swept away as uncompetitive relics of a bygone era, "labour market rigidities" that constrain our domestic productivity.

It is naïve, then, to claim, as some have, "policies to combat social exclusion offer the hope of increasing employment opportunities and reducing poverty" (Guildford, 2000, p. 16). These poverty-reducing jobs will be created in one of three sectors: the public, the private or the informal/underground. Informal sector work is highly insecure, private sector employment increasingly so, and the public sector has been under two decades of right-wing attack to reduce its expenditures by trimming its labour force. Only "strong state" regulatory and redistributive policies might re-allocate employment opportunities in some more durably inclusive way. Yet it is these very policy instruments that are being traded away in free trade negotiations, in such accords as the General Agreement on Trade in Services (which could further privatize public services, and under foreign ownership and even provision), the Agreement on Trade-Related Investment Measures (which prevents governments from putting equity-oriented "performance requirements" on foreign investment), and the Agreement on Government Procurement (which could bind government contracting-out to purely commercial criteria, including "national treatment" of foreign bidders) (Labonte, 2003).

## Social justice: Equality of opportunity or equality of outcome?

What pulls these concepts of social inclusion/social exclusion in sometimes contrary directions, strange as it might first appear, is social justice. This is because there are two broad norms of social justice, defined by their emphases on equality of opportunity or equality of outcome. Both norms are ideal types. There can never be equality of opportunity because different individuals or groups have vastly differing resources or capacities that automatically disadvantage the less well endowed. There can never be equality of outcomes because there are differences between people that cannot be, or should not be, bludgeoned into similitude. But equality of opportunity, the mantra of neo-liberalism and, it seems, central to the U.K. and other countries' approach to social inclusion, is a grossly insufficient norm if some degree of distributive fairness is our goal.

A pithy illustration of the conflict between these two norms is a cartoon from a newspaper in Aotearoa, New Zealand from 1991. This was the year that country began its radical dismantling of labour and welfare rights and entitlements, as part of a program begun in 1984 of embracing free trade and neo-liberal economic policies. (It has since partially reversed this trend, which gave that country one of the highest growth rates in poverty—doubling between 1988 and 1996—and poorest records of economic growth amongst the wealthy nations making up the Organization for Economic Cooperation and Development; Kelsey, 2002). The cartoon showed a massive giant and a little pipsqueak in a wrestling ring. The match: rich and powerful vs. poor and powerless. As one of the ringside commentators enthused: "It should be a good match. They're playing on a level playing field." The "level playing field"—equality of opportunity—is exactly what is allowing our new global trade regime to ensure that the rich will get richer and the poor, even if they are successful in gaining ground materially, will fall further behind the rich in the economic power game. In strictly economic terms, the biggest winners of the past 20 years of increased global market integration has been the world's wealthiest nations, reversing the trend of the previous two decades (1960–1980) when economic growth in poor countries outpaced that in rich ones (Weisbrot et al., 2001; Milanovic, 2003). The biggest struggle in the World Trade Organization today is not between civil society protestors and trade negotiators. It is between poor and rich countries. Poor countries want stronger "special and differential" exemptions to trade rules so that they can grow their economies by expanding their exports while protecting their domestic markets from imports; by directing foreign investment to where it will do the most developmental good; and by copying technological innovations without threat of trade sanctions. Despite having "developed" their economies using precisely these strategies, rich countries now want the "level playing field" to deny poorer countries the same opportunity (Labonte, 2003).

Equality in outcome demands inequalities in opportunity. Full stop. "Inequalities in opportunity" does not mean targeted programs at the expense of universal programs. But universal programs without some targeting within them (some deference to greater disparity, greater need, greater historic *exclusion*) can heighten inequalities in outcome because of who is better able to avail of such programs.

## The need for a global lens

Consider, finally, that social inclusion/ exclusion requires a global and not simply a national or local lens. Given the same or largely unchanged economic and political rules or structures that are *socially excluding*, does success in including one group come at the expense of excluding another? Are we at risk, not of redistributing wealth and opportunity, but of redistributing poverty and marginalization?

Globally, for example, increasing numbers of women in developing countries are now being "included" in the economic wage-labour system, partly because capital has "excluded" from the same system the semi-skilled, blue collar, primarily male, primarily white labour force in developed countries. For many women, this foreshadows a shift in their empowerment. Yet much of women's employment remains low-paid, unhealthy, and insecure in "free-trade" export zones that often prohibit any form of labour organization and employ only single women. Often, the income they earn still goes to male household members. Women are favoured in such employment because they can be paid less. Most developing countries lack pay equity laws; the gender income gap in many countries is widening (Gyebi et al., 2002). Public caring supports for young children have been declining in many trade-opened countries, portending future health inequalities. There is also evidence of a global "hierarchy of care." Increasing numbers of women from developing nations are getting employment as domestic workers or other service providers in wealthy countries. They become "socially included," at least in an economic sense. They send much valued currency back home to their families, which helps in their social inclusion back home. Some of this money is used to employ poorer rural women in their home countries to look after the children they have left behind. These rural women, in turn, leave their eldest daughter (often still quite young and ill-educated) to care for the family they left behind in the village (Hochschild, 2000). In the absence of changes in the rules by which we trade and govern, the process of including some will almost inevitably exclude others.

## Conclusion

Our concern, then, should not be with the groups or conditions that are excluded, but with the socio-economic rules and political powers that create excluded groups and conditions and the social groups who benefit by this. Borrowing from similar cautions I made about last season's first blush with social capital (Labonte, 1999), I offer a focal question for practitioners, researchers, and policy-makers.

For practitioners, social inclusion/exclusion may be a useful idea in their ongoing struggles to keep some resources flowing into that part of their work that aims to see the less powerful become more powerful, the disorganized more organized, the less capable more resourced and confident in their capacities. Like ideas of community empowerment and capacity before it, social exclusion should give practitioners pause to question: How has their work improved the situation for the least well off within the ambit of their communities? And how has it avoided "excluding" other, perhaps almost as least well off from the support and resource access they might require?

For researchers, social inclusion/exclusion could represent a new opportunity for research funding grants, peer-reviewed publications, theoretical refinements, and invitations to health determinants conferences in nice places around the world. The problem is that the term becomes more a vehicle for career advancement than for social change. The question for those in the academy, then, is: How will theorizing and researching social inclusion/exclusion create differently new knowledge and argument useful to community workers and citizens, media sound-biters and policy-makers, in redirecting public governance towards the end of a "good life" for all, to which the market is necessarily subordinate? That is, does this idea prompt us to pose important questions for which we do not already have adequate answers?

For policy-makers, those unenviably straddling political discourses that have captured the noun by eroding the adjective, the question may be: How can the arguments elicited by social inclusion/exclusion convince the free market ideologues of the necessity of disciplining economic practices towards fairness in the distribution of wealth and sustainability in the use of natural resources? Can a social inclusion argument be extended to what we know are important health determinants residing in our economic practices (adequate income and its equitable distribution, access to education and health care), forcing the evidence-based policy conclusion that these conditions require a return to the strong, redistributive state policies we have seen eroded over the past twenty years? Can a social exclusion argument be used to challenge the orthodoxy of equal opportunity with the ideal of equal outcome?

I sow these questions in this chapter as seeds rather than transplanted agendas. I encourage debate upon them, since disagreement is usually more enlightening than prescription.

And I conclude this chapter by drawing attention to how I titled it: "dancing the dialectic." A dialectic is a form of reasoning or argument based on "a contradiction of ideas that serves as the determining factor in their interaction" (www.hyperdictionary.com). I don't want to discard the hopefulness that infuses the social inclusion/social exclusion concept. The dialectic dances between seeking to include more people into social systems stratified by exclusion even while trying to transform these systems. It's an old dialectic, one that never fully resolves but remains at best a grapple-able task; one that straddles the imperatives of revolution with the pragmatics of reform. It would be hubris to deny that many excluded groups simply want the same chance to climb the ladders of wealth and power that others have before them. It would be unethical to criticize the existence of such ladders in the first place, or to join in struggles to shrink their height.

I also like the idea of dancing. I recently returned from Brazil, where I learned the samba and where every year during Carnival the social incohesion of that country's skewed wealth distribution—rivalling South Africa's as the worst on the planet—is momentarily obliterated in the world's biggest dance festival. Or, as Emma Goldman, the early 20th century anarchist, feminist, and trade unionist, inspirationally aphorised: "If I can't dance then it's not my revolution."

## Notes

1.   There is a long history of critique of the romanticized community. Good overviews are provided by Lyon (1989), who points out that every century produces its own laments for the lost halcyon community of earlier, simpler times; Hunter and Staggenborg (1988), who chide many community workers for failing to distinguish between "communities of limited liabilities"—our de-centred opportunity networks—and "communities of enforced locality"—the ghettoes into which we would like to lock up the threatening poor; and Friedmann (1992), who urges a development paradigm in which state/civil society, globalism/ localism and many of the other dualities encountered in community theory and practice literature (such as inclusion/exclusion) are problematized rather than dichotomized.
2.   Income inequalities *per se* may be less a direct threat to health than the more stubborn poverty and loss of social solidarity that such inequalities create.
3.   I am sympathetic to the aim of many of today's social capital and health researchers, who should not take my critique of the construct as undermining the importance of understanding better, why, *ceteris paribus* (which they never are), some communities are healthier than others. But rather than working towards a better theorization and operationalization of social capital to study how or why it is a determinant of health, I would urge that studies examine the cultural history and political economy of nations and communities to understand better the determinants of social capital, i.e., to link social capital conceptually and analytically to the structured inequalities created by economic capital and capitalism.
4.   The A-Way story is adapted from a report, *Equity in action*, Ontario Premier's Council on Health, Wellbeing and Social Justice (Labonte et al., 1994).

## Recommended readings

The Policy Research Initiative Horizons—www.policyresearch.schoolnet.ca/keydocs/horizons/ horizons-e.htm

The February 2001 issue on social inclusion highlights various aspects and concepts associated with social inclusion, including access to work, education, poverty and social inequalities, social and cultural diversity, and new emergent inclusion challenges for public policy development.

Making the Case for Social and Economic Inclusion—www.hc-sc.gc.ca/hppb/regions/atlantic/documents/
e_abs1.html#14

This report examines the development of policies and programs to combat social exclusion in Europe over the past decade, and the potential of social inclusion for contributing to the development of healthy social policy in the Atlantic region. It includes a 19-page annotated bibliography of articles, reports, and books relating to the concept of social inclusion.

(The above two descriptions are taken from the Health Canada website: www.hc-sc.gc.ca/hppb/phdd/ news2001/pdf/social_exclusion_en.pdf)

Clutterbuck, P. and M. Novick. (2002). *Building inclusive communities: Cross-Canada perspectives and strategies*. Draft Discussion Paper prepared for the Federation of Canadian Municipalities and the Laidlaw Foundation. Online at www.laidlawfdn.org/

This report draws together the findings from a cross-Canada series of "community soundings" that engaged 250 city leaders, agency professionals, and social advocates in ten urban centers in 2002 to assess social vulnerabilities and civic capacities. It develops a vision of inclusive communities and cities, and outlines the institutions, strategies, and resources for successful implementation. The report identifies a number of priorities: inclusive planning perspectives, inter-governmental co-ordination, balancing national standards and local initiative, and the formation of cross-Canada civic panels to mobilize community and municipal input for "strong" local infrastructures that integrate physical, economic, and social development. Civic panels on Children, Youth and Families and on Urban Diversity are proposed.

Atkinson, T., Cantillon, B., Marlier, E. and Nolan, Brian (2002). *Social indicators: The EU and social inclusion*. London: Oxford University Press.

This book describes the Action Plan on Social Inclusion submitted to the EU by national governments in June 2001, and critically assesses the indicators that can be used to measure social progress in key areas such as poverty, homelessness, and low educational attainment.

Earnes, M. and Adebowale, M. (2002). *Sustainable development and social inclusion: Towards an integrated approach to research*. York: Joseph Rowntree Foundation.

This edited volume explores conceptual and policy linkages between social inclusion and environmental justice, making an argument for engaging the insights and experience of excluded communities in the emerging agenda for sustainable development research.

(The above three descriptions are taken from the CPRN *Nexus* Newsletter "Urban Nexus No. 4—Cities and Social Inclusion," January, 2003.)

## Related websites

The Laidlaw Foundation—www.laidlawfdn.org/

The Laidlaw Foundation web site contains numerous documents and reports on social inclusion, as part of its program on Children and Youth:

Building Inclusive Cities and Communities is the new focus of the Children's Agenda Program of the Laidlaw Foundation. It follows a two-year process whereby the Foundation adopted social inclusion as a tool for evaluating and advancing social policy in support of children and families. As part of the process, the foundation has commissioned 12 working papers that have contributed to understanding social inclusion and pointed to the importance of cities and communities as places where inclusion and exclusion are first experienced by children and families.

Publications include:
*Dynamics of social inclusion: Public education and Aboriginal people in Canada*
    Terry Wotherspoon
*The role of recreation in promoting social inclusion*
    Peter Donnelly and Jay Coakley
*Poverty, inequality and social inclusion* (PDF format)
    Andrew Mitchell and Richard Shillington
*Social inclusion, anti-racism and democratic citizenship*
    Anver Saloojee
*Thumbs up! Inclusion, rights and equality as experienced by youth with disabilities*
    Catherine Frazee
*Immigrant settlement and social inclusion in Canada*
    Ratna Omidvar and Ted Richmond
*Social inclusion as solidarity: Rethinking the child rights agenda*
    Michael Bach
*Social inclusion through early childhood education and care*
    Martha Friendly and Donna S. Lero
*Feminist perspectives on social inclusion and children's well-being*
    Meg Luxton
*Ethical reflections on social inclusion*
    Dow Marmur
*Leave no child behind! Social exclusion and child development*
    Clyde Hertzman
*Does work include children? The effects of the labour market on family income, time and stress*
    Andrew Jackson and Katherine Scott
*Literature review on social inclusion*
    Pedro Barata
*Social cohesion bibliography*
    David Welch

The Policy Research Initiative of Canada—www.policyresearch.gc.ca
    The Policy Research Initiative of Canada, a branch of the federal government, has several policy programs involving research studies, conferences and scholarly opinion pieces.
    Two of these directly bear on social inclusion/exclusion and other ideas addressed in this chapter:

*New approaches for addressing poverty and exclusion*
*Social capital as a public policy tool*

The first program is described as follows:

Canadian policies for addressing poverty and social exclusion were designed to support the social contract of the 1960s, and, as a result of incremental adjustments, have adapted reasonably well to the radical changes in society that have taken place since then. In the 1990s, due to the worsening economic situation, and cuts to social spending, Canada's efforts to address poverty and exclusion fell behind. Since the recovery of the mid-90s, many indicators related to poverty have improved, but earnings and income among poorer families have declined.

In recent years, there has been a great deal of change in the way developed countries perceive issues of poverty and exclusion. New data have allowed a better understanding of the dynamics of poverty, its persistence over the course of life, and the identification of groups at risk. The PRI is collaborating with other federal departments in a systematic exploration of the potential implications for policy-making of these newer ways of perceiving poverty and exclusion.

The PRI journal, *Horizons,* is available in both online and print format and has featured articles and book reviews on social capital and social inclusion.

Centre for Economic and Social Inclusion—www.cesi.ork.uk
The U.K.-based Centre for Economic and Social Inclusion:

> is an independent, not-for-profit organisation working with Government, the voluntary sector, business and trade unions. *Inclusion* promotes social justice and tackles disadvantage. We want to help individuals, families and communities achieve economic independence and access more and better opportunities.

> The site contains several policy and research papers and a monthly journal, titled "Working brief." The site underscores the UK approach to social inclusion as fostering labour market attachment.

The Social Exclusion Unit—www.socialexclusionunit.gov.uk/
The UK Social Exclusion Unit, operating out of the office of the Deputy Prime Minister, is a governmental body charged "by the Prime Minister to help improve Government action to reduce social exclusion by producing 'joined-up solutions to joined-up problems.'" The website offers this definition:

> Social exclusion is a shorthand term for what can happen when people or areas suffer from a combination of linked problems such as unemployment, poor skills, low incomes, poor housing, high crime environments, bad health and family breakdown.

Intended to inform government action through policy studies and reports:

> since it was set up in 1997, the SEU has published 28 reports in the following major policy areas: truancy and school exclusion; rough sleeping; teenage pregnancy; 16–18 year olds not in education, employment or training; neighbourhood renewal and reducing re-offending by ex-prisoners.

European Union program to combat social exclusion—www.europa.eu.int/comm/employment_social/soc-prot/soc-incl/index_en.htm
The European Union adopted a program of action to "eradicate poverty and social exclusion by 2010" by "sustained economic growth, more and better jobs and greater social cohesion." This site, titled "The Social Inclusion Process," describes and contains documents, including reports, studies and monitoring of national action plans, related to this 10-year goal.

# Chapter Eighteen

———————⬤———————

# THE HEALTH OF ABORIGINAL PEOPLES[1]

## Chandrakant P. Shah

## Introduction

According to the census, Aboriginal peoples, also known as the First Nations peoples or Native Canadians, fall into four groups; Status Indians, non-Status Indians, Métis, and Inuit. "Status Indian" has specific legal connotations and is defined as Aboriginal peoples registered under the *Indian Act* (Government of Canada, 1995). This group has signed treaties with the federal government that accord them certain privileges to be compensated for having relinquished certain land rights. Four centuries of colonization—being subjugated and stripped of their land, religion, culture, language, and autonomy—have taken their toll on the physical, mental, emotional, spiritual, and cultural health of the Aboriginal communities. Today's determinants of health reflect these injustices.

Aboriginal people define health and illness in terms of balance, harmony, holism, and spirituality rather than in terms of the western concepts of physical dysfunction and disease within the individual (Kirby and LeBreton, 2002). Some First Nations refer to this concept as the "medicine wheel," a holistic wheel consisting of the four quadrants or components of health: physical, mental, emotional, and spiritual. For achieving health, there must be harmony among all these components.

Unless otherwise indicated, the information in this section comes from *A second diagnostic on the health of First Nations and Inuit people in Canada* (First Nations and Inuit Health Branch and Health Canada, 1999). Interested readers are advised to read other publications listed in the end notes (Kirby and LeBreton, 2002; MacMillan et al., 1996; Manitoba Centre for Health Policy, 2002; Waldram, Herring, and Young, 1995).

Because of limitations related to health determinants and status information on the Métis and non-Status Indian populations, this section will focus primarily on the health information available for those registered as First Nations and Inuit. There is generally less information available about off-reserve Aboriginal people except for recent publications by Statistics Canada and others, which indicate the health and health determinants of these populations to be poor compared with other Canadian populations (Hanselmann, 2001; Richards, 2001; Shah and Dubeski, 1993; Tjepkema, 2002).

## Demography

The beginning of the 20th century represents the lowest point in the size of the population of Aboriginal people in Canada, with subsequent steady recovery since then, so that today it is at its highest level post-Confederation (Siggner, 1986). The 2001 census, which asked respondents to specify whether they were North American Indian, Métis, or Inuit, found that 976,305 or 3.3% of Canadians reported that they were Aboriginal compared with 2.8% or 799,010 five years ago (Statistics Canada, 2003). Of these, 608,850 (62%) people were North American Indian, 292,310 (30%) were Métis, and 45,070 (5%) were Inuit, and the remainder 3% identified themselves with more than one Aboriginal group. This population growth is due to a natural increase.

The crude birth rate per 1,000 population declined from 44.3 in 1965 to 27.3 in 1993, but in 2000 the fertility rate among the Aboriginal population was still 50% higher than the general Canadian population. Similarly, Aboriginal death rates remain higher than the rates for other Canadians. In 1996–97, First Nations and Inuit people throughout Canada had mortality rates at about 1.5 times the national mortality rate. Although life expectancy increased about 10 years between 1975 and 2000, life expectancy at birth was 68.9 years in 2000 for Registered Indian males and 76.3 years for females, substantially lower than the life expectancy of 76.3 years for Canadian males and 81.5 years for females.

The high birth rate of Aboriginal people, coupled with a consistently lower life expectancy, ensures a relatively young population compared to the general population. In 2001, the median age of the Aboriginal population was 24.7 years compared with 37.7 years in the general population: 33.2% were aged 0 to 14 years and 4.1% were aged 65 years and over, compared to 19.1% and 12.9%, respectively, for the general Canadian population. Although the Aboriginal population accounted for only 3.3% of Canada's total population, Aboriginal children represented 5.6% of all children in Canada. The gender distribution (a ratio of 49 men to 51 females) is approximately the same as for all Canadians.

Of the total Aboriginal population in 2001, 19.3% lived in Ontario, 8.1% in Quebec, 5.4% in the Atlantic region, and 67.3% lived in the four western provinces. Ontario had the highest absolute number (188,315) of Aboriginal people accounting for less than 2% of its total population followed by British Columbia with 170,025 people or 4.4% of its population. However, when viewed as a percentage of the total provincial or territorial population, Aboriginal peoples constituted 85% of Nunavut, 51% of the Northwest Territories, and 23.0% of the Yukon Territory. Ontario had more North American Indians than any other province. Alberta had the largest Métis population, while Nunavut had the largest Inuit population. In 2001, almost half (49.0%) of the Aboriginal people lived in urban areas; 31% lived on Indian reserves and settlement and the remainder (20%) lived in rural non-reserve areas. There are approximately 2,284 reserves in Canada. In 2001, 25% of all Aboriginal people lived in 10 of the nation's 27 census metropolitan areas; Winnipeg had the greatest number (55,755), followed by Edmonton, Vancouver, Calgary, Toronto, Saskatoon, Regina, Ottawa-Hull, Montreal, and Victoria.

## Determinants of health

### Psycho-social and socio-economic environment

Family violence is an important psycho-social issue faced by many Aboriginal communities. Results of four studies show that at least 75% of Aboriginal women have been victims compared with 7% of Canadian women. Up to 40% of children in some northern First Nations communities have been abused by a family member and elder abuse has also been identified as a serious problem in some First Nations communities.

The socio-economic environment, indicated by education, employment and income, is an important predictor of the health status of a population. In 1996, 54% of the Aboriginal population, compared with 35% of the non-Aboriginal population, had not completed high school. Compared to 16% of the non-Aboriginal population, only 4.5% of the Aboriginal population had a university degree. However, there has been some improvement among those at younger ages: for those in their 20s, an increased percentage of people have completed a non-university post-secondary diploma or degree (from 19% in 1981 to 23% in 1996); for on-reserve students, there has been an increase in the number remaining until Grade 12 for consecutive years of schooling (from 37% in 1987–88 to 74% in 1997–98).

Among First Nations people living on reserves, the unemployment rate was 29% in 1997–98, triple the national unemployment rate at the time. Forty-six percent of First Nations people on reserves rely on social assistance, a rate four times higher than the general Canadian population. As has been discussed elsewhere in this book, incomes on social assistance typically fall far below the low-income cut-off (LICO) set by Statistics Canada.

In addition to high unemployment rates, in 1995 one third of employed Aboriginal people 15 and older (compared to 25% of non-Aboriginal Canadians) worked in some of the lowest paying occupations, and the percentage of those employed in management positions was 1.5 times lower than those who were non-Aboriginal. In 1995, the mean income of employed Aboriginal people was 50% lower than the national average. Average earnings of Aboriginal people on reserves were lower than those of Aboriginal people not living on reserves. Forty-four percent of Aboriginal people have incomes falling below LICO, compared with 20% of the total Canadian population. Twice as many Aboriginal children live in single-parent or low-income families as other Canadian children (32%). Although they constitute only 3% of the Canadian population, Aboriginal people account for 16% of the sentences to correctional facilities.

On and off reserves, relative homelessness has been well documented by both government and other sources including the Royal Commission on Aboriginal Peoples (Royal Commission on Aboriginal Peoples, 1996). With high prevalence of the risk factors for homelessness—high unemployment, welfare dependency, poverty, substance abuse, physical and mental health problems, and domestic and sexual abuse—Aboriginal people have been identified to be the group perhaps most at risk for becoming homeless in Canada. Many Aboriginal people alternate between living on the reserve in the summer and in the city in the winter, leading to problems associated with consistent housing in the city.

Crowded living conditions are associated with increased risks of transmission of a number of infectious diseases including tuberculosis, hepatitis A, and shigellosis. In 1991, the average number of people per occupied private dwelling for on-reserve Registered Indians was 4.1, compared to 2.7 for the total Canadian population. Only 1% of Canadian dwellings had more than one person per room compared with 22% of on-reserve dwellings.

Housing condition is also an important determinant of health. Inefficient ventilation systems and high humidity can promote the growth of moulds, which has recently been identified as a problem in Aboriginal housing, that can induce respiratory and immune system illnesses. The availability of adequate water supplies and sewage disposal is important in the control of infectious diseases. Housing on reserves appears to be improving; however, nearly half the houses are still inadequate in terms of needing major repairs, having poor ventilation, and being overcrowded.

Environmental contaminants such as polychlorinated biphenyls (PCBs) and mercury can accumulate in fish and marine mammals, and ingestion of high levels of these compounds within such food sources can pose health risks to children (particularly the developing fetus and newborns). First Nations and Inuit people are considered at higher risk for exposure because of their traditional diets. In studies on Inuit from Quebec and Nunavut and on the Montagnais in Quebec, the amount of PCBs and mercury in infants' bodies has been found to be much higher than in other infants from similar areas and to be above the thresholds for cognitive and neurological impairments. In another study amongst the Cree in James Bay, mercury levels were high in a much smaller proportion of the population in 1993 (2.7%) than in 1988 (14.2%).

The issue of environmental contaminant exposure through traditional food sources is complex because game meat and fish are important sources of nutrients, are a healthier diet (compared to processed non-traditional foods), and contribute to cultural and spiritual bonds for the Aboriginal people.

## Lifestyle and behavioural risk factors

### Smoking
In 1997, First Nations and Labrador Inuit people 15 years old and over smoked at a rate of 62%, more than double the general smoking rate of Canadian population (29%). First Nations and Labrador Inuit smokers began smoking very early in life (at six to eight years of age) and show a rapid increase in initiation at ages 11 and 12.

### Alcohol and substance abuse
Alcohol and substance abuse, including the abuse of solvents, is considered a major problem within many Aboriginal communities. Information from addiction treatment centres, hospitalizations for alcohol-related causes, and violent deaths (e.g., suicides) have shown that alcohol is the abused drug of choice in Aboriginal Canadians. There are also more severe consequences of alcohol and substance abuse. Risks for alcohol-related problems are two to six times higher in Aboriginal youth than non-Aboriginal Canadian youth. Binge and chronic drinking is a problem among Aboriginal people and leads to risks of fetal alcohol syndrome (FAS) or fetal alcohol effects (FAE) in pregnancy. The incidence of FAS and FAE are variously reported in range of 100 cases per 1,000 births in Aboriginal communities, compared with 0.33 for FAS in Western countries. Aboriginal men may be more likely to abuse alcohol; Aboriginal women may be more likely to abuse other drugs alone.

Social Determinants of Health

Drug abuse also constitutes an important problem. In the Northwest Territories, Aboriginal people 15 and older were 3 to 3.5 times more likely than non-Aboriginal people to have used illicit drugs such as marijuana, hashish, LSD, speed, cocaine, crack, or heroin. Use of solvents and non-beverage alcohol (such as rubbing alcohol) is also a major problem among Aboriginal youths, with 20% having used solvents and with one third of users under 15 years of age. In the Northwest Territories, Aboriginal people 15 and older had 11 times the risk of having used solvents compared to the non-Aboriginal population and 24 times the risk compared to the general Canadian population.

### Problem gambling

Problem gambling may be an increasing problem among Aboriginal youth and adults. In Alberta, almost half of the Aboriginal students in grades 5 to 12 who participated in a study were either problem gamblers or at risk of becoming one. Another Alberta study in 1994 found that 22% of Aboriginal people aged 15 and older were problem gamblers, 40% were moderate pathological gamblers, and 15% were severe pathological gamblers.

### Nutrition

Many Aboriginal people in Canada, particularly in remote communities, experience all or most aspects of food insecurity due to low incomes, safety risks due to pollutants in the traditional food supply, quality problems associated with inappropriate shipping, handling, and home preparation of commercial foods, and disruptions to access caused by interruptions in shipping or changes in animal migratory patterns. More and more Aboriginal people are turning to commercial foods, which are more expensive and not always as nutrient-dense as traditional foods. The cost of commercial food is high, as is the cost of supplies for fishing and hunting (Food Security Bureau, 2001).

### Physical activity

With the reduction in fishing, hunting, and trapping that has accompanied acculturation and the loss of traditional ways of life, Aboriginal people now lead much more sedentary lives. According to the 1994–95 National Population Health Survey, 20% of Aboriginal residents in Northern Canada had active leisure time activities, compared to about 28% of non-Aboriginal northern residents (Diverty and Perez, 1998).

### Body mass index

The combination of genetic factors, changes in diet, and physical inactivity has led to a high prevalence of overweight among First Nations people. In a study of Northern Ontario residents, 29% of those of youth aged 5 to 19 and 60% of adult women were obese. Another study of adult Cree and Ojibwa in Northern Canada found a higher prevalence of overweight in the Aboriginal compared to non-Aboriginal population; almost 90% of women aged 45 to 54 had a body mass index of 26 or over. Fat distribution in Aboriginal peoples tends to occur primarily in the abdominal area, which is associated with increased risks for a number of chronic diseases including hypertension, coronary heart disease, stroke, premature death, breast cancer, and type 2 diabetes and its complications such as renal failure and blindness (Luepker, 1998).

### Sexual practices

According to the Ontario First Nations Healthy Lifestyle Survey (Myers et al., 1993), two out of every five males and one out of every five females reported multiple sexual partners in the 12 months prior to the survey; 15.4% of respondents reported having sexual partners both within and outside the community; 56.9% of respondents reported having unprotected sexual intercourse at least some of the time, and only 13.3% of respondents reported protected intercourse only. About two thirds of Aboriginal women surveyed by the Aboriginal Nurses Association of Canada indicated that they did not use condoms (Aboriginal Nurses Association of Canada, 1996). Condom use and the consistency of use were associated with learning about sex from family and through health services (Myers et al., 1999).

*Immunization*
First Nations 2-year-olds living on reserves were found to have lower vaccination coverage compared to the 2-year-olds in the rest of Canada in 1997. Immunization rates in 2- and 6-year-old Aboriginal children have also been found to be well below the national immunization target rates of coverage. This is an important issue, especially when combined with some of the issues related to housing and living conditions (e.g., crowding) on reserves that facilitate infectious disease transmission.

# Healthcare organizations

Different legislative acts, federal reports, and Supreme Court decisions have shaped the federal health policy for Aboriginal people and are well outlined in the Kirby report (Kirby and LeBreton, 2002). The federal government is responsible for the health care of Aboriginal peoples on reserves, and the provincial government for those off the reserves. The First Nations and Inuit Health Branch (FNIHB) of Health Canada is responsible for providing health services to those Aboriginal peoples with whom the government of Canada had signed treaties and are living on reserves. At present, there are approximately 976,300 eligible First Nations and Inuit people in Canada. The mandate of FNIHB is to assist First Nations and Inuit communities and people to address health inequalities and disease threats through health surveillance and population health interventions; to ensure the availability of, or access to, health services for First Nations and Inuit people; and to devolve the control and management of community-based health services to First Nations and Inuit communities and organizations.

There are three main programs. The Non-Insured Health Benefits Program (NIHB) provides registered Indians and recognized Inuit and Innu peoples with a range of medically necessary goods and services, which supplement benefits provided through other private or provincial and territorial programs. Non-insured health benefits include drugs, dental care, vision care, medical supplies and equipment, short-term mental health services, and transportation to access medical services.

The Community Programs Directorate (CPD) works in partnership with First Nations and Inuit peoples to deliver a wide range of programs in key community health sectors. All CPD activities have the goal of maintaining and improving the health of First Nations and Inuit, and facilitating First Nations and Inuit control of health programs and resources. CPD is organized as follows: Children and Youth Division; Mental Health and Addiction Division; Chronic Disease Prevention Division, and Addiction programs.

The Primary Health Care and Public Health Directorate (PHCPH) is responsible for primary healthcare delivery in partnership with First Nations and Inuit health authorities. All PHCPH activities strive to support knowledge and capacity building among First Nations and Inuit people, and to facilitate First Nations and Inuit control of health programs and resources. The PHCPH has the following divisions: the Primary Health Care Division, the Infectious Disease Control Division, the Environmental Health Division, and the Dental and Pharmacy Programs Division.

Nurse practitioners or physicians provide primary care in remote and isolated communities. In certain provinces and territories, several universities provide medical personnel and students on rotation. Since Aboriginal peoples live all over Canada, there is a network of 567 specially designed health facilities that operate in all provinces and territories (82 nursing stations, 189 health stations, 94 health offices, 202 health centres, five hospitals, 54 alcohol and drug abuse inpatient treatment centres, and 10 solvent abuse inpatient treatment centres for youth). Provincial departments of public health do not provide services on reserve. Unlike the provincial and territorial healthcare systems, public health programs for reserve residents are not mandated by legislation. A comprehensive public health program provides dental care for children, immunization, school health services, health education, and prenatal, postnatal, and healthy baby clinics and it provides care on reserves that other residents of Canada would receive from provincial and territorial governments, such as home care.

As residents of a province or territory, First Nations people are entitled to the benefits of the cost-shared provincially operated plans for medical and hospital insurance on the same terms and conditions as other Canadians. As many of the First Nations communities are small and often located in remote and isolated areas, these insured benefits are supplemented by the FNIHB, which assists First Nations bands to arrange transportation and to obtain drugs and prostheses. The FNIHB is in the process of transferring control of health services to the First Nations.

The FNIHB's Program Policy, Transfer Secretariat, and Planning Directorate facilitates the transfer of authority for community-based health programs and services to First Nations and Inuit control. This involves the development of policies, health-funding arrangements, planning strategies that support that role, and activities leading to the negotiation and conclusion of self-government agreements with First Nations. At the time of writing, of the total 602 First Nations and Inuit communities, 286 communities have signed transfer agreements with the Program Policy, Transfer Secretariat, and Planning Directorate. The branch, which serves as a national clearinghouse, has also established programs on Aboriginal diabetes, prenatal nutrition, home and community care on reserves, injury prevention and control, and alcohol and drug abuse, and has also initiated a national First Nations telehealth project.

Two thirds of Aboriginal peoples live in rural or remote areas, where healthcare services are often provided by nurses or community health workers supplemented by visits from physicians. In the 1994–95 NPHS, only 50% of those from the Northwest Territories and the Yukon had seen a general practitioner, compared with 77% from the provinces. Aboriginal northerners were much more likely to have seen a nurse (41% versus 18%). Aboriginal northerners were also less likely to have seen a dentist than non-Aboriginal northerners (Diverty and Perez, 1998). Admission rates for general and mental hospitals, usually located at great distances from the communities themselves, are high compared with other Canadian rates. In 1996–97, data from the Prairies indicated that First Nations people had a hospitalization rate 2.5 times that of the general Canadian population.

Geographic isolation also makes it difficult to provide appropriate services to northern communities. The priorities set by Aboriginal people are frequently at variance from those developed by the government, and many strategies for delivering health programs are inappropriate. However, in recent years, many Aboriginal communities have assumed the administration and management of health care in their own communities.

## Health status and consequences

### Mortality
Despite a decline in Aboriginal mortality, the gap in mortality between the Aboriginal and the general Canadian population remains wide. In 1996–97, mortality rates among First Nations and Inuit people from Eastern and Western Canada and the Prairie provinces were almost 1.5 times higher than the national rate (First Nations and Inuit Health Branch and Health Canada, 1999).

*Infant Mortality*
In 1995–97, infant mortality rates among First Nations people in Eastern and Central Canada, the Prairie provinces, and British Columbia were up to 3.5 times the national infant mortality rates. Neonatal death rates were up to double the general Canadian rates, while post-neonatal mortality rates were up to almost four times higher, contributing to high infant mortality rates. The common post-neonatal mortality causes are infectious diseases, respiratory diseases, and sudden infant death syndrome (SIDS) and injuries.

Relative risk of Indian children dying of SIDS is approximately three times higher than non-Indian children (MacMillan et al., 1996).

*Causes of death*
In 1996, for Canada as a whole, the four leading causes of death were circulatory diseases, neoplasms, respiratory diseases, and injuries (Federal Provincial and Territorial Advisory Committee on Population Health, 1999). The leading causes vary among different Aboriginal populations in Canada: in the Atlantic provinces and Quebec, the leading causes were circulatory system diseases followed by cancer, then injuries and poisonings. In the Prairies and British Columbia, the leading causes were injuries and poisonings, followed by circulatory system diseases and then cancer. Overall among all Aboriginal peoples in Canada, between 1979 and 1993, the four leading causes of death in order of decreasing frequency were unchanged: injury and poisoning, diseases of the circulatory system, cancer, and diseases of the respiratory system.

Although there has been an overall improvement in mortality rates from injury and poisoning, in 1996–97 First Nations and Inuit people were 6.5 times more likely to die of injuries and poisoning than the total Canadian population. The suicide risk among Registered Indians also varies by age and community, but is generally 2.5 times that of the general Canadian population (Federal Provincial and Territorial Advisory Committee on Population Health, 1999). In 1994, the suicide rate for Aboriginal people aged 15 to 24 was up to eight times higher than that of other Canadian youth (Task Force on Suicide in Canada, 1994).

*Potential-years-of-life-lost*
In 1996, the main causes of potential years of life lost (PYLL) among the Canadian

Social Determinants of Health

population were cancer followed by injuries and then cardiovascular diseases (Task Force on Suicide in Canada, 1994). In 1997, data from Western Canada show injuries and poisonings to be the leading causes of PYLL among the Aboriginal population. In 1993, Aboriginal PYLL was two times higher than that of the general Canadian population. In addition to injuries and poisonings, sudden infant death syndrome, congenital anomalies, and perinatal conditions were important causes of PYLL among Aboriginal people in 1993.

## Morbidity

### Infectious diseases

A variety of infectious diseases are found at higher incidence and prevalence in the Aboriginal population. Botulism, sometimes fatal, occurs in Aboriginal (and more frequently, Inuit) communities due to ingestion of fermented marine mammal meat, raw or parboiled fish, or salmon eggs. Since 1994, AIDS cases have been declining in the general Canadian population; in the Aboriginal Canadian population, however, the number of AIDS cases has risen dramatically. In 1997, the prevalence of AIDS in Aboriginal Canadians (33.2 per 100,000) was 11 times the national rate of 3.1 per 100,000. Injection drug use was responsible for 19% of AIDS cases in Aboriginal men and 50% in Aboriginal women.

Tuberculosis (TB) is also an important issue in the Aboriginal population. Although incidence rates have decreased between 1991 and 1996, with an average decline of 7% per year, the age-standardized incidence rate in Status Indians (35.8 per 100,000) greatly exceeds that of Canadian-born non-Aboriginal persons (2 per 100,000) (FitzGerald et al., 2000). In 1996, the incidence rate of TB among persons living on reserves was 40 per 100,000. In 1996, the highest provincial TB incidence rate in the Aboriginal population was in Saskatchewan (105 per 100,000).

The increase in AIDS cases seen among Aboriginal persons has important implications for TB because infection with HIV is a risk factor for active TB. Crowded living conditions, which are prevalent on reserves or in homeless shelters, aid the transmission of infectious diseases including TB. Data from Western Canada show that 42% of TB cases in Aboriginal people are due to recent infection compared to 12% of cases in the general Canadian population (with the remainder of active cases due to reactivation of old infection). The movement of many Aboriginal people between reserves and inner city locations adds to the challenges of control in terms of spread of disease geographically and because such movement has been identified as a risk factor for defaulting on treatment (FitzGerald et al., 2000).

### Chronic conditions

Table 18.1 shows the prevalence of a number of self-reported chronic diseases and conditions in Aboriginal people compared to the non-Aboriginal Canadian population. In 1997, those chronic diseases and conditions at higher prevalence in the Aboriginal population included heart problems and hypertension (about 2.5 to 3 times more likely to be reported than the general Canadian population), diabetes (almost four times more likely to be reported in Aboriginal men and more than five times more likely to be reported in Aboriginal women compared to the general Canadian population), and arthritis and rheumatism (about 1.5 to 2 times more likely to be reported than the general Canadian population) (First Nations and Inuit Health Branch and Health Canada, 1999).

**Table 18.1: Comparison of age-adjusted prevalence of chronic conditions in First Nations and Inuit and general Canadian population**

| Chronic condition | Gender | Age-adjusted prevalence (%) | | |
|---|---|---|---|---|
| | | First Nations and Labrador Inuit (FN&I) | General Canadian population | FN and I to Canadian population ratio |
| Heart problems | Male | 13 | 4 | 3.3 |
| | Female | 10 | 4 | 2.5 |
| Hypertension | Male | 22 | 8 | 2.8 |
| | Female | 25 | 10 | 2.5 |
| Diabetes | Male | 11 | 3 | 3.7 |
| | Female | 16 | 3 | 5.3 |
| Arthritis and rheumatisim | Male | 18 | 10 | 1.8 |
| | Female | 27 | 18 | 1.5 |

Before 1940, there was no evidence of diabetes among Aboriginal Canadians (D'Cunha, 1999). Today, however, the age-standardized prevalence of type 2 diabetes among Aboriginal peoples is at least three times that of the general population. Approximately two thirds of the First Nations people with a diagnosis of diabetes are women. The incidence of type 2 adult-onset diabetes in children as young as six years old appears to be increasing at a rapid rate (Diabetes Division Bureau of Cardio-Respiratory Diseases and Diabetes, 1999). The combination of genetic predisposition with a high prevalence of obesity (particularly central obesity) and physical inactivity contribute to the increased risks of diabetes. Although dietary acculturation has occurred in many Aboriginal communities, the association between diabetes and dietary factors has not been demonstrated consistently (Young et al., 2000).

*Disability*

Studies from the late 1990s indicate that disability rates among Aboriginal people aged 15 and over were high compared with the total Canadian population. According to the 1999 First Nations and Inuit Regional Health Survey (FNIRHS) (First Nations and Inuit Regional Health Survey National Steering Committee, 1999), 25% of those aged 55 and older had activity limitation in the home and one third had hearing problems. Overall, 15% of the Aboriginal population surveyed had hearing problems, a rate twice as high as the general Canadian population. The National Advisory Council on Aging has reported that the length of disability experienced by Aboriginal Canadians is about twice that of non-Aboriginal Canadians. According to the FNIRHS, chronic conditions were associated with activity limitations. As indicated above, incidence of FAS/FAE are higher among aboriginal communities leading to physical, mental, and emotional disabilities among children.

# Conclusion

The continued improvement of Aboriginal health will require attention to be paid to the determinants of health. The poor psycho-social, socio-economic, and physical environments within which many Aboriginal people live contribute greatly to the difficulty in achieving healthy lifestyles and to the much poorer health status in the Aboriginal population. Cultural insensitivity has often led to the paternalistic imposition of ineffective interventions. Five basic areas must be addressed to improve Aboriginal health, namely health research, a greater sensitivity to Aboriginal culture, a continuing process of control of health service and other aspects of local government services transfer to the communities, increased opportunities for the success of Aboriginal peoples in various healthcare professions, and an overall improvement in the socio-economic status of Aboriginal Canadians (Waldram et al., 1995). To achieve these ends, several efforts have been put in place to establish areas of Aboriginal self-government, and the federal government is transferring control of healthcare services to the local level of Aboriginal government or band councils. Ultimately, self-determination remains one of the hopes for improving the health of Aboriginal peoples.

In 1996, the Royal Commission on Aboriginal Peoples delivered the most comprehensive report on all aspects of the Aboriginal peoples' life, including their health, and made a number of recommendations related specifically to Aboriginal health (Royal Commission on Aboriginal Peoples, 1996). The Royal Commission recommended that the Aboriginal health and healing system should embody the following characteristics: equity in access to health and healing services and in health status outcome; holism in its approach to problems and their treatment and prevention; Aboriginal authority over health systems and, where feasible, community control over services; and diversity in the design of systems and services to accommodate differences in culture and community realities.

The federal government responded in 1998 by stating four objectives: to renew partnerships, strengthen Aboriginal governance, develop a new fiscal relationship, and support strong communities, people, and economies (Royal Commission on Aboriginal Peoples, 1997). It pledged $350 million to support the development of community-based healing for the legacy of psychological and physical abuse endured in the residential schools to which Aboriginal children were sent until 1969. Also in 1998, the Aboriginal Healing Foundation, an independent non-profit corporation, was established to address the healing needs of all Aboriginal peoples.

A number of health sciences programs now have programs to recruit Aboriginal students, and many regional health authorities seek Aboriginal participation in their governance. Professional organizations provide their members with cross-cultural awareness and the Society for Obstetrics and Gynecologists has published *The guide for health professionals working with Aboriginal peoples* (SOGC Policy Statement, 2000). Models of traditional healing practices along with western medicine are being developed in number of provinces. The Aboriginal Canada Portal is a useful site with links to national Aboriginal organizations, 12 federal government departments with Aboriginal mandates, all provincial governments, and organizations with Aboriginal responsibilities, as well as related Aboriginal community information (Government of Canada, 2002).

## Box 18.1: Encouraging signs for aboriginal people living off reserves

Carmelina Prete
*The Hamilton Spectator*

Aboriginal people living off reserves are improving their quality of life but still lag behind the average Canadian when it comes to health care, education and housing.

The 2001 Aboriginal Peoples Survey, released yesterday by Statistics Canada, shows health is worse among older female aboriginals and best among the young. This is encouraging since aboriginals under 25 are a growing segment of the population and now make up nearly half of the off-reserve Aboriginal population in Canada.

The survey is significant because it updates the statistical portrait of the well being of aboriginal people in Canada. The last one was done in 1991. Survey questions were answered by 117,000 Indian, Inuit and Métis people—of mixed Native and European descent—including 86,000 living off reserves.

Yesterday's survey dealt solely with Aboriginal people living off reserves, who make up 70 per cent of the total Aboriginal population in Canada.

"Things are getting better but we still have a long way to go," says Bruce Peterkin, executive director of the Aboriginal Health Centre in Hamilton.

Overall, 56 per cent rated their health as good or excellent compared with 65 per cent of all Canadians. The gap was negligible among young natives and widened among elder natives.

For example, four in 10 Aboriginal women aged 55–64 reported fair or poor health, more than double the number of non-Native women who said the same.

"I'm not surprised. They're the poorest of the poorest of the poor. They're the bottom rung," says Peterkin.

He says elder Natives have greater difficulty gaining access to mainstream medical services, which often means they seek help when they are already quite ill.

Nearly half of Aboriginal adults reported having a chronic illness. Arthritis, rheumatism, high blood pressure and asthma were most common. In every case, Ontario Natives reported a higher rate of chronic illness than the national aboriginal average.

For example, 19 per cent of Native Canadians reported suffering from arthritis.

The number was 26 per cent in Ontario.

Heather Tait, an author of the report, isn't sure why.

"We're just starting to scratch the surface with these numbers," she said.

The survey also sheds light on why 48 per cent of young Aboriginals off reserves drop out of high school compared with about one-third of non-Natives. One-quarter of Native

con't

Social Determinants of Health

con't

girls aged 15 to 19 said they left school because of pregnancy or child-care issues. Twenty-four per cent of boys in the same age group blamed boredom.

Catherine Brooks, an indigenous student counsellor at McMaster University, says roadblocks such as poverty and family responsibilities prevent aboriginals from completing their education. She said Aboriginals are more likely to start their post-secondary education after they've started a family, which make the pressures more intense. Statistics from the survey also show Aboriginals are more likely to complete their schooling later in life.

Roxanne Miller considers herself privileged.

The 30-year-old Mohawk is finishing an undergraduate degree at McMaster University with plans to start a masters degree in occupational therapy next year. Her goal is to become a doctor and serve the Aboriginal community.

She also works part-time at a Native health centre while raising her two children, aged 10 and 3, with the support of her fiancé.

"I know I'm not the norm," she says. "I'm privileged. I had a decent upbringing and a lot of support ... My push is that I want to provide a better life for my children."

Miller is among 100 Aboriginal students at McMaster, which has an enrolment of more than 17,500.

The survey also suggests overcrowding is a serious problem for Aboriginals living off reserves. In 2001, 17 per cent lived with more than one person to a room compared with seven per cent of other Canadians. Crowding was most serious for Aboriginal people in Winnipeg, Regina, Saskatoon and Edmonton where Native populations are larger.

The survey didn't offer statistics specific to Hamilton. According to the 2001 census, about 7,300 people living in Hamilton, Burlington and Grimsby identified themselves as Aboriginal—a 33 per cent jump from 1996.

—With files from Canadian Press

Source: *The Hamilton Spectator*. Thursday, September 25, 2003, p. A04

## Note

1.   Health of Aboriginal People is reprinted with the permission of Elsevier Canada from Shah, C.P., "Health of vulnerable groups," in *Public health and preventive medicine in Canada*, 5th edition, p. 163-173, and Shah, C.P. (2003), "Federal and provincial health organizations," in *Public health and preventive medicine in Canada*, 5th edition, p. 397–398.

## Recommended readings

Waldram, J.B., Herring, D.A., and Young, T.K. (1995). *Aboriginal health in Canada: Historical, cultural, and epidemiological perspectives*. Toronto: University of Toronto Press.

*Aboriginal health in Canada* is about the complex web of physiological, psychological, spiritual, historical, sociological, cultural, economical, and environmental factors that contributes to health and disease patterns among the Aboriginal peoples of Canada. This is a single, concise source of information about the different aspects of health and health care of the Canadian Aboriginal peoples.

Royal Commission on Aboriginal Peoples. (1997). *People to people, nation to nation: Highlights from the report of the Royal Commission on Aboriginal Peoples.* Ottawa: Minister of Supply and Services Canada.

This book introduces the reader to some of the main themes and conclusions in the final report of the Royal Commission on Aboriginal Peoples. That report is a complete statement of the Commission's opinions on, and proposed solutions to, the many complex issues raised by the 16-point mandate set out by the government of Canada in August 1991.

Society for Obstetricians and Gynecologists of Canada Policy Statement. (2000). "Guide for health professionals working with Aboriginal peoples: The sociocultural context of Aboriginal Peoples in Canada," *Journal of Society for Obstetricians and Gynecologists of Canada* 22(12), 1070–1081.

There are eight excellent recommendations for health professionals who work with Aboriginal Peoples supported by pertinent facts and literature review. These guidelines were developed by Aboriginal health care professionals and others working with the aboriginal organizations.

## Related websites

Aboriginal Canada Portal—www.aboriginalcanada.gc.ca

This is a site that links with 16,000 other sites and is provided by the Government of Canada and all Aboriginal organizations across Canada. It provides information for all aboriginal groups on health, education, social and legal issues/services, treaties, residential schools, directories of Aboriginal services, etc.

Health Canada—www.hc-sc.gc.ca/english/search/a-z/a.html

This site provides entry to the First Nations and Inuit Health Branch thorough A–Z index. It provides details about Aboriginal health and programs offered by the branch.

U.S. Department of Health and Human Services, Indian Health Service—www.ihs.gov

This is an official site for the U.S. Indian Health Services. It provides the various programs run by the government and also provides rationale for the program and services and statistical information on health of U.S. Indians.

Social Determinants of Health

# Part Five

———— ⬤ ————

# SOCIAL POLICY

I<small>N ALL OF THE PRECEDING SECTIONS</small>, there has been a clear recognition that the quality of social determinants of health is profoundly influenced by social policy decisions made by governments. In this section, specific focus is upon social policy developments in Canada and how these influence the social determinants of health. Social policy is primarily concerned with social welfare issues. More specifically, Vaillancourt and colleagues see social policy as involving, in part, state and government interventions that have the potential to contribute to the well-being of individuals and communities and foster full citizenship. These interventions could permit the redistribution of income, the offering of collective human services, and the development of individual and collective citizenship. A common theme running through discussions of social policy are the economic and other structural forces that drive policy change. As noted by other contributors, increasing globalization profoundly affects how governments consider and implement social policy. These social policies affect the quality of numerous social determinants of health, and by extension, the health of Canadians. And as documented in this volume, women, working, low-income, new, racialized, and Aboriginal Canadians are especially vulnerable to the effects of regressive social policy.

**David Langille** offers an analysis of the political forces influencing the social determinants of health. The erosion of many social determinants of health—verified by numerous indicators of social well-being in Canada—results from Canadian public policy being increasingly shaped to the needs of business. The ideology of neo-liberalism—driven by owners and managers of major transnational enterprises—has wielded an enormous influence over public policy. Langille sees the main levers affecting policy related to the social determinants of health as being macroeconomic policy that sets constraints on the role and scope of government. While Canada has never been richer, and never had so many resources as it does now, Canadians have been led to believe that social and other programs are not affordable. The solution to this crisis is a better balance between equality and freedom. Equality must be reclaimed as a positive social value.

**Michael Rachlis** explains how health care services can become a social determinant of health by being reorganized to support health. He provides many examples of effective— but all-too-rarely implemented—means of preventing deterioration among the ill through chronic disease management and rehabilitation. Screening that has been carefully assessed for its effectiveness can support health. And most important is preventing disease in the first place by promoting the social and living conditions that support health. Policy-makers and the health care communities have neglected prevention issues. There are significant political barriers to implementing the effective primary care that links communities to primary health care, continuing care, and public health services. The goal of Medicare should be keeping people well rather than just patching them up when they become sick.

**Yves Vaillancourt, François Aubry, Muriel Kearney, Luc Thériault, and Louise Tremblay** show how evolving social policies in Canada are major determinants of the health and well-being of the population. They trace recent developments in Canadian social policy and see the decline of the welfare state as resulting from economic forces associated with increasing globalization and adoption by governments of neo-liberal ideology. They then consider how social economy (or third sector) initiatives can contribute to positive social policy reforms, in the context of the changing welfare state. Vaillancourt and colleagues document how the social economy sector in Quebec has contributed to progressive policy development and program implementation in employment integration, early childhood education, and care, community home care, and social housing policy. Implications of the social economy for future policy development are outlined.

**Pat Armstrong** considers how Canadian women are being affected by recent social policy changes and by social economy sector initiatives. Changes in the funding and provision of services, including caring services—usually involving reductions and increasing privatization— most affect women. Women are more likely to use caring services, to be employed by the public sector to provide them, and to be called upon to provide care on a non-paid basis when funded services are not available. Her analysis of the social economy indicates that these initiatives may provide opportunities for community organizations to provide services in more democratic, transparent, and community-sensitive ways. These initiatives may also be unable to meet emerging needs without further burdening caregivers in the community, many of whom are women, or inadequately compensating them.

**Dennis Raphael and Ann Curry-Stevens** consider the role ideology plays in whether a nation assigns a high priority to strengthening the social determinants of health. The status of the Canadian welfare state is compared to other nations. They then direct attention to various actions that can strengthen the social determinants of health in Canada. These involve actions at various levels to implement policies and programs to strengthen the social determinants of health. Finally, they provide an intensive analysis of some of the psychological, social, and political forces that lead to the social determinants of health being so low on the policy agenda. How does the public view health and its determinants? Why are social determinants of health so neglected by health-related institutions and authorities? Are governments reluctant to raise the issues of the social determinants of health because of the role they play in weakening these health determinants?

# Chapter Nineteen

———◆———

# THE POLITICAL DETERMINANTS
# OF HEALTH

### David Langille

## Introduction

It has been demonstrated that social factors play an enormous role in determining the health of Canadians. And it is also clear that many of the indicators of social well-being have eroded over the past couple of decades. Why has there been this erosion in our social fabric? How can we explain or understand this deterioration?

This chapter shows that over the last three decades Canadian public policy has been moulded to the needs of business. It shows how the ideology of neo-liberalism has been applied in the Canadian context, and how global competition has influenced politics and public policy.

The driving forces shaping our social determinants of health have been the owners and managers of major transnational enterprises—the men who have defined our corporate culture and wielded an enormous influence over public policy. Their main instrument has been macroeconomic policy which they have used to set constraints on the role and scope of government. They have pushed for Canadian governments to adopt a free market or neo-liberal approach to macroeconomic policy.

The analysis shows that the corporate offensive of the last two decades was a response to democratic pressure for regulation and redistribution. It also shows democratic politics might once again put the public interest ahead of corporate interests. By identifying the political actors behind what are often seen as impersonal market forces, citizens can come to understand that progressive change is possible—and how they might improve the social determinants of health.

## Explaining recent socio-economic trends

Out of respect for the complexity and diversity of modern life, we often lose sight of the primary forces driving our society. Perhaps this is deliberate: "Although the knowledge that social and economic inequality produces inequities in health status has long been available, policy-makers avoid their root causes" (Hofrichter 2003, p. xvii). We need to explain a host of policy changes by federal and provincial governments, policies that not only took apart the social safety net erected by the welfare state in previous decades, but contributed to a fundamental reduction in the role and scope of the state.

There is a tendency to cite economic factors—e.g., lack of funding—as if the economy was some inexorable or omnipotent force that dictated social outcomes. There might be some merit to such an argument if our economy had collapsed, but our gross domestic product (GDP) has increased by 79% over the last two decades (1983–2002), from $599 billion to $1,075 billion (in constant 1997 dollars). On a per capita basis, GDP increased 45% during this period (Centre for the Study of Living Standards, 2004; See Figure 19.1). The country is now far richer and could have sustained or increased expenditures on social programs.

Rather than keep pace with economic growth, overall program spending by all levels of governments fell during the period 1983–84 to 2002–03. At the federal level, total program expenditures fell by 37.5%, from 18.4 to 11.5% of GDP (Canada,

Department of Finance, 2003, p.16) (See Figure 19.1). Provincial and territorial expenditures decreased by 18%, from 19 to 15.5% of GDP (Canada, Department of Finance, 2003, p. 36). Declining program expenditures cannot be blamed on the costs of servicing public debt. Total spending (program expenditures plus public debt charges) followed a downward trend regardless of whether debt charges went up or down (Canada, Department of Finance, 2003, p. 16, 36). Given that our governments could have spent more on program spending but chose to spend less, we are more likely to find our explanation in the realm of politics than economics.

There is no doubt that changing ideology has had an enormous impact, as manifested in the triumph of neo-conservatism or neo-liberalism (Coburn, 2000; McBride, 2001; Navarro and Shi, 2001). Both these ideologies celebrate the merits of free enterprise, but the neo-conservatives are more likely to retain a strong state in order to defend religious values, national security, and domestic law and order. Classic examples of neo-conservatism include Ronald Reagan, Margaret Thatcher, and George W. Bush. In contrast, neo-liberalism

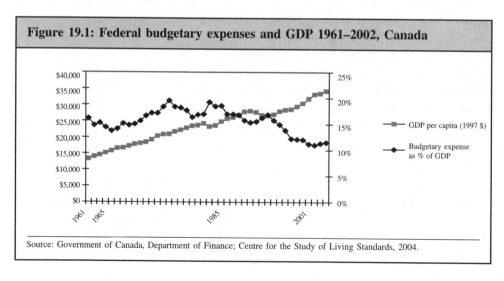

**Figure 19.1: Federal budgetary expenses and GDP 1961–2002, Canada**

Source: Government of Canada, Department of Finance; Centre for the Study of Living Standards, 2004.

Social Determinants of Health

allows more scope for individual rights—it means being fiscally conservative, keeping government spending and taxation to minimal levels, and taking a conservative approach to monetary policy, with strict control over interest rates and the money supply so as to protect capital against inflation—even if it means slowing down growth and job creation. The ranks of the neo-liberals include Carter and Clinton in the U.S., Blair in Britain, and Mulroney, Chretien, and Martin in Canada. While changes in ideology are important, we need to probe a little deeper to uncover the sources of these ideas and how they are being transmitted—the carriers, bearers, or communicators that propagate the ideology of free markets and less government. Typically, the words of academics only have political impact when they are championed by a think-tank and passed on to the mass media, prompting us to ask who sponsors the think-tanks and who owns the media.

There are political analysts who ascribe reduced social spending to a change in public priorities and a preference for tax cuts over public goods. Some credence must be given to this notion because the welfare state failed to sustain the support of many who depended on its largesse (Albo et al., 1993). But public opinion polls show Canadians routinely prefer public spending to tax cuts. Although some corporate spokespeople blame the public for changing their values or priorities (and do everything within their power to promote such changes), there is strong evidence that Canadians remain a compassionate, caring society that places a high value on public goods and services (Adams, 2003). Why then are they not getting policies to reflect their priorities? Perhaps the answer is not so much corruption of politicians as the corruption of our political process.

Let us exorcise another suspected culprit, globalization. Apologists for reduced social spending often invoke the need to be competitive and surrender to the dictates of the world economy (D'Aquino and Stewart-Patterson, 2001). As we will see, the same interests have also been working hard to remove whatever protected us from the vagaries of world markets and expose us to more competitive pressures (Clarkson, 2002; Dobbin, 2003; McBride, 2001). Globalization is increasingly understood as a political project or process that exploited new technologies of communication and transportation to weaken national barriers and create a world market for the transnational corporations.

## An historical perspective

It helps to understand the current corporate offensive against the welfare state and the political role of the popular sector if we retrace some history. Although there has been an ongoing struggle between classes inspired by their conflicting interests, our story begins after the Industrial Revolution when the free enterprise of those dark satanic mills was gradually regulated by the slow extension of the franchise and the exercise of democratic or popular power. Reforms and concessions were made not only to foster capital accumulation but to maintain the legitimacy of capitalist rule. The welfare state rested on a tension between two systems of decision-making: democratic government and the capitalist marketplace. When the conditions were right, the welfare state was a powerful mix and able to beat off challenges from fascism and communism.

The Canadian welfare state was slow to emerge given the powerful influence of business, which enjoyed a very close and influential relationship with the federal state no matter whether Conservative or Liberal governments were in power (Dobbin, 2003; McBride, 2001; Moscovitch and Albert, 1987; Teeple, 2000). Under the rubric of economic development, the state provided business with its infrastructure, its funding guarantees, bailouts, and subsidies. The state also helped to raise the qualifications and reduce the expectations of the labour force, as required. The Canadian political system was described as a confraternity of power, or a system of elite accommodation (Panitch and Leys, 2003). Of course, there was a period from the 1940s to the 1970s when the Canadian state gained relatively more autonomy from capital than it has enjoyed before or since. But as we will see, the corporate community launched a political offensive to reassert their control over the state.

Comparisons with the United States often help to clarify what is distinct about Canadian politics. Despite the elaborate system of checks and balances that circumscribe the power of the American state, it has more often served as a tool of populist sentiment—witness the trust-busting era at the turn of the century, and Roosevelt's New Deal during the Dirty Thirties. Canadian business was never subjected to the sort of strict anti-combines legislation as found in the United States—perhaps we place less faith in the merits of free competition. The American state was also more supportive of organized labour, at least for a time in the 1930s and 1940s, and it adopted a stricter set of environmental controls in response to the public interest movement of the 1970s (McCann, 1986). Although Canadians have enjoyed a more extensive welfare state, the Canadian state has at the same time been more supportive of or beholden to business. This may be on

account of the fact that the state has been dependent on the support of a very concentrated corporate community that has been more closely tied to capital in London and New York than to their Canadian workers. Given our high dependence on foreign trade and investment, Canadian business leaders have always had a "global consciousness" and have used it to lever support from the Canadian state (McBride, 2001; McBride and Shields, 1997; Panitch and Ley, 2003).

Clearly, the state was a terrain of political struggle. Corporate influence was being contested by social movements struggling to exert democratic control—a struggle in which artisans and craft unions, suffragettes, farmers, and industrial unions all played critical roles (Brodie and Jenson, 1988). In fact, the growing strength of the labour movement posed a challenge to business leaders. As labour institutionalized and developed its trade union bureaucracy, so too the business community created its trade associations and chambers of commerce.

We ended up with two systems of representation: political parties and "interest groups," which was the term used by liberal-pluralist political theorists to legitimize the influence wielded by these new participants in the political process. It was obvious that individual citizens wielded less influence, and a plurality of groups was preferable in their eyes to a polarization between classes. So these theorists redefined democratic politics as a struggle between competing groups. However, it was misleading to assume any sort of inherent equality or balance between these groups—between business associations and day care supporters for instance—and to assume that the state would play the role of a neutral arbiter between them, giving equal attention to all and rendering a balanced decision in the public interest. This was unlikely given that our liberal democracy exists within a capitalist economy, an economic and social system that is structurally imbalanced, dominated by powerful economic interests able to translate their economic power into political influence.

## Democracy delivered! We won—for a while ...

Under these conditions ordinary working people have to be mobilized and organized to act in a collective fashion if they are to have political power, i.e., if democracy is to work. That is what happened—people mobilized and democracy delivered—for a while. There was an upsurge in democratic activity following the Great Depression and the Second World War. First, the labour movement was able to secure their rights to collective bargaining and enjoy a share of increasing productivity. Unfortunately, the Canadian government's commitment to a Keynesian system of economic regulation began to falter soon after the war when pressure from the political left began to ease.

Due in part to the open nature of the Canadian economy, the government was never able to maintain steady growth, full employment, and rising incomes. However, by the time stagflation hit in the mid-Seventies and the Keynesian tools were finally abandoned, a social safety net had been erected that helped to protect workers from the worst effects of the economic crisis. Meanwhile, the civil rights struggle had erupted, followed by the anti-war movement, the environmental movement, and the struggle for women's rights. It was a time when businessmen were vilified as polluters and corporate welfare bums, and citizen participation via public interest groups helped increase state regulation and redistribution.

Corporate leaders became concerned. A report to the Trilateral Commission in 1975 warned about "an excess of democracy" that was placing too many demands on government (Crozier et al., 1975). It complained about too much welfare, too much protection for workers, a top-heavy bureaucracy and too many critics in academe and the media. The answer was to strengthen government's commitment to economic growth by centralizing authority and reducing its susceptibility to democratic inputs from citizens whose diverse demands undermined "efficient planning" (Marchak, 1991). This call was taken up by corporate leaders in all of the industrialized countries where state intervention and labour demands were threatening corporate profits. They organized a political counter-offensive to regain full control of the state (Frank, 2000; Monbiot, 2000; Phillips, 2002).

## Capital strikes back: A new era of corporate rule

The corporate offensive against the Canadian welfare state was led by the Business Council on National Issues. Over the last twenty-five years, the BCNI has become well known to those familiar with Canadian politics. It was founded in 1976 by corporate leaders anxious to exert more influence over a state that they felt had grown too large and interventionist. They organized 150 chief executives from the major, transnational corporations so as to be able "to contribute personally to the development of public policy and the shaping of national priorities" (Dunbar and Derry, 1984). As their website notes, these companies administer over $2.3 trillion in assets, earn revenues of more than $550 billion per year, and account for a significant majority of Canada's private sector

---

**Box 19.1: The institutions of neo-liberalism in Canada: How corporate priorities are realized**

---

**BUSINESS ASSOCIATIONS**

**Canadian Council of Chief Executives**—The voice of big business, representing the 150 CEO's of the major transnational corporations, formerly know as the Business Council on National Issues. Tom D'Aquino is President and CEO.

**Canadian Chamber of Commerce**—A coalition of local Chambers of Commerce representing the interests of many large and small businesses. Nancy Hughes Anthony is President and CEO.

**Canadian Bankers Association**—The leading lobby group for the chartered and foreign banks. Raymond Protti is President.

**Canadian Manufacturers and Exporters**—Canada's oldest business lobby group represents large manufacturers and exporters. Perrin Beatty is President and CEO.

**THINK TANKS**

**C.D. Howe Institute**—The voice of the Bay Street business elite, led by President and CEO Jack Mintz.

**Fraser Institute**—Founded in 1974 by Michael Walker to represent the "new right" devotion to free markets.

**Institute for Research on Public Policy**—A liberal response to the economic challenges of the Seventies, allowing more scope for government. Hugh Segal is President.

**"CITIZEN" FRONT GROUPS**

**National Citizens Coalition**—Funded by business leaders to defend individual freedom against government intervention.

**Canadian Taxpayers Federation**—A watchdog for the well-to-do against the "special interests" responsible for "runaway spending."

**LOBBYISTS**

"Government relations consultants" hired to help firms increase their influence and gain favours from government. A growth industry in recent years as dozens of firms enter the market. Examples include Earnscliffe Consulting, Executive Consultants, GCI, and Hill and Knowlton.

---

investment, exports, training and research and development. Although they had always subordinated the national interest in the pursuit of world markets, in keeping with their global mandate, they changed their name in 2001 to the Canadian Council of Chief Executives—when "it became clear that 'national issues' increasingly had global dimensions" (CCCE, 2004). Although there are other actors involved in implementing the neo-liberal agenda, as shown in Box 19.1, the BCNI/CCCE has exerted a greater impact on Canadian public policy than any other interest group, social movement, or non-governmental organization (Langille, 1987). Given that all but two or three of its 150 members are men, it is also the strongest institution of patriarchy in the country.

The Business Council is an inter-sectoral business association that has become the senior voice of business within Canada. It is also a participant in the new right political offensive which transnational corporations helped inspire throughout the industrialized countries. Discussions of such capitalist restructuring are often conducted at such a level of abstraction that we risk losing sight of the political actors. However, political theorists such as Antonio Gramsci, Robert Cox, Stephen Gill, Giovanni Arrighi, Emmanuel Wallerstien, and Sidney Tarrow help us appreciate how such structures are socially constructed—to see how social forces make history. It is important to expose in this way what are otherwise seen to be impersonal market forces—all powerful forces which move inexorably and cannot be resisted. Once we appreciate how political actors emerge and trace their struggles over time we gain a better sense of their vulnerabilities and of the possibilities for opposition forces.

Guided by their primary objective of curbing the role and size of the state, the Business Council has helped maintain the fight against inflation, cut back public spending, and restore corporate profits. The BCNI's greatest success to date has been to engineer support for high-level agreements facilitating world trade and investment, beginning with CUFTA and NAFTA, agreements which do not guarantee free trade but serve as a new economic constitution for the Americas—guaranteeing an investment climate conducive to the prosperity and expansion of transnational corporations. These agreements further undermine the sovereignty of the Canadian state and the policy capacity of our provincial

governments, which find themselves forced to compete in a process of downwards harmonization, offering less services to their citizens in an effort to sustain business confidence. The net effect has been a serious erosion of support for government and a loss of faith in democratic possibilities.

## Taking stock of the political dynamics and assessing the balance of forces

As we have seen, Canada's social movements and citizens groups exerted pressure on the state to constrain the corporate sector and redistribute wealth. Threatened with a loss of control and the erosion of profits, the corporations launched a counter-offensive. Quite self-consciously, they have been waging a class struggle and winning. Economic trends, many of them politically inspired, have reinforced the power of capital while weakening the social movements: unemployment (often induced by technological change or other corporate restructuring initiatives), the increase in part-time work, the erosion of social security, international competition, the mobility of capital and of production, and the deregulation of trade, financial, and labour markets. Consequently, the organizations of capital have not had this much political, economic or social power in 50 years.

But the popular sector is certainly not powerless or ineffectual. If further evidence is required, one can look at the fluctuations in corporate political activity over the past few decades as they have been forced to respond to threats from below. Although the Business Council on National Issues prefers to maintain a rather low profile and not wield their weight in public, to avoid squandering their political capital or wasting other resources, they have been forced to take public stands on several issues over the past 20 years. In fact, their very origins stemmed from an outbreak of public concern over "corporate welfare bums," and their first action was to collaborate with organized labour in a quest to remove wage and price controls. The BCNI mobilized in the early 1980s in response to the outbreak of economic nationalism associated with the NEP and FIRA. The organization was then able to lay low during the first Mulroney years confident that the Conservatives were doing their best to implement the BCNI's agenda. However, in the run-up to the federal election of 1988 they were galvanized to defend the Canada–U.S. free trade agreement when it appeared that opposition forces might derail the deal. The Business Council had to organize the Canadian Alliance for Trade and Job Opportunities and raise many millions of dollars for its advertising campaign in order to win that battle. Also in that decade, the BCNI's Task Force on Defence and International Security responded to pressure from the peace movement that called for Canada to "Refuse the Cruise" and reduce military spending. Instead, they kept flogging the threat of the Soviet Union as an aggressive superpower in order that a few high-tech manufacturers could profit from the arms race. Similarly, the Business Council created its Task Force on the Environment to develop their own interpretation of "sustainable development", and subsequently came out as a leading opponent of the Kyoto Accord, an international effort to reduce the gas emissions that contribute to global warming.

## Manufacturing the debt and deficit mania

BCNI/CCCE President Tom D'Aquino used to consider the free trade fight to be his greatest victory, and the failure to reduce the deficit his greatest liability. But as soon as the 1988 election confirmed the Canada-U.S. trade agreement, the BCNI launched its campaign to reduce the deficit by cutting government spending. Although the Ontario NDP Government tried to use conventional Keynesian techniques to ride out the recession of the early 1990s, they eventually succumbed to the (business) pressure for restraint. The only serious threat to corporate priorities came from within the Liberal Party as it sought to be elected on a commitment to job creation. After the Liberal victory in 1993 there was a further period of uncertainty about which direction the new government would take, and the BCNI resurfaced as vocal champions of deficit reduction until Finance Minister Paul Martin's first budget confirmed the defeat of the reform liberals. Since then the combined efforts of business and government have had a considerable impact on public opinion, generating a deficit mania and a fixation with balanced budgets. Worse still, there have been ideological zealots in both Canada and the U.S. so obsessed with reducing government and cutting taxes they have been willing to induce a revenue crisis and manufacture a deficit—helping to de-legitimize any collective response via public policy.

By focussing on the fiscal framework, the Canadian Council of Chief Executives have not dictated all aspects of public policy but have set the boundaries or constraints on what governments can do. So what will it mean to have one of their former members, the former CEO of Canada Steamship Lines, at the helm as Prime Minister? Professor Robert MacDermid points out that "Corporations and corporate executives gave over 9 million dollars to Paul

Martin's leadership campaign, often giving $100,000 or more" (Centre for Social Justice, 2003). He questions whether Martin's connections to business will affect his commitment to middle and lower income Canadians and the poor. It is worth reflecting on his record as Finance Minister.

## The Martin legacy: Minimal government and enhanced trade

The legend about Paul Martin designing and delivering an amazing economic recovery in Canada while ridding the nation of chronic deficits is largely myth. Murray Dobbin has shown that his enormous cuts to health and education did not eliminate the deficit, but rather it was the Bank of Canada's decision to dramatically lower interest rates that sparked a burst of economic growth and generated nearly $100 billion in surpluses from 1997 to 2003.

> Canada's performance in the 1990s was the worst of any decade in the 20th century except the 1930s. By virtually every economic measure of importance—GDP growth, employment, new investment, productivity, standard of living, wages and salaries—the 1990s were a flat-out disaster ... Paul Martin's fiscal and economic policies didn't work—and they're still not working. The productivity gap with the U.S. is growing, not shrinking. GDP growth is still anemic, wages and salaries have increased only marginally, job growth is weak and we still have the second-highest number of low-wage jobs among all industrialized countries. We still attract less

foreign investment per capita than the U.S., and most of it is used to buy up existing assets. (Dobbin, 2003b)

Consistent with corporate priorities, Finance Minister Paul Martin was primarily committed to improving trade. He made cuts of 50 to 60% to the many departments that were long associated with nation building—agriculture, fisheries, transportation, natural resources, regional and industrial development, and the environment. There was such a faith that trade would drive the economy that the government abandoned its traditional tools of industrial and regional development, tools that had built the domestic economy. In fact, less than 20% of our real GDP is accounted for by trade. The policies designed to facilitate trade benefitted a relatively small number of Canadian businesses. Just 4% of all exporting establishments accounted for 82% of the total value of merchandise exports, while 80% of Canadian enterprises do not export at all (Dobbin, 2003b).

The wisdom of the corporate agenda in increasingly in doubt. As Jim Stanford points out:

> The world can change quickly in the era of globalization and we have seen such changes in just the past two years. The U.S. economy is precarious, with its balance-of-payments deficit at the unsustainable level of five per cent. The U.S. budget deficit this year will be a staggering $500 billion. The U.S. dollar is falling and ours is rising, posing a real threat to our export market. If Washington raises interest rates to finance its deficit, it could dampen their already

precarious growth—and further undermine our exports. (Stanford, 2003)

## The social implications

It is noteworthy that the average compensation received by the chief executives of the 68 largest publicly-traded companies in 2002, including salary, benefits and stock options, was $7.2 million. CCCE Vice-Chairman Gordon Nixon, CEO of the Royal Bank was paid $12.8 million. "Such excessive payments contributes to growing income inequality in Canada," notes Professor Robert MacDermid, "especially when you consider that minimum wage workers earned an average of only $14,102 that same year—it would take them 912 years to earn that much" (Centre for Social Justice, 2003).

Although there is clear evidence that poverty and inequality reduces health outcomes, there is good reason to question the corporate commitment to address the problem. The CCCE leaders have pledged to "ensure that the real disposable incomes of the worst-off 20 percent of Canadian families—their incomes after taxes, government transfers and inflation—should grow over the next ten years at least as quickly as that of the average Canadian" (D'Aquino and Stewart-Patterson, 2001, p. 300). That would increase the incomes of poor people by one-third over the decade, which the authors suggest "would clearly represent real progress by any definition," but it would in fact mean they fall further behind other Canadians and it would widen the gap between rich and poor. While a one-third increase in an income of $9,000 would add $3,000, a one-third increase in an income of $90,000 amounts to $30,000. The

corporate executives aren't calling for a substantial reduction in poverty, and they are not even offering to reduce inequality. It just is not on their agenda.

Instead, the CCCE is pushing for increased continental integration. "Canadian business leaders believe that the time has come for the next big step forward in the Canada–United States relationship" (CCCE, 2004). The North American Security and Prosperity Initiative was launched in January of 2003, and calls for action on five fronts:

- *Reinventing borders*—removing barriers to trade between Canada and the U.S., and harmonizing our immigration policies.
- *Maximizing economic efficiencies*—harmonizing regulations.
- *Negotiation of a comprehensive resource security pact*—ensuring free access.
- *Reinvigorating the North American defence alliance*—putting more troops and weapons systems under US control.
- *Creating a new institutional framework*—creating a stronger partnership.

Integrating more closely with the United States could not fail to put further pressure on Canada's frail social safety net and further exacerbate inequalities in income, wealth and power (Grinspun, 2003).

## Corporate power and democratic resistance

Citizens need to know why the corporate leaders have so much power and are able to exert so much influence if they are to challenge their hegemony. As Box 19.2

---

**Box 19.2: Why the chief executives are so powerful—and how citizens can regain democratic control**

1. **POWER IN NUMBERS**
   Their power comes from 150 corporations with:
   - Assets of $2.3 trillion (up from $440 billion in 1982)
   - Earning revenues of over $550 b./yr (up from $170 billion in 1982), and
   - Employing 1.3 million Canadians (down from nearly 2 million in 1982)

   What can citizens do...?

   **HAVE POWER IN NUMBERS**
   - 30 million Canadian citizens
   - 6 billion global citizens

2. **GOOD POLITICAL ORGANIZATION**
   (a) They are pre-emptive and pro-active. They have a long-term vision and seize the initiative. Citizens can do that.
   (b) They focus on a few critical areas, and do good research. Citizens can do that.
   (c) They speak everyday language in an effort to define what is common sense. Citizens can do that.
   (d) They form "task forces" that shadow government departments and offer new policy initiatives. Citizens can form networks of academics and activists to shadow corporations and government—and offer their own citizen's agenda, alternative budgets, and legislation.
   (e) They champion the national interest—pretending that what's good for the corporations is good for Canada. *But they're the real special interests.*

---

shows, the power of the Canadian Council of Chief Executives rests primarily on their control over enormous economic assets. But they have also demonstrated very effective political organization, recruiting their members into task forces that served as virtual "shadow cabinet" for the government, covering the national economy, social policy, political reform, environmental policy, the international economy and foreign affairs, defence, and corporate governance. The Council does not typically engage in lobbying and influence peddling to boost the profits of a particular company or sector, but makes an orchestrated effort to create a favourable climate for business—to privilege private, for profit, activity.

In promoting its agenda, the CCCE has been aided by a network of research institutes, including the C.D. Howe and the Fraser Institute. Most of the corporations that fund and support these institutes are also members of the CCCE. Together, these corporate "think tanks" organize conferences, seminars, retreats and briefings on major public policy concerns to which they invite politicians, journalists, academics, and other community leaders or elites. To maintain a common front in the business community, the Business Council recruited the heads of the Canadian Chamber of Commerce, the Canadian Manufacturers and Exporters, and le Conseil du patronat in Quebec. While they did not have formal alliances with the National Citizens' Coalition or the Canadian Taxpayers' Association, these right-wing networks helped spread their message to the general public.

Although having a CEO as Prime Minister symbolizes the growing corporatization of Canadian politics, Box 19.2 also shows how citizens can learn a great deal from the CCCE about how they might mobilize an effective resistance. If citizens are to reassert their power and restore democracy they will first have to raise public awareness about the threat of corporate control. They will have to elect politicians ready to put citizens first, and that requires not only banning corporate contributions to candidates and parties, but eliminating tax deductions for lobbying or other political activities. We will have to reimpose stronger regulations at both domestic and international levels and withdraw from agreements that put corporate interests ahead of citizens.

## Conclusion

This chapter has demonstrated how politics over-determines the social determinants. It has put a human face to the abstract notions about capital, corporate power, and economic restructuring. We need to know in concrete terms with whom we are dealing with if we hope to regulate in the public interest. And regulate we must. There are countless opportunities to address the many social determinants of health, and concrete gains can be achieved via local initiatives, but it is clear that overall conditions are continuing to deteriorate because the state is being run according to the needs, interests, and priorities of transnational corporations. Despite their rhetoric to the contrary, the corporate policies stand in fundamental and concrete opposition to the public interest—they are not conducive to improving the health of Canadians.

Canadians need a monetary policy and fiscal policy that encourage the growth of the domestic economy.

> That means endorsing the now widely accepted monetary view that inflation levels of six per cent or less are not harmful to the economy, but in fact promote healthy economic growth. The same is true of fiscal policy: rather than use most of our future budget surpluses to pay down the debt, we need to renew social spending. (Dobbin, 2003b)

Although exports are critical, export markets can be precarious and unpredictable, so we must also ensure that our domestic economy is strengthened and that Canada maintains a high-wage economy. Improving public services by spending on nurses and teachers contributes directly to our domestic economy. A national child-care program would enable tens of thousands of women to enter the workforce just as Canada is starting to face a labour shortage. The Alternative Federal Budget process shows that it is feasible to improve the social determinants of health within a realistic fiscal and monetary framework.

At a philosophical and personal level, the solution is to find a better balance between equality and freedom—to reclaim equality as a positive social value. Equality has gone out of fashion in recent decades, having been squelched in the pursuit of free enterprise. The values of the marketplace—individual greed, fear, insecurity—triumphed and our rich legacy of social values—compassion, caring, sharing—was demeaned. In concrete terms, reversing these priorities calls for a change in government.

# Recommended readings

Canadian Council of Chief Executives. (2004). *A Canadian agenda for progress and prosperity: Where Canada's business leaders stand.* Ottawa: Canadian Council of Chief Executives.

A comprehensive summary of the CCCE's positions across the full spectrum of economic and social policy, at home and abroad. It is organized along seven strategic themes: setting the fiscal framework, encouraging innovation and competitiveness, fostering human and community development, etc.

Clarkson, S. (2002). *Uncle Sam and us: Globalization, neoconservatism, and the Canadian state.* Toronto: University of Toronto Press.

While Clarkson focuses on how Canada has always been strongly influenced by its southern neighbour, he offers a good guide to understanding how public policy in this country is being affected by the corporate pressure for further continental integration.

Dobbin, M. (2003). *The myth of the good corporate citizen: Democracy under the rule of big business, 2nd edition.* Toronto: James Lorimer.

An account of how corporate globalization has affected Canadians by undermining our democracy and eroding our social and economic well-being.

Doern, B. (Ed.) (2003). *How Ottawa spends: 2003–2004: Regime change and policy shift.* Toronto: Oxford.

This annual series offers chapters analyzing the politics and public policy of particular sectors such as education, health care, housing, pensions, poverty, and deregulation.

Hofrichter, R. (Ed.) (2003). *Health and social justice: Politics, ideology, and inequity in the distribution of disease.* San Francisco: Jossey-Bass.

This collection offers a broader analysis of the politics of health inequalities, covering the effects of racism, social class, and gender discrimination. It also examines the political implications of various perspectives used to explain health inequities and explores alternative strategies for eliminating them.

McBride, S. (2001). *Paradigm shift: Globalization and the Canadian state.* Halifax: Fernwood.

McBride reveals how the pressure to remove obstacles to global trade and investment has contributed to growing inequality and insecurity, as well as undermining Canadian sovereignty and democratic governance.

# Related websites

Canadian Council of Chief Executives—www.ceocouncil.ca/

Given how the most powerful pressure group in the country manages to set the agenda for government, watch this site in order to keep abreast of emerging trends in Canadian public policy.

Centre for Social Justice—www.socialjustice.org

The CSJ undertakes research, education and advocacy in an effort to narrow the gap in income, wealth, and power. It offers a range of materials covering the social determinants of health.

Canadian Centre for Policy Alternatives—www.policyalternatives.ca

The CCPA conducts research on issues of social and economic justice and produces a range of publications, including a monthly digest of progressive research and opinion.

Canadian Policy Research Network—www.cprn.com

The CPRN's mission is to create knowledge and lead public debate on social and economic issues important to the well-being of Canadians.

Institute for Research on Public Policy—www.irpp.org

The IRPP seeks to improve public policy in Canada by generating research, providing insight and sparking debate on public policy.

# Chapter Twenty

———●———

# HEALTH CARE AND HEALTH

## Michael Rachlis

## Introduction

Historically, health care or more specifically, illness treatment services, have not been a major determinant of population health. McKeown (1979) traced the decline of several major communicable diseases in developed nations and showed that the bulk of mortality had already been eliminated by the time an efficacious therapy had been developed.

Advances in health status in the future will depend upon preventing illness through more policy attention to the broader determinants of health. Over 80% of cases of coronary heart disease, diabetes, and lung cancer could be prevented. While major health gains require broad-based prevention, re-engineered illness treatment services could make health care a more important determinant of health.

This paper outlines how better engineered health care services could implement more effective tertiary, secondary, and primary prevention. Primary prevention promises the most health gains but primary prevention has largely proven beyond the grasp of health services, even public health services. This chapter outlines some of the barriers to primary prevention and then discusses how to surmount them.

## Re-engineered health care could be a more important determinant of health

### Tertiary prevention: Preventing deterioration in function

The federal government first funded hospital services and then physician services leading to a system heavily tilted towards treatment. Coronary heart disease (CHD) is one of the major causes of death in Canada. Death rates fell by over 50% between 1969 and 1997, due in part to changes in risk factors such as hypercholesterolemia, smoking, and hypertension (Heart and Stroke Foundation, 2000). But improved living conditions during Canadians' formative years are also strongly implicated (Raphael and Farrell, 2002). The prime methods of treatment for CHD are surgery and medication but comprehensive rehabilitation using diet, exercise, and stress reduction has been proven to be as effective as these modalities for selected patients (Ornish et al., 1998). Unfortunately, cardiac rehabilitation is available to a minority of Canadian CHD sufferers.

A recent review concluded that most studies of "lifestyle" rehabilitation had positive results (Wagner, 1997). Exercise has been found to improve cognitive function in the elderly (Fabre et al., 2002), improve mood for patients with fibromyalgia (Gowens et al., 2002), and improve function and endurance in patients with chronic obstructive pulmonary disease (Ortega et al., 2002).

An example of a comprehensive approach to rehabilitation for people with multiple chronic health problems is the Program for All-Inclusive Care of the Elderly or PACE programs (see www.onlok.org/stats.html). The first PACE program was the On Lok Senior Health Services which opened its non-profit operation for the frail elderly in 1973 with a day health centre located in a renovated nightclub in downtown San Francisco. Today On Lok serves 860 high-risk seniors, whose average age is 83. Clients of this program are very frail. Three-quarters of On Lok's participants are incontinent and over 60% have some type of cognitive problems, mostly Alzheimer's Disease.

In addition, many are at special risk because of poverty and isolation. Sixty percent of its participants live alone and 40% are poor enough to qualify for SSI (Supplemental Security Income). Located in San Francisco Chinatown, most of On Lok's enrollees are Chinese, although Filipinos, Italians, other Caucasians, and Blacks also use its services.

On Lok became the prototype for PACE. There are now over 40 in the United States.[1] The model appears to work. PACE residents typically cost 5% less than traditional care but they use a dramatically different array of services (King, 1992). PACE spends only 22% of its dollars on hospitals, long term care facilities, lab tests, X-rays, medications, and medical specialists. This leaves almost four fifths of the program's dollars to be spent on day programs, home care, and family doctors. The program's participants use less hospital care than the average for the entire U.S. over 65 population, even though On Lok's participants are all very frail and have an average of seven chronic illnesses.

## Secondary prevention

### Screening and early detection
Screening and early detection of disease has shown more promise than results. Screening has been shown to improve survival from cervical (Nygard et al., 2002), breast (Sox, 1998), and bowel cancer (Ransohoff and Sandler, 2002). However, the issues are not as clear as the public usually sees them. The public tends to imagine that when one is screened for a cancer, it provides 100% protection. And the public tends to assume that screening has no risks to the patient. Neither supposition is correct.

Cancer screening programs have both false negatives (where people with cancer erroneously test negative) and false positives (where people without cancer erroneously test positive). The first group will go on to develop their cancer despite the screening program. The second group will be subjected to further (and sometimes) dangerous testing after the screen positive test. The pros and cons for cancer screening have recently been reviewed (Barratt et al., 1999). Barratt et al. concluded that screening can cause the following harms:

- Complications arising from investigation.
- Adverse effects of treatment.
- Unnecessary treatment of persons with true-positive results who have inconsequential disease.
- Adverse effects of labelling or early diagnosis.
- Anxiety generated by the investigations and treatment.
- Costs and inconvenience incurred during investigations and treatment.

## Chronic diseases: Big problems for the Canadian health care system

The complications of and the acute manifestations of chronic illnesses are responsible for most deaths and a substantial majority of hospitalizations (Hoffman et al., 1996):

- Chronic diseases account for 70% of all deaths.
- Chronic diseases account for more than 60% of medical care costs.
- Chronic diseases account for one third of the years of potential life lost before age 65.

The Canadian health care system does a poor job of managing chronic illnesses. Depending upon the disease studied, 40-80% of patients are inadequately treated.

- Less than 30% of Canadians with high blood pressure have their blood pressure properly controlled (Wolf et al., 1999; Joffres et al., 1997).
- In B.C. at least 40% of diabetics have not had a HgA1C determination within the last year, 60% have not had a lipid profile in the past 3 years, 60% have not had

an eye examination in the past year, and 70% have not had their urine checked for protein (Gibbs, 2000).
- A B.C. study of asthma showed that only 20% met the criteria for appropriate medication management (Anis et al., 2001). A national survey showed that 60% of Canadian asthmatics did not have their disease properly controlled (Mellor, 2000).
- A McMaster University study found that Ontario family physicians offered only 40% of the preventive manoeuvres recommended by the Canadian Task Force on the Periodic Health Examination (Hutchison et al., 1998).
- Over 20% of patients discharged from hospital with congestive heart failure are re-admitted within 60 days (Lee et al., 2001; Vancouver Richmond Health Board, 2001).
- At least 35% of Ontario elderly patients who should have taken beta-blocker drugs after a heart attack did not get them (Rochon et al., 1999).

## Chronic disease management: Great potential

While Medicare was designed to provide acutely ill patients with access to hospitals and physicians, managing chronic illness and an aging population requires community-based care and a focus on maintaining function and health. A system designed mainly for acute care will be overwhelmed with chronic patients who develop complications. Some provinces and communities have developed innovative chronic disease management programs.

For example, a pilot project in British Columbia provided 4–12 hours of health promotion to patients who were applying for long-term care. After 36 months, those in the health promotion group were 39% less likely than members of the control group to have died or to have been placed in a long-term care institution (Hall et al., 1992).

Diabetes affects only about 6% of the population but diabetics have 32% of the heart attacks, 51% of the new cases of kidney failure, and 70% of amputations (ICES, 2002). Better control of diabetes can greatly reduce these complications (U.K. Prospective Diabetes Study Group, 1998). The Sault Ste Marie Group Health Centre is Canada's largest alternatively funded group practice and has 44,000 enrolled patients, 60 doctors, and over 100 nurses. It also has an electronic medical record with a registry of over 2,200 diabetic patients. Since January 2000, the Centre has documented major improvements in all aspects of diabetes control (Bragaglia et al., 2001).

Congestive heart failure (CHF) is the number one cause of non-reproductive hospital admissions in adults. The Sault Ste Marie Group Health Centre uses specially trained nurses to follow their CHF patients after discharge. This project decreased the rate of readmissions by over 60% within the first six months (Lee et al., 2001).

## The Chronic Care Model

Dr. Ed Wagner is the director of Group Health's McColl Institute for Healthcare Innovation. Dr. Wagner and his colleagues at Group Health in Seattle have worked with others to develop new approaches to improve health organizations' management of chronic illnesses. The McColl Institute is also the national program office for the Robert Wood Johnson Foundation's program on Improving Chronic Illness Care. Improving Chronic Illness Care (ICIC) has three underlying provisos:

1.  There are highly effective clinical and behavioural interventions for most chronic illnesses.
2.  There is good evidence on how to change the delivery system to improve care.
3.  There is a need to develop action-oriented improvement strategies to accomplish the changes.

The following principles guide the system re-design:

1.  *Comprehensive*: reorient the organization and individual practices to provide planned care.
2.  *Evidence-based*: rely on high-grade evidence of improvement in outcomes.
3.  *Client-centred*: build services around meeting client needs for confidence and skills in self-management.
4.  *Population-based*: design to assure the delivery of effective interventions to all patients with particular needs.

Dr. Wagner's group developed the Chronic Care Model, which is shown in Figure 20.1. The Chronic Care Model (or CCM) outlines diagrammatically an organizational approach for chronic disease management. The model identifies the essential elements of a system that encourages high-quality chronic disease management. These are: the community, the health system, self-management support, delivery system design, decision support, and clinical information systems. Appropriate action at these levels should lead to more productive interactions between patients who are actively involved in their care and providers who have the resources and skills needed for the attainment of improved functional and clinical outcomes. These methods can be applied to a variety of chronic illnesses, health care settings, and target populations.

Group Health has achieved considerable success internally using the CCM. Wagner reported that using the CCM for program planning, Group Health's diabetic patients had sustained improvements in glycemic control. The health plan realized cost savings within 1–2 years of improvement (Wagner et al., 2001).

## Primary prevention

A population health approach appreciates that the most effective strategy to deal with most health problems is to understand their root causes and then take preventive action. For example, adult onset (or type II) diabetes was very rare in first nations people prior to contact with Europeans.[3] Now, more than 25% of adults over 50 years of age in some aboriginal communities suffer from this condition (Young et al., 2000). A healthy lifestyle consisting not only of improved diet, non-smoking, exercise, etc., but also reduced exposures to material deprivation and income, housing, and food insecurity could also prevent over 80% of coronary heart disease cases, as well as up to 90% of cases of lung cancer (Stampfer et al., 2000; Raphael and Farrell, 2002). However, it is a challenge for health care systems to translate these theoretical gains into tangible outcomes.

While the health system can directly improve the clinical outcomes in patients with chronic illness by preventing deterioration, it is much more limited in its ability to effect primary prevention.

For example, diabetes in Aboriginals could be mainly prevented with a more traditional culture and lifestyle, and one that was not distinguished by material and social deprivation. Several communities have developed prevention programs, which reinforce First Nations culture. The Kahnawake Schools of the Mohawk Nation has led to improvements in diet and rates of physical exercise in children (Macaulay et

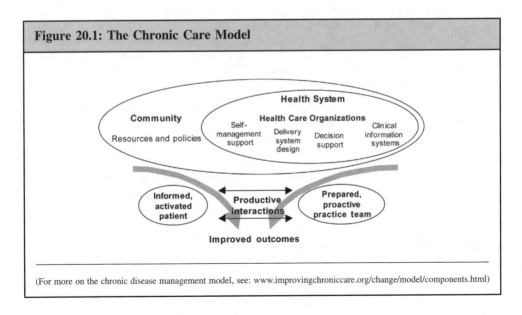

**Figure 20.1: The Chronic Care Model**

(For more on the chronic disease management model, see: www.improvingchroniccare.org/change/model/components.html)

The Chronic Care Model identifies the essential elements of a health care system that encourage high-quality chronic disease care. These elements are the community, the health system, self-management support, delivery system design, decision support, and clinical information systems.

Evidence-based change concepts under each element, in combination, foster productive interactions between informed patients who take an active part in their care and providers with resources and expertise. The model can be applied to a variety of chronic illnesses, health care settings, and target populations. The bottom line is healthier patients, more satisfied providers, and cost savings.

**The development of the Chronic Care Model**

The staff at the MacColl Institute for Healthcare Innovation developed the model drawing on available literature about promising strategies for chronic illness management, and organizing that literature in a new more accessible way. The model was further refined during a nine-month planning project supported by The Robert Wood Johnson Foundation, and revised based on input from a large panel of national experts. It was then used to collect data and analyze innovative programs recommended by experts. RWJF then funded the MacColl Institute to test the model nationally across varied health care settings: the national program being "Improving Chronic Illness Care" (ICIC).

**Refinements to the Chronic Care Model**

In July of 2003, ICIC and a small group of experts updated the Chronic Care Model to reflect advances in the field of chronic care both from the research literature and from the scores of health care systems that implemented the model in their improvement efforts.

We list more specific concepts under each of the six elements. Based on more recent evidence, five new themes have been incorporated into the Chronic Care Model:

- Patient safety (in health system);
- Cultural competency (in delivery system design);
- Care coordination (in health system and clinical information systems):
- Community policies (in community resources and policies); and case management (in delivery system design).

The model element pages have been redesigned to reflect these updates. Each page describes the overall strategy for each element, and the health system change concepts necessary to achieve improvement in that component.

Source: *Overview of the chronic care model 2004* (includes 50 minute talk on the model), online at www.improvingchroniccare.org/change/model/components.html

al., 1997). A community-wide project in an Aboriginal community in West Australia improved diet, increased exercise, and reduced fasting insulin levels in group of high-risk individuals (Rowley et al., 2000). However, there were few changes in the overall community risk factor profile. A community health promotion project in the Okanagan Valley found little change in diabetes status between the intervention and control communities (Daniel et al., 1999).

These programs show potential, but they also highlight the limitations in the health care system's ability to engineer the massive social change required to effect population lifestyles. For example, the Kahnawake intervention involved bans of "junk food" from the school (Walker, 2002). This might not be a popular policy with fast food chains, which presently sell their products in 30% of American high schools (Markel, 2002). It might not be popular with school funders increasingly looking to private partnerships. Reducing the costs of healthy, low-fat foods, increases their consumption at schools and workplaces (French et al., 2001). Food subsidy programs would improve the consumption of healthy foods in northern and remote areas. Perhaps this would save overall health care costs in the medium term. But, the new money would still have to be found in the short term and where would it come from when most voters live in urban areas?

There are numerous examples of successful health promotion programs for those who are ill or at very high risk for heart disease (Ornish et al., 1990; Ornish et al., 1998; Kokkinos et al., 1995; Schuler et al., 1992). However, most cases of coronary heart disease occur in the large number of persons at moderate risk rather than the small minority at high risk (Rose, 1985; Rose, 1981). And, unfortunately, community-wide heart health promotion programs have been more limited in their impact.

The Stanford Five Cities study implemented a number of programs directed at risk factor modification (diet, exercise, smoking, cholesterol, and high blood pressure) in two test cities in Northern California, while 3 other cities served as controls. Over 14 years, there were major changes in all communities but there was no greater change in the intervention communities (Fortmann and Varady, 2000).

Another heart health project was initiated in 1972 in North Karelia, a province of Finland that had one of the highest death rates from coronary heart disease of any area in the world (Puska et al., 1998). As in California, there were major reductions in coronary disease, but the results in North Karelia were only slightly greater than in other parts of the country.[4]

## Barriers to primary prevention

It often seems only good sense to health professionals to concentrate on preventing illness. However, not all citizens agree that the value of improving health should trump other values or interests. Furthermore, too often health professionals assume that good information automatically makes better policy.

## Rudolf Virchow and Typhus in Silesia

In 1848 Rudolf Virchow was only 26 years of age but he was already one of Germany's greatest scientists. In that year, the Berlin City council asked Virchow to investigate an epidemic of typhus, which had broken out in Upper Silesia (currently part of Poland). Virchow concluded that the cause of the epidemic was "mismanagement of the region by the Berlin government" (Taylor and Rieger, 1985). Virchow's recommendations included full democracy for Silesia, allowing Polish as the official language of the region, the separation of church and state, shifting the burden of taxation from the poor to the rich, a program of road construction, the improvement of agriculture, and the establishment of farming cooperatives. The Berlin council was very unhappy with Virchow's report. The Council criticized Virchow for producing a political document rather than the scientific report, which they had thought they had commissioned.

Virchow then made his famous statement, which still resonates 150 years later:

> Medicine is a social science and politics is nothing but medicine writ large!

Virchow further claimed that if medicine were to be successful then it must enter political and social life because diseases were caused by defects in society. He claimed that "if disease is an expression of individual life under unfavourable circumstances, then epidemics must be indicative of mass disturbances."

## Health is politics

As Virchow so eloquently described over 150 years ago, a society's pattern of health and illness reflects its values, culture, and institutions. In other words, health is politics. North Americans have very high rates of coronary heart disease and lung cancer because we eat too much of the wrong food, too many of us smoke, and too many of us are exposed to conditions of material deprivation and stress. We have low rates of water and food borne illness because of the safe disposal of sewage and the safe supply of food and drinking water. On the other hand, African peasants have low rates of coronary heart disease and lung cancer and high rates of water and food borne illnesses. A particular population's health status is as unique to that society as fingerprints are to an individual. If we accept the rule that health is a political construct then there are several important points that follow:

1.  Major change in a society's pattern of health and illness usually requires change in that society's values and customs.

2.  Some powerful groups will be threatened by this change and will use their positions of privilege to oppose them. Some citizens will be offended by the new values implied by healthy public policies.

3.  These threats to interests and values will inevitably cause some political backlash. This backlash will alter intersectoral action and healthy public policies so that they will be less offensive to mainstream interests and values. The eventual policies implemented will usually focus on communities or individuals rather than larger populations and will almost always be less effective than they would have been without this political intervention.

## Surmounting the barriers to primary prevention

It is easier to gain the cooperation of different sectors for effective action at the local or community level than at the national or even provincial level. Hancock notes that there are a variety of reasons for better results at the local level (Hancock, 1992):

1.  The smaller, more human scale allows for closer ties amongst participants in local projects.

2.  Policy-makers live where they work so they are both more accountable for their decisions but also more likely to be affected by their decisions.

3.  Community and municipal bureaucratic structures are smaller and relatively more accessible.

However, while it is easier to start intersectoral action at the local or community level, action at higher levels (e.g., federal, provincial) tends to have more impact on population health (Hertzman, 1996). Unfortunately, intersectoral action at higher levels causes more political conflict, especially around different values and competing interests.

A good example of this phenomenon is the problem of drinking and driving. Typical Canadian campaigns have focussed on education and criminal penalties. However, in Finland, policies to reduce drinking and driving have included actively discouraging the ownership of private automobiles (Ross, 1989). In Canada this approach would be seen as beyond the "boundary" of the issue.

The most effective intersectoral action combines activity at all levels, creates positive feedback loops to sustain itself, and uses the media and other sources to spread key messages.

## Creating a positive feedback loop for health

Intersectoral action is more likely to be successful at the local or community level than at higher levels (e.g., Federal or international level). However, local intersectoral action tends to have less impact on population health than action at higher levels. The ideal would be to use action at the local level to promote action at higher levels and then have higher levels provide further support for community activity.

Successful local action can create pressure to advance higher action on the broader determinants of health. Community development can also mobilize people and helps to create a more civic and democratic society. Successful community activity can promote higher level intersectoral action for health. As noted by Robert Putnam in *Making democracy work*, in Italy, national level action (e.g., the establishment of health

clinics and day care centres) both reflected and stimulated local democracy and intersectoral action for health (Putnam et al., 1993). Health promotion, intersectoral action, and population health all thrive in more civic societies (Marmot, 1998).

Intersectoral action for health works best when the health sector acts in a coordinated fashion across different levels. Neil Pearce of New Zealand recently noted:

> … community interventions frequently fail, or have limited success because they do not recognize the population-level factors that limit what can be achieved at the community level. (Pearce, 1997)

Pearce offers as an example how different levels can work together on tobacco control. He suggests that action at the community level will be more effective if there is higher level intersectoral action for health, e.g., tighter regulation of tobacco production, distribution, and advertising.

Some of Canada's success with intersectoral action on tobacco control has occurred when each level of the health system has assisted the action of the others. Public health workers, community health centres, regional health care staff, and voluntary health organizations have established local coalitions in many provinces to push for municipal smoking bylaws. But they have also put pressure on their federal and provincial politicians for action at those policy-making levels. For example, local action by Quebec's public health departments and community health centres helped to consolidate political support for federal gun control legislation and for the province's Tobacco Control Act of 1998.

## Box 20.2: Teamwork can improve public health care

DEANNA WILK

On April 5, 2001, at 1 p.m., daunted by the reported shortage of doctors in Waterloo Region and still holding onto my family doctor in Mississauga, I went to the Grand River Hospital emergency room for the first time.

I woke up that day looking the same as usual. Two hours later, my lower abdomen was growing, fast, and for no apparent reason. My main fear was internal bleeding or an abscess. By 2 p.m. I was admitted. By 8 p.m. I was home.

During my lengthy seven-hour stay, my first doctor left for the day, apparently not telling anyone I was still there. My second doctor had no information about me and it appeared we were going to start from scratch with a blood test, something I'd already done four hours prior. After a search, the results of the blood test were found. My blood was normal and it was concluded that a previously pulled groin muscle was aggravated. After four days with an ice pack, the swelling started to recede. Annoying but harmless.

To me, this service left much to be desired. My experience could be seen as a cry for help from the private sector. It could also be seen as proof our universal public health care system has room for improvement through reforms.

Many decision-makers are enamoured with creating more room for private health care alongside our public system. They have a fondness for making doomsday proclamations regarding public health care.

But a better public health care system can be had through innovation, not unsustainable funding. The dogma that going private is the only way of being innovative in health care delivery should be put to rest. Keeping public also has the benefit of being cheaper because it's non-profit and has more buying power, while remaining equitable.

In 1998, total expenditure on health care (public and private) in Canada as a share of gross domestic product was 9.5 percent. In the U.S., it was 13.9 percent, with 40 million citizens uninsured. U.S. citizens also have a higher degree of dissatisfaction with their health care than Canadians, according to a recent Commonwealth Fund study.

Recently, I went to my dentist's and saw the efficiency of a well-run, private dental office. I had the impression three people knew where I was: the hygienist, the receptionist, and the dentist.

While an emergency room will never run like a dental office, a family physician's practice certainly could by reducing its waiting lists and giving patients better service and preventative education, by utilizing nurses and co-ordinators to their full potential.

In Beechy, Sask., we have such an example. A physician and three nurses provide primary care to 4,000 residents, enabling the physician to look after more than twice as many patients as the average family doctor.

"Specialists, like family doctors, can be more efficient if they work in teams with doctors, nurses and other care providers," state Dr. Michael Rachlis, Robert G. Evans, Patrick Lewis, and Morris. L. Bauer in their January 2001 study, Revitalizing Medicare.

Their study looks at partnerships. Pharmacists working with physicians would improve the quality of prescription services by giving doctors non-biased information on the most cost-effective drugs. Other health care professionals working with doctors would be able to offer lifestyle change and alternative therapies instead of drugs for appropriate cases, helping to control skyrocketing drug costs.

Even in our publicly funded system, we have encouraged for-profit health care by our fee-for-service payments to physicians and specialists who rush to get patients in and out of their office.

con't

Social Determinants of Health

con't

Other public health care innovations include the Cardiac Care Network in Ontario which co-ordinates cardiac surgery and catheterization waiting lists and ensures the most serious cases get treated first. By having a registered nurse only a phone call away, Telehealth often prevents a trip to the emergency room. There are many examples across Canada.

Revitalizing Medicare states: "All successful models of primary care share at least two common characteristics: comprehensive care is provided to a clearly defined population, and funding is other than just fee-for-service . . . the challenge is to move from pilot, or local success, to mainstream practice, so that all Canadians may benefit from best practices."

Accepting innovation, while keeping the principles of the Canada Health Act and renewing federal support, will hold it securely together.

Source: Wilk, Deanna. (2002). "Insight," *The Record* (Waterloo Region), May 31, 2002, p. A13.

## Box 20.3: Health care administrative costs: Canada vs. U.S.

There's a prevailing assumption that any government-run enterprise is financially inefficient and most private companies are not. It was a recurring theme during the public debates when the Clinton Administration attempted to introduce universal health care coverage. The belief held sway in that era, despite the existence of a 1991 government-initiated survey showing that the administrative costs of Medicare were 3%, as opposed to 25% for private insurance companies.

In the same year, Steffie Woolhandler, MD, MPH, and David U. Himmelstein, MD, reported in *The New England journal of medicine* that people in the U.S. spent about $450 per capita on health care administration in 1987, as compared with Canadians who spent one third as much. (Canada has a national health insurance system that covers virtually everyone.) Now Dr. Woolhandler and Dr. Himmelstein have joined forces with Terry Campbell, MHA, of the Canadian Institute for Health Information, Ottawa, to conduct a comparison study of the costs of health care administration in the U.S. and Canada. They wanted to see whether the introduction of computers, managed care, and more businesslike approaches to health care delivery have decreased the administrative costs in the U.S. The results, published recently in *The New England journal of medicine* (August 21), were not encouraging. In 1999, health administration costs in the U.S. were $1,059 per capita, as compared with $304 per capita in Canada. As for individual doctors, their administrative costs were far lower in Canada.

Steffie Woolhandler, MD, MPH, and colleagues concluded, "The gap between U.S. and Canadian spending on health care administration has grown to $755 per capita. A large sum might be saved in the U.S. if administrative costs could be trimmed by implementing a Canadian-style health care system."

Interestingly, Dr. Woolhandler and colleagues wrote that their estimates actually understate the overhead costs of both nations because they excluded the marketing costs of pharmaceutical firms, the value of patients' time spent on filling out medical forms, and most of the cost of advertising by providers, health care industry profits, and lobbying and political contributions. They note that their analysis also omits the costs of collecting taxes to fund health care and the administrative overhead of such businesses as retail pharmacies and ambulance companies.

Source: *Healthfacts* (October 2003), available at www.findarticles.com/cf_dls/m0815/10_28/108994048/p1/article.jhtml

When health ministers have the political strength of effective local action behind them, they can then bring forward policies of their own.

Finally, the circle can be completed if higher levels of the health system can facilitate more effective community action through establishing local institutions or providing resources to local coalitions. This creates a positive feedback loop for health. Successful local action promotes effective higher level action, which, in turn, provides resources for more effective local action.

A key step in this process is to link public health personnel with their communities. The origins of public health in Canada, like Britain, and the U.S. lie with social reformers who were leaders in their local communities (Rosen, 1958). Analyses of successful healthy community projects in Quebec have concluded that involvement of public health and community health centre personnel is key to successful local projects (Fortin et al., 1994). Many health advocates argue that community action is the lifeblood of public health. Toby Citrin from the School of Public Health at the University of Michigan claims that "... communities are essential to the future of public health" (Citrin, 1998). New Zealand epidemiologist Dr. Robert Beaglehole claims that the empowerment of local communities is "a necessary step in the rejuvenation of public health" (Beaglehole and Bonita, 1998).

A useful metaphor that describes this process is the lighting of a bonfire. You can't start a large fire by holding a match to a pile of logs. The fire must be started with small sticks, the kindling. As the kindling catches fire, bigger sticks are added until, finally, the large logs are laid on the fire. Community level action is the kindling that starts the fire. However, without larger logs (higher level action) the fire will soon burn out (Rachlis, 1999).

## Conclusion

This chapter makes the point that health services have historically not been an important determinant of health. However, re-engineered services could help make health care a bigger influence on our health status. There is the opportunity to decrease morbidity and mortality by providing more rehabilitation and better managing chronic illness. The health system also has a potential to play a part in the primary prevention of illness. However, there are significant political barriers to implementing effective primary prevention. The key to unlocking the potential of primary prevention is to better link communities to primary health care and public health services.

With the release of the Romanow Royal Commission on Health Services reports, many Canadians are focussed on the renovation of our country's health care system. It would be wise to remember the words of Tommy Douglas, arguably the father of Medicare:

> Therefore I'm suggesting that when you're fighting this battle, as I hope you will to maintain Medicare, you'll not forget that the ultimate goal of Medicare must be the task of keeping people well rather than just patching them up when they're sick. (Douglas, 1982)

# Notes

1. For more information on PACE in the U.S. see: www.natlpaceassn.org, or for On Lok, see: www.onlok.org.
2. See the Improving Chronic Illness Care website: www.improvingchroniccare.org.
3. For that matter, adult-onset diabetes was also rare amongst Europeans until the last 100 years or so.
4. There was a 73% reduction from coronary heart disease in North Karelia and a 65% reduction in Finland as a whole.

# Recommended readings

Rachlis, M.M. (2003). *The federal government can and should lead the renewal of Canada's health policy*. Published by the Caledon Institute of Social Policy, February 2003, online at www.caledoninst.org/PDF/55382038X.pdf

Rachlis, M.M., Evans, R.G., Lewis, P. and Barer, M. (2001). *Revitalizing medicare: Shared problems, public solutions*. Published by the Tommy Douglas Research Institute, January 2001, online at www.tommydouglas.ca/reports/revitalizingmedicare.pdf

Rachlis, M.M. (2000). *Modernizing medicare for the 21$^{st}$ century*. Published by the British Columbia Ministry of Health, June 2000, online at www.hlth.gov.bc.ca/cpa/publications/innovation/medicare.pdf
    All three of these reports provide in-depth analysis of the means by which the Canadian health care system could be reformed to improve the health of Canadians.

Rachlis, M.M. (2004). *Prescription for excellence: How innovation is saving Canada's health care system*. Toronto: HarperCollins Canada.
    Dr. Rachlis' latest book focuses on examples of "best practices" which make the health care system a more effective determinant of health.

The U.S. National Institute of Medicine. (2001). *Crossing the quality chasm: A new health system for the 21$^{st}$ century*. Washington: National Academy Press, online at www.nap.edu.
    This landmark US document outlines the challenges and opportunities to improve quality in the health care system.

# Related websites

The Tommy Douglas Research Institute—www.tommydouglas.ca/
    The Institute is an independent non-profit Canadian economic and social research and educational organization. Named after T.C. Douglas, the former Premier of Saskatchewan and acknowledged father of Medicare in Canada, the Institute's main objective is the redirection of public attention to the respective role of both the large business sector and governments in providing for the well-being of Canadians.

The Caledon Institute of Social Policy—www.caledoninst.org/
    Established in 1992, the Caledon Institute of Social Policy is a private, non-profit organization with charitable status supported primarily by the Maytree Foundation, located in Toronto. The site contains many reports on health and the health care sytem including *The Federal Government can and should lead the renewal of Canada's health policy* by Dr. Rachlis.

Centre for Health Services and Policy Research—www.chspr.ubc.ca/index.htm
    The mission of the Centre for Health Services and Policy Research (CHSPR) is to stimulate scientific enquiry into issues of health in population groups, and ways in which health services can best be organized, funded and delivered. CHSPR is based at the University of British Columbia; the website contains many research publications on the Canadian health care system.

Canadian Centre for Policy Alternatives—www.policyalternatives.ca

The website of this non-profit non-partisan progressive think tank has many articles and reports about the Canadian Health Care System. Once there, click on "Health Care" in the "Hot Topics" section.

Commission on the Future of Health Care in Canada—www.hc-sc.gc.ca/english/care/romanow/index1.html

This website contains the full report, commissioned research papers and numerous news articles about the Commission and its aftermath. The report contains recommendations on sustaining a publicly funded health system in Canada.

# Chapter Twenty-One

---•---

# THE CONTRIBUTION OF THE SOCIAL ECONOMY TOWARDS HEALTHY SOCIAL POLICY REFORMS IN CANADA: A QUEBEC VIEWPOINT[1]

Yves Vaillancourt, François Aubry, Muriel Kearney,
Luc Thériault, and Louise Tremblay

## Introduction

This chapter is largely inspired by various studies conducted at the *Laboratoire de recherche sur les pratiques et les politiques sociales* and at the *Community-University Research Alliance on the Social Economy* (Université du Quebec à Montréal), as well as in Saskatchewan at the Social Policy Research Unit (University of Regina). It has two aims. The first is to highlight how changing social policies in Canada are a major determinant of the health and well-being of the population. The second is to explain that social economy initiatives (or "third sector" initiatives) can contribute to make social policy reforms, in a context of transformation of the welfare state, more apt at ameliorating the health and quality of life of individuals, families, and communities in Quebec and in the rest of Canada.

For us, these two aims are very closely linked. In fact, in the current context of a transformation of the social policies inherited from the welfare state, it seems both from a theoretical and practical viewpoint that a partnership arrangement between the State and social economy stakeholders can contribute to the creation of reforms that will improve social policies and, in turn, enable these policies to have a more positive impact on the health and well-being of the population. To put forward this vision of things, we have analysed some European and Quebec examples of social policy initiatives during the last ten years. We know that these experiences are still frail and that they emerged in a global and continental context marked by the enormous influence of neo-liberalism, which encourages all public authorities to transform downward the social programs that emerged during the golden era of the welfare state in Canada (i.e., 1950–1980). These experiences deserve our attention, nevertheless, because the nostalgia for the golden era of the welfare state will not suffice to block neo-liberal proposals in favour of the privatization and commodification of human services. To use the terminology of the Caledon Institute of Social Policy, we can say that the improvement of tomorrow's social policy requires a "new policy architecture" (Battle and Torjman, 2002). As says Ken Battle: "We need a new 'architecture' for social policy ... to invigorate both the redistributive and human capital development capacities of Canadian social policy" (Battle et al., 2002, p. 2).

However, contrary to the Caledon Institute and to the mainstream of social policy research in English-Canada, we are not content with analyzing the social policy initiatives of the federal government. While we take these into account, of course, we place a much greater emphasis on the initiatives of the provincial and territorial governments, and in particular on the case of Quebec. In fact, it is too often forgotten that in the Canadian federal system social policies are the responsibility of both *orders* (not *levels*) of government: the federal government on one side and the provincial and territorial governments on the other. Also often forgotten is that the latter have, according to the Constitution, stringent duties regarding social policy. Another oversight is that social policy innovations often originate in the provinces rather than in Ottawa (Noël, 2003; Vaillancourt, 2003b; Bach, 2002).

The chapter is comprised of three parts. The first part offers a theoretical examination of the links between social policy, the social economy and the determinants of health. The second part looks at the re-engineering of federal social policy conducted during the 1990's with a focus on the impact of this process on provincial policies. In the third part, we look at the specific contribution of social economy organizations and enterprises in some recent Quebec social policy reforms. We then focus on four particular areas of social policy: occupational integration, early childhood/daycare services, social housing, and home care services.

## Part 1: Social policy, social economy, and social determinants of health

Our argument suggests that the improvement of social policy at this time can and should be made via a new alliance between the State and the stakeholders from the social economy (or third sector). To clarify this argument, it is important to look back at the definitions of *social policy* and the *social economy* within a theoretical framework that goes beyond the bipolar "Market vs. State" approach.

### A multipolar versus a bipolar model

The mainstream trend in Canadian and Quebec literature (be it progressive or conservative) on social policy and on health reform is caught up in this bipolar framework. Despite the fact that the third sector is now referred to in the literature with genuine interest and often in a positive fashion, we do not observe a real recognition

of the sector as a significant capacity builder to be taken into account in health and well-being policy-making. In Canada as in Quebec, the important work of community organizations is still too timidly acknowledged (Gouvernement du Quebec, 1992; Forum national sur la santé, 1997a, 1997b; Commission Clair, 2000; Groupe Arpin, 1999; CSBE, 2002).

Many actors in the public health sector in Quebec, although convinced of the importance of the social determinants of health and well-being such as poverty, housing, education, and employment are, to this day, unable to comprehend fully that the actors of the social economy are key allies especially when non-medical determinants of health and well-being must be taken into account. Consequently, the social economy is still far from having full recognition as a potential partner in a new development model.

With a growing number of analysts we find that this dual State/Market framework is old fashioned for it ignores important parts of our social and economic reality such as the social economy, but also the domestic sphere where women, unfortunately, still play the major role in the area of health and social care. In our work, we regularly put forward the idea that the social economy is one pillar of a plural economic development model. As does Polanyi (2001), we consider that the economy must be envisioned as plural and must be articulated around three major poles (the market economy, the non-market economy and the non-monetary economy) and four governing principles that interact with each other and whose relative importance varies in time and place. These economic principles are efficiency, territorial redistribution, reciprocity, and household management (i.e., home economics). Four sectors of economic activity, each dominated by one of the three poles specified earlier, can thus be identified: the market, the State, the social economy, and the domestic sector.

## A definition of social policy

Social policy can be viewed as State and government interventions that contribute to the well-being of individuals and communities and foster full citizenship. Social policy programs permit, through State interventions, redistribution of income, offer collective human services and individual and collective citizenship. With Esping-Andersen (1999, 2000), we insist upon the fact that these State and governments interventions are aiming to counterbalance the negative effects of the market economy rules (hence these policies are working toward "de-commodification") and to avoid the possibility of transferring too many responsibilities to the domestic sphere which are mainly on women's shoulders. In that respect, social policy is also working toward

"de-familiarization." In other words: "Social policy begins where the laws of the market and the virtues of family and domestic solidarity cannot guarantee to individuals and communities the quality of life to which every citizen has a right" (Vaillancourt, Caillouette, and Dumais, 2002, p. 30; Vaillancourt, 2003a).

Social policy is a question of well-being and citizenship, of financial resources and dignity, of income distribution and access to services and, most importantly, of participation or empowerment of people and communities. In a post-welfare State period, it is important to insist on this "support to full citizenship" aspect in a definition of social policy. Of course, social policies are about income support and services that the State should provide to citizens, especially the most socially and economically vulnerable ones, but they must be about more than that. Otherwise, the citizens being served will remain only at "the receiving end," as recipients or beneficiaries (Beresford and Holden, 2002). In our definition of social policy, we would like to break the wall that separates the producers and the users of social policy in the welfarist model. We aim at a new architecture that enables the citizen-users to participate in the production, management and evaluation of social policy and, in so doing, to develop as citizens capable of self-determination and empowerment (Roeher Institute, 1993; OPHQ, 1984; Fuchs, 1983; Jetté et al., 2000; Vaillancourt et al., 2000; Jetté et al., 2001). It is precisely because full citizenship is at stake that social policy cannot solely rely on State intervention; an alliance must be struck with the initiatives of the social economy. To visualise this link between the social economy and social policy we have to remember that policy reforms can produce system configurations in which the State assumes key responsibilities in terms of setting standards and funding, without always having to be directly involved in the management and provision of services. In other words, having social economy organizations as service providers does not mean that the State has to abandon its regulation and funding roles. This model is found, for instance, in the reform of early childhood day care centres (CPE) in Quebec.

Therefore social policy is about State and government intervention, but not exclusively. While the theoretical approach of Esping-Andersen takes the state, the market and the family into account, it unfortunately neglects to consider the contribution of the social economy (or third sector), that is to say the initiatives of the civil society that can collaborate with State intervention for the common good. In Jean-Louis Laville and Marthe Nyssens' (2001) recent book on social services for the elderly, we find an interesting theoretical contribution explaining that social policy is increasingly in interaction with social (or solidarity-based) economy initiatives. These authors emphasize that the history of the welfare state and that of the non-profit sector are closely intertwined, the two having contributed to the "de-commodification" of social services, including services to senior citizens.

This fact is important if one wants to understand the evolution of social policy. The decrease of the importance of the market and of the family in the sphere of social services and social policy cannot be attributed only to the increase in the role of the public sector. It also stems from an increasing presence of the non-profit sector and a growing recognition of its contribution by the State that manifests itself by a growing cooperation between the State and the third sector. Historically the interaction of the State with the social economy has contributed widely to the development of social policy. Our particular interest with the social economy lies in its capacity to democratize social policy through the double empowerment of workers and users of personal services.

## A definition of social economy

In this chapter, we use the terms social economy and third sector as more or less synonymous even though we are aware (see Vaillancourt, 1999) that we can find in the literature some fine distinctions between the notion of social economy and other concepts like voluntary sector or non-profit sector that are probably more familiar to English-Canadian readers (see CCP, 2003; Jolin et al., in CCP, 2003: Appendix D).

In Quebec, the term *social economy* is now widely used and refers to a vast array of enterprises and initiatives, mostly from the non-profit sector, including advocacy groups, voluntary organizations, other community-based organizations (CBOs), as well as cooperatives. The definition of the social economy that has been adopted in Quebec since 1996 is broad, with an emphasis on values, and is inspired by Belgium. This definition encompasses older forms of social economy realities dating back to the 19th century as well as new forms of initiatives that emerged in the 1970s, often referred to as the "new social economy" (Lévesque et al., 1999; Lévesque and Ninacs, 1997). Since the middle of the 1990s, the term *social economy* has thus been widely used in Quebec. At the Economic and Employment Summit of 1996, attended by representatives of government, business, labour, the women's movement and community-based organizations, consensus was achieved over a five-element definition of the social economy (Chantier de l'économie sociale, 1996 and 2001).

This definition is appealing because it makes room for both community-based organizations and social enterprises that sell some goods and services on the market (D'Amours, 2002). The term *social economy* is not widely used in the English-speaking countries. Until recently, it was rarely used in English Canada although some literature acknowledges the term (Quarter, 1992; Quarter et al., 2003; Shragge and Fontan, 2000). More often used concepts in Canada are that of third, voluntary or non-profit sectors. A major problem with these concepts is that they exclude cooperatives, as in the case of the prestigious international research program led by Lester Salamon (Salamon et al., 1999). If we were to choose an expression used in the English language literature that better befits our definition, we would, with Taylor (1995, p. 214) and some Irish authors (Donnelly-Cox et al., 2001), prefer the term *voluntary and community sector* to the expression *voluntary sector* used in English-Canada, or *non-profit sector* frequently used south of the border. In our view these terms are too limited in their scope, the first one insisting on organizations relying mostly on voluntary or unpaid work, while the second term excludes social enterprises such as cooperatives.

Social economy organizations are distinctive because of their values and rules. Their approach to social policy issues can be of great interest to policy-makers as partners in service delivery and as a model of user, worker, and community empowerment. Be it through the democratic rules that govern them (one person, one vote), through the values of solidarity, autonomy, reciprocity, and self-determination that inspire them, the ends that they pursue, their contribution to social and economic networking, through their capacity to create jobs (paid or voluntary) or through the empowerment of users and workers that they favour, social economy initiatives are capable of contributing positively to the health and well-being of individuals, families, and communities.[2]

Whatever the terms used—*social economy*, non-profit sector, third sector, voluntary sector—the reality that is covered "is deeply rooted in the social, economic, political and cultural history of a society, the conditions in which it emerges and the role

---

**Box 21.1: Defining features of social economy organizations**

Social economy organizations produce goods and services with a clear social mission and have these ideal-type characteristics and objectives:

- The mission is services to members and communities and non-profit oriented
- Management is independent of government
- Democratic decision-making by workers and/or users
- People have priority over capital
- Participation, empowerment, individual, and collective responsibility

Source: Chantier de l'économie sociale. (1996). *Osons la solidarité*. Rapport du groupe de travail sur l'économie sociale, Sommet sur l'économie et l'emploi, Québec; Chantier de l'économie sociale. (2001). *De nouveau nous osons*. Document de positionnement stratégique, Montréal.

that it currently plays will necessarily vary from one province to another" (Vaillancourt and Tremblay, 2002, p. 164). Hence, we must focus on both quantitative aspects (e.g., the scope of the sector) and qualitative aspects (e.g., relationships with the State) when looking at the role of the social economy in social policy reforms.

Today's social economy organizations play a major role in many spheres of economic and social life. Box 21.2 offers a list of activity areas in which the social economy is present. Table 21.1 suggests that the social economy family defined broadly in Quebec involves more than 11,151 enterprises and organizations and more than 159,000 jobs.

## Double empowerment of users and workers

What is particularly interesting in social economy organizations is the possibility offered by their legal attributes to empower users and to democratize work organization and the way services are organized in order to empower workers. We do not want to infer that for-profit and public sector organizations are by nature not able to empower workers and users or to put forth

a democratic work organization, nor do we want to infer that such practices can be found, in a perfect form, in all community-based organizations. However, we believe that community-based organizations and other social economy organizations have a comparative advantage over public and for-profit organizations in this area since their rules and values are better adapted to and favour such practices. Hence the notion of double empowerment is key in our analysis.

## Social economy and users' empowerment

Social economy encourages individual and collective empowerment of users of social policy and services. The case of disabled people is particularly enlightening in this area and the work of the *Independent Living Movement* is most conclusive in this regard. In fact, the empowerment of these people as consumers of services was developed through a trend that can substantiate reflection on social policy-making in general.

The *Independent Living Movement* that started in the U.S. in the late 1960s puts forward the rights of disabled people to live an "ordinary life" as do people without a handicap and insists on treating people with

---

**Box 21.2: Social economy areas of activities**

- Health and social services
- Labour market integration
- Media and information technologies
- Popular education
- Sports and recreation
- Tourism
- Advocacy
- Cultural activities
- Land management
- Environment and recycling
- Local and regional development
- Fair trade
- Financial services (credit unions)

## Table 21.1: The social economy in Quebec—2001

| Type of activity | No. of organizations | | | No. of employees | | |
|---|---|---|---|---|---|---|
| | COOPs | NPOs | TOTAL | COOPs | NPOs | TOTAL |
| Commercial[1] | 3,210 | 3,941 | 7,151 | 79,222 | 45,080 | 124,302 |
| Non-commercial[2] | - | 4,000 | 4,000 | - | 35,000 | 35,000 |
| TOTAL | 3,210 | 7,941 | 11,151 | 79,222 | 80,080 | 159,302 |

1. Partly or wholly commercial. Chantier de l'économie sociale. (Novembre 2003), *L'Économie sociale en mouvement*, p. 6.
2. Wholly non-commercial. Estimates prepared by the Laboratoire de recherche sur les pratiques et les politiques sociales (LAREPPS).

disabilities as citizens (Ramon, 1991). The movement aims at increasing the autonomy of disabled persons in order that they make the decisions that concern them. The philosophy of the *Independent Living Movement* rapidly became an example for other advocacy groups defending the rights of vulnerable segments of the population: native groups, women's groups, ex-offenders, drug addicts, gay/lesbian rights groups, welfare rights groups (Fuchs, 1987; Boucher in Vaillancourt et al., 2002: chap. 2 and 3).

In Canada, the Roeher Institute and the network of Independent Living Resource Centres have contributed to put in place and popularize this approach which has been cited in different federal and Quebec publications since the beginning of the 1980s (Office des personnes handicapées du Quebec, 1984; Federal/Provincial/Territorial Ministers Responsible for Social Services, 1998). The *Independent Living Movement* encourages self-management. As Don Fuchs says:

> Disabled people through their experience in being disabled, best know the needs of disabled persons: support services should be based on consumer-controlled policies; the focus of services is to change

the environment and not the individual; the goal of services is integration into the community; the disabled individual can help him/herself through helping other disabled people. (Fuchs, 1987, p. 193)

When disabled persons take charge of the organization of services at the user end, the empowerment is individual and collective. Disabled persons that join and engage become social actors capable of developing and investing CBOs to defend their interests and influence social policy.

This vision and way of doing is totally different from the old progressive framework of "welfarist" policy reforms that consider users solely as recipients of social policy. The new approach shatters the traditional structure where the user "demands" and the provider "supplies" social policies. It convenes users and providers to co-operate in a mutual elaboration of supply and demand (Laville, 2000).

### Social economy and workers' empowerment

It is today recognized that a certain number of conditions that affect life and work, such as social and economic exclusion, unemployment and poverty, have a negative impact on the health and well-being of individuals and can lead to lower life expectancy. On the other hand, having a job, doing meaningful work, having a certain amount of autonomy in one's work and benefiting from varied and rich social relations in the workplace and in the community generally have a positive impact on the health and well-being of individuals and families.

It is generally admitted that work has a complex influence on the health and well-being of men or women whether they have a job or are deprived of one. Although work may have downsides and contradictions, it is a fundamental activity that facilitates time structuring, and creates opportunity for social relations. It consolidates self-esteem, gives access to identity, security, and human contact (Mercier et al., 1999; Lauzon and Charbonneau, 2001; Charbonneau, 2002, 2004). Even though it has been demonstrated that these factors play a very important role in the case of people suffering from mental illness, they can also contribute positively to improve the health and well-being of individuals who do not suffer from any specific medical problems.

Moreover, the empowerment of workers is a factor that improves the quality of life in the workplace. Anti-democratic relations increase chances of burnout and undermotivated personnel. These relations are at the origin of a growing number of health and safety issues in the workplaces of modern societies. When, in a workplace, the organization of production relies on the intelligence and the responsibility of workers, these workers will tend to mobilize their imagination, their efforts and their know-how in order to meet production goals. In such a system, work is healthier, profitable, and productive.

Evidence shows that stress at work plays an important role in contributing to the large differences in health, sickness absence and premature death that are related to social status. Several workplace studies in Europe show that health suffers when people have little opportunity to use their skills, and low authority over decisions. Having little control over one's work is particularly strongly related to an increased risk of low back pain, sickness absence and cardio-vascular disease. (World Health Organization, 1998, p. 16)

On the other hand, when the organization of production is characterized by an increasing number of controls and regulations, by a reduction of workers' autonomy and freedom, by process fragmentation and standardization, there is a loosening of solidarity and identity ties within the workplace. In this context, the organizational culture of the social economy can form a basis that will help to democratize workplaces and, at the same time, make them safer and healthier for those who work in them.

## Part 2: The re-engineering of federal social policy during the 1990s

We are not going to attempt to draw a complete picture of federal social policy here. We will, however, identify a few characteristics in the transformation of these social policies during the 1990s in order to better understand their impacts on Canadian citizens and on the public finances of provincial and territorial governments. Taking into account federal initiatives is particularly important to get a sense of the margin of manoevre available to Quebec and the other provinces in their own social policy reform during the 1996–2003 period. By looking broadly at some elements of the federal government's strategy to balance its budget, we can observe that a number of federal social programs underwent a significant overhaul.

The federal government's strategy to eliminate the deficit was announced unilaterally in Paul Martin's Budget speech of February 27, 1995. We say "unilaterally" because the announced decisions were not the result of any federal-provincial consultation process. To the contrary, they had been hidden during 1994 by official discussions on the Axworthy reform "for improving social security in Canada." This publicly debated reform, supported by the publication of official documents, had occupied the mind of citizens and advocacy groups while the real reform was being prepared, under wrap, in the Department of Finance.

In the Lloyd Axworthy Green Paper of the Fall of 1994, the federal government had identified programs that were not targeted for revisions: "Old Age Security (OAS), the Guaranteed Income Supplement (GIS), the Canada Pension Plan (CPP) and federal support to health care which are outside the scope of this review" (Axworthy, 1994, p. 12). The targeted programs included the Unemployment Insurance (UI), the Child Tax Benefit (introduced in 1993 with the end of universal family allowances), the Canada Student Loans Program, the Established Programs Financing (EPF), the Canada Assistance Plan (CAP), and the Vocational Rehabilitation of Disabled Persons (VRDP) program (Axworthy, 1994, p. 12). The Axworthy Green Paper was mute on the abolition, since 1993, of federal grants to

share the cost of provincial programs aimed at establishing new social housing units. This federal abandonment in the field of social housing was going to be extremely painful for the provinces during the 1990s and be a major disincentive for them to enter into new social housing initiatives (Vaillancourt and Ducharme, 2001).

We know now that the list of non-targeted programs was respected as far as the CPP and social security programs for the elderly (OAS, GIS, and spousal benefit). These important direct intervention federal programs largely remained the same during the period. Accordingly, benefits provided to Canadians by the CPP reached $20.5 billion in 2003, and $27 billion for the three other federal programs for the elderly. However, contrary to what had been announced by Axworthy in 1994, the federal support to health care was going to be affected by Martin's reform. As for programs identified by Axworthy as targeted by his reform, these were in fact affected. But the modus operandi to be followed by the Department of Finance in social policy reform in 1995 was considerably different than that proposed in 1994 by Human Resources Development Canada (HRDC).

The deficit reduction strategy announced by Finance Minister Paul Martin in February 1995 was to take effect April 1, 1996. The application of this very harsh medicine one year after its announcement, gave only a brief respite to Canadians. The aim of this strategy was to gradually reduce the deficit from $42 billion in 1995 to zero within a four-year period (i.e., from April 1996 to March 2000). The goal was in fact reached as early as 1997–98 when the federal government posted a $3.8 billion surplus. The strategy operated in three main ways:

- A reduction of the size of the federal public service.
- A drastic transformation of Unemployment Insurance (now Employment Insurance) that tended to increase the amount of premiums collected and to decrease the benefits paid. This permitted the E.I. fund to move away from its $6 billion deficit position at the start of the 1990, to the accumulation of a $40 billion surplus between 1996 and 2002! This transformation helped in balancing the budget two years earlier than expected and turned the E.I. into a revenue-generating machine to fight the deficit on the backs of unemployed workers. The reform was to do much good to the finances of the federal government and create major heartaches for the Canadian workers most exposed to the risk of unemployment, such as women, youth, casual workers, and Maritimers (Vaillancourt, 1996; Vaillancourt, 2003b).
- A transformation of social transfer payments to the provinces and territories. In terms of scope, this transformation meant a reduction of cash transfers of about 30% over two fiscal years (from April 1996 to April 1998) (Vaillancourt, 1996). It is only in 2003 that cash transfers have got back to where they were in 1994! These transfers serve to co-finance provincial and territorial programs in the areas of health, post-secondary education, income security, and social services. The end of CAP (a classic *cost-sharing* program funding income security and social

services) and the EPF (a *block funding* program funding health services and post-secondary education) gave birth to the Canadian Health and Social Transfer (CHST). With the CHST, block funding (a type of demo-grant approach) has won the day over the cost-sharing method that was based on the real expenditures made by the provinces.

This federal strategy was tremendously effective, bringing a balanced budget early and easily. Surpluses have been realized during six consecutive years, from 1997–1998 to 2002–2003. However, the strategy adopted has caused major problems to the provinces and territories. Hence, the current debate on the fiscal imbalance when the federal government tries to hide large surpluses while the provinces experience great difficulties in balancing their own budgets (Noël et al., 2003; Noël, 2003; Vaillancourt, 2003b).

Attending to its own deficit objective while placing the provincial governments in a difficult posture, the federal government has also maintained its image as the keeper of the national standards in discussions regarding health care and social services reforms. In time, the federal contribution to the health expenditures of the provinces has decreased to about 15% according to estimates presented by Monique Jérôme-Forget (1998), formerly of the Institute for Research on Public Policy. The federal-provincial health funding agreements of September 2000 and February 2003 will ease the problem, without solving it (Noël et al., 2003).

In this context, it is paradoxical to see the federal government multiply attempts since 1997 to launch (often unilaterally) new targeted social policy initiatives in high-visibility areas of provincial jurisdiction. These initiatives are sometimes indirect (as in the area of homelessness), but most often take the form of direct interventions (Millennium Scholarships Program, Canada Research Chair, Canadian Institute for Health Research, Canadian Foundation for Innovation, compassionate leaves under E.I.).

It is in this context also that the federal government has, starting in 1997, transformed the Child Tax Benefit into the National Child Benefit and doubled (since 2000) the amount available to a maximum of $2,422 per child in November 2002. The Caledon Institute has often saluted this reform "as the most promising social policy innovation" of the current period, while arguing that the amount should be increased to $4,400 per child to offer an adequate answer to child poverty (Battle et al., 2002) Battle and Torjman, 2002; Mendelson and Battle, 2003).

To complete an overview on the transformation of federal social policy in the last decade, we would need to touch upon programs for First Nations people, veterans, and persons with disabilities. We would also need to talk about the Social Union Framework Agreement (SUFA) as we have done elsewhere (Vaillancourt, 2003b) which would enable us to emphasize the innovative character of the federal discourse in the area of social policy of persons with disabilities. This originality is found, for instance, in the document *In Unison* (Federal/Provincial/Territorial Ministers Responsible for Social Services, 1998). There, much attention is given to the issues of full citizenship and participation, as is the case in our definition of social policy presented in Part 1 of this chapter. Yet, it is difficult to implement this new vision both in federal and provincial

social programs, as can be seen by the traditional approach taken in the Employability Assistance for People with Disabilities (EAPD) that has replaced the Vocational Rehabilitation of Disabled Persons (VRDP) since 1998.

In a general fashion, we can say that federal social policy has not been very innovative. Of course, some major programs for the elderly, veterans, retired people, and poor children have continued to offer an important social protection to individuals and families. But the architecture of these programs remain rather welfarist and characterized by central State planning and hierarchical management with little attention paid to the democratization process based on the double empowerment mentioned earlier in Part 1. In sum, the governance model for federal social policy remained impervious to the empowerment of users and employees directly concerned by the services offered. Moreover, the re-engineering of social transfer payment programs, of the E.I. system, and in the area of social housing is framed into a neo-liberal model. This tends to act as a negative determinant on the health of citizens and on the fiscal reality of the provinces.

## Part 3: Contribution of the social economy to Quebec's social policy reforms

In this part of the chapter, we examine recent Quebec social policy reforms with an emphasis on the contribution of the social economy. By so doing, we want to show that the federal re-engineering discussed in Part 2 has an influence on the social policy initiatives of the provinces and territories, but without controlling them totally.

This observation would be better empirically established if we had the space here to pay attention to contribution of the social economy to social policy reforms in many provinces, as we had done elsewhere (Vaillancourt et al., 2000; Vaillancourt and Tremblay, 2002). We could better see then the variations in the role of the social economy in social policy reforms across Canadian provinces.

Because we do not have the space required to use inter-provincial comparisons, we are limiting ourselves to the Quebec case to demonstrate how social policy can be reformed outside a neo-liberal framework. While we recognize that neo-liberalism has been influential in Quebec long before the arrival of the government of Jean Charest, our argument is that recent reforms in the province are indicative of the tentative emergence of a more democratic and solidarity-based model of social policy. Here are briefly four concrete examples of social policy innovations to which the social economy has contributed greatly.

## Occupational integration

We have stated previously that having a job is one of the most significant social determinants of health (World Health Organization, 1998). Work gives structure to one's life and enhances social relations. Following the economic crisis of the early 1980s, unemployment became a critical social and economic issue in Canada that devastated the more vulnerable groups of the population such as school drop-outs, single mothers, physically or mentally disabled persons, and individuals dealing with mental health problems.

In Quebec, social policy in this area is operationalized through public agencies such as *Emploi-Quebec* that offer programs to promote learning, occupational integration and employment services. In reaction to the job crisis and echoing the State policies,

many community-based organizations are involved in creating jobs and developing employment services targeted to victims of social exclusion. These new social economy organizations often offer products or deliver services at the local level and provide social services with a different set of skills, objectives, and rules than those of the State or the private, for-profit sector (Larose et al., 2003). In this area, the contribution of community economic development is increasingly acknowledged. For example, the well-known federal-provincial paper *In Unison* explicitly underlines the contribution of community economic development (a component of social economy) to labour market integration of persons with disabilities:

> Opportunities for enhancing the integration and employment of persons with disabilities also could be explored through support for community economic development (CED) and self-employment. CED is an approach to local economic development that combines economic and social goals. (Federal/Provincial/Territorial Ministers Responsible for Social Services, 1998, p. 24)

In the area of job integration, the case of people with mental health problems in Quebec is interesting. Since 1987, research by *Santé Quebec* indicates that psychological despair and problems related to drug or alcohol addiction have increased. It is estimated that 500,000 people suffer from mental illness in the province—notably depression, manic depression, and schizophrenia (CSMQ, 1997). These problems are critical for youth, and many of them face major obstacles integrating into the labour force.

For over a decade the Quebec Health and Social Services Department has indicated in its policy objectives the crucial importance of work for people with mental health problems: "[…] integration to a socially productive activity such as work is, among other things, a process toward building an identity, a status, a role and finally a reconciliation with the social sphere that is identified as carrying certain determinants of health" (Charbonneau, 2004, p. 87).

*Accès-Cible (Santé Mentale et Travail)* is a good example of a new social economy organization that offers various job integration activities to individuals that have mental health problems. Over the last 14 years, *Accès-Cible (SMT)* welcomed over 800 persons in group workshops, office skill learning, employment services, and professional training practice. Some 60% of participants found a job that helped them take better control of their life and health (Dumais, 2001).

As with other organizations of the social economy, the innovative practice that stemmed from the community contributes to the well-being of citizens with a different approach to that of public institutions. However, their objectives are similar and a partnership between the State and the social economy appears natural and fundamentally constructive.

Despite the positive returns of their efforts, organizations like *Accès-Cible* often deplore the lack of recognition of their role in supporting social policy. To continue to work adequately they require a long-term financial contribution from the government. Social economy initiatives in the fields of health and welfare constitute part of the solution to the crisis of the Welfare State and of the labour market (Vaillancourt, 1999). However this innovative part of the solution cannot be implemented alone. A

plural social development model, in our view, is one where society is built upon all the components or pillars aforementioned.

**Early childhood daycare services**

The social economy model has been essential to the construction of Quebec's day-care services for preschool children. Today's universally subsidized program is the result of numerous experimentations and struggles conducted by social movements and community-based organizations since the end of the 1960s (Aubry, 2001). These grassroot groups argued that a locally-run, but centrally financed, daycare structure was the best approach to allow women to pursue professional activities and to ensure that all preschool children evolve in a healthy and stimulating environment.

In the 1960s and 1970s, "subsidized daycare services were viewed as a social welfare measure and were restricted to underprivileged recipients, unrelated either to a woman's right to work or to educational planning for young children" (Vaillancourt et al., 2002, p. 38). As the number of women joining the labour force increased, the demand for daycare services also grew substantially. On one hand, the private for-profit sector was active in responding to the needs of parents who could pay for daycare services while, on the other hand, civil society established a number of affordable neighbourhood daycare centres based on the social economy model of non-profit and democratic rules.

In 1979, the Quebec Government recognized the principle of collective responsibility for daycare and granted a two dollars per day subsidy for each authorized daycare space. This opened the door to further universalizing daycare services.

In the 1980s and 1990s more institutionalization took place in Quebec with the development of spaces and public funding. By then, most of the services were provided by independent non-profit organizations. The 1997 Quebec Family Policy constituted a major reform in this field. At that time, the State confirmed its preference for non-profit daycare and announced that daycare services would become universally available for a minimal fee of five dollars per day per child to be paid by parents (Vaillancourt et al., 2002). This innovative program stimulated an increase of daycare spaces from 58,000 in 1997 to 150,000 in 2003. Early childhood daycare centres employ 24,000 people in 2003 compared to 12,000 in 1997, making them the third larger employer in Quebec outside of the public sector.

The non-profit orientation of these daycare centres is a distinguishing feature of Quebec's program. Another distinctive feature of the system is the control of parents through the board of directors of each community daycare centre. Worker representatives are also present on these boards. The democratic participation of users ensures that the service corresponds to the needs of the children and remains independent from the State. In our view, this empowering environment is a positive determinant of well-being not only for children and parents but also for the entire community.

Concerning health and well-being, it appears that early involvement of pre-school children in day-care programs has a positive impact on their future. The World Health Organization (WHO) notes that: "important foundations of adult health are laid in early childhood" (WHO, 1998, p. 12). The WHO indicates that early-life policy should (among other things) aim to "introduce pre-school programmes not only to improve reading and stimulate cognitive development but also to reduce behaviour problems in childhood and promote educational attainment, occupational chances and healthy behaviour in adulthood" (WHO, 1998, p. 13). The importance of these programmes is particularly crucial in the case of vulnerable populations.

A consensus now exists that daycare and its costs are not a responsibility of parents alone but of society as a whole. The daycare system in Quebec is made up mainly of non-profit organizations providing services in the public interest that are controlled by local stakeholders and financed by the State (85%) and by contributions of parents (15%). This is an eloquent example of social economy principles that attain various social policy objectives.

## Homecare services

The Quebec Government recognizes that remaining in one's natural living environment constitutes a positive factor towards health and well-being (MSSS, 1992). For people experiencing temporary or permanent incapacities, staying at home implies numerous support services to ensure good living conditions. Generally these home support services are provided by public sector actors—Centres locaux de services communautaires (CLSC)—and private sector agencies. However, social economy agencies now play a growing role, particularly in dispensing homecare services such as home maintenance and meal preparation.

Community-based organizations that are active in domestic services have evolved significantly in recent years. Since 1997, social economy organizations account for a large part of home service provision. The sector now consists of 6,000 workers in 103 community-based organizations that offer services to 62,400 clients across the province. With a non-profit or a co-operative status, these entities operate according to the rules and principles of the social economy, namely democratic management, user and worker empowerment, and priority of people and work over capital. While they generate revenue through billing their clients, they depend largely on State funding. In this context, a 36 million dollar State financial assistance program for home services offers citizens a revenue-linked financial support to pay for domestic services offered by a recognized social economy organization (ministère de l'Industrie et du Commerce, 2002).

Social economy enterprises in this area provide specific domestic services (light and heavy cleaning and maintenance, non-diet meal preparation, etc.) to an aging population or people with temporary or permanent incapacities. Partnership relations are established with local public sector agencies (CLSCs) in all regions, which ensure exclusivity to social economy home services organizations on their territory. Moreover, the CLSC personnel refer clients that require such services.

However, social economy organizations providing domestic services, like many social economy organizations, must deal with a certain number of difficulties often related to inadequate funding: staff shortage, low wages, and high turn-over (Vaillancourt et al., 2003). Nevertheless, the services they offer respond to an increasing need.

For this reason, the State must ensure them an even greater role as partners in this social policy area. The segment of the population over 65 years of age will continue to increase significantly over the coming years. Further considerations should be given to the financial commitment the State is ready to make in the domestic service area. If the government considers that the home environment is most adequate in view of its health and well-being policy, and if it believes that community-based organizations can ensure quality services in which users and producers have a say, then more resources must be allocated for them to do so.

## Social housing

Housing is a major determinant of health and well-being (MSSS, 1992). As Pomeroy (1996, p. 42) noted: "Health and welfare are connected to the presence of support networks, opportunities to participate, controlling the elements that affect one's life and the ability to stay in a stable community. These elements are closely linked to the housing environment."

Social housing policy is an element of any integrated social policy. In Quebec, the social economy's input in the transformation of social housing policy and practices has been significant. In the field of housing, three types of actors are involved on the Quebec scene (Vaillancourt and Ducharme, 2001). First, there is the private sector comprised of the owners of rental properties, boarding houses, and apartment buildings. Second, there are the actors related to public institutions such as the Canada Mortgage and Housing Corporation (CMHC), the Société d'habitation du Quebec (SHQ), and the municipal housing offices. Finally, we find the actors of the social economy. These are community-based organizations such as advocacy groups, co-operatives, and non-profit organizations that are responsible for a growing number of social housing units. There are also associated actors who provide services or community support to vulnerable residents in their own buildings. There are technical resource groups that offer services such as setting up a non-profit organization, helping residents form a co-operative, providing expert advice and skills, etc.

These social economy actors are very active in Quebec in the construction of new social housing units and in redefining social practices in this area. Since the 1960s, 49,000 cooperative and non-profit housing units have been created in Quebec, including 7,000 new units developed since 1996 thanks to the Accès-Logis program (Ducharme and Vaillancourt, forthcoming). In comparison, the public housing stock comprises 65,000 units. Of the 20,000 public housing units owned by the Montreal Municipal Housing organization, some 600 are administered by non-profit organizations and cooperatives, and provide community support services (Vaillancourt and Ducharme, 2001).

Innovative practices have expanded during the 1990s in Quebec. It is the crisis of the Welfare State that has exposed the limits of the social security system and has forced public sector and third sector managers and practitioners to find new approaches to enhance the quality of life of their tenants and to develop, within public institutions, more democratic practices of governance (Ducharme and Vaillancourt, 2004).

Social housing with community support is a good example of innovative practices developed by actors of the social economy. Community organizations and cooperatives have been working with the Municipal Housing Office of Montreal to offer support, personal attention and services to their vulnerable groups of residents. These services are intended for semi-independent seniors, people with mental disabilities or psychiatric problems and victims of domestic violence, for example (Vaillancourt and Ducharme, 2001; Thériault et al., 2001).

Another interesting case is the supplier relation between the Municipal Housing Office of Montreal and the *Fédération des Organisations d'habitation sans but lucratif (OSBL) de Montréal*. In the first year of its creation in 1987, the Housing Office contracted the social economy actors to manage non-profit rooming houses. These housing organizations now administer 192 social housing complexes with community support, and five non-profit organizations offer services to nearly 2,000 housing units in Montreal (Jetté et al., 1998). The community support consists of on-site janitor-supervisors and follow-up visits by community service workers for individuals who have problems of housing instability, substance abuse, mental health, or are HIV-positive. This approach has an impact on the tenants' quality of life. According to Jetté et al. (1998) such social housing with community support can produce positive impacts for residents in terms of physical environment, safety, social relations, and self-esteem. Indeed, social housing with community support represents "a viable alternative to institutionalization in a context of the redefinition of the Welfare State, provided that the people who are marginalized receive the support they need in order to be integrated into society" (Jetté et al., 1998, p. 187).

## Conclusion

In this chapter we have taken as a given that social policies are an important social determinant of health. The point is not to ask whether social policies have an impact on health, but if this impact is positive or negative. Those who still doubt the link between social policy and health should study the Great Depression of the 1930s when very few, if any, social programs were in place. It is obvious that the quality of life of hundreds of thousands of individuals experiencing unemployment was very negatively affected by the absence of social policy.

Hence, the issue of how social policy impacts the health of individuals and communities. This is why we focused on the architectural design of current social policy when the welfarist model is undergoing transformation. In Part 1, we touched upon the theoretical definition of social policy by making a prominent place for State intervention. We also asserted that leaving the State to do everything, like leaving everything to market forces, is a dead end. Instead, we put forward a multi-polar perspective that argues that the emergence, within the civil society, of social economic activity mindful of citizens' participation can contribute significantly to the satisfaction of needs that tend not to be satisfied by the market or the State.

Then, we hypothesized that the initiatives of the social economy, given their great potential for democratization, are capable of an alliance with public service initiatives to counter both the over *commodification* and *familiarization* of human services. This alliance would give a new dynamism to the development of full citizenship of women and men in society, starting with those that are more at-risk.

In Part 2, based on the theoretical foundations presented in Part 1, some key characteristics of the re-engineering of federal social policy were examined. This examination showed that some important programs of direct federal government intervention were left mostly untouched, for instance, the income security programs for the elderly, retired persons, and veterans. On the other hand, social housing programs, employment insurance, and transfer payment in cash to the provinces were affected. These reforms produced a diminution of social protection against risks for Canadian citizens and de-stabilized the budgets of the provinces by reducing their margins of manoeuvre to operate their own social policy reforms. In our analysis of federal social policy reforms, we skipped over the contributions of the social economy or third sector. We could have spoken, for instance, of the federal government's interest in the *Voluntary Sector Initiative* (VSI) since 1999. But, thus far, we cannot say that this new vision has translated itself in operational terms into the social policy reforms proposed by Ottawa.

Finally, in Part 3, we stood by our general view that more attention must be paid to the social policy initiatives of the provinces and territories by examining four recent examples of reforms in Quebec. Some innovative characteristics were identified, notably the service delivery and administration roles played by the social economy in parallel to the program planning, funding, and regulating roles assumed by the State. Of course, the many new provincial governments elected in 2003 will, along with the new leadership in Ottawa, initiate changes that will, again, affect both the directions taken by social policy and the health and well-being of individuals and communities.

## Notes

1.  The authors would like to acknowledge that the research for this chapter has been made possible thanks to funding provided by two SSHRC grants (842-201-0006 and 410-2002-1039).
2.  We insist here on the *capacity* of the social economy to contribute to progressive social policy reforms. We do, however, recognize that the social economy can also be used in neo-liberal or even neo-welfarist transformations (Vaillancourt and Favreau, 2001; Vaillancourt, 2003b, p. 162–168; Vaillancourt, Aubry, and Jetté, 2003, p. 30–31). The possibility to use the social economy in a neo-liberal fashion has been

clearly demonstrated by the government of Mike Harris in Ontario (see Browne and Welch in Vaillancourt and Tremblay, 2002, chapter 4). Alternatively, a neo-welfarist use of the social economy is emerging in the case of Saskatchewan (see Thériault and Gill in Vaillancourt and Tremblay, 2002, chapter 5).

## Recommended readings

Vaillancourt, Y. and Tremblay, L. (Eds.). (2002). *Social economy, health and welfare in four Canadian provinces.* Montreal/Halifax: LAREPPS/Fernwood.

This is the first book to analyze the reality of some social economic practices in several provincial jurisdictions, with a focus on issues of health and well-being. It presents the results of a 3-year long collaboration between university researchers from Montreal, Moncton, Ottawa, and Regina.

Vaillancourt, Y., Aubry, F. and Jetté, C. (Eds.). (2003). *L'économie sociale dans les services à domicile.* Quebec: Presses de l'Université du Quebec.

This new book analyzes in detail the initiatives of the social economy in Quebec in the area of home support services. Eleven experts contribute to an in-depth look at this emerging sector, which is providing services that are key for the quality of life of both the elderly and disabled populations.

Fortin, S., Noël, A. and St-Hilaire, F. (Eds.). (2003). *Forging the Canadian social union: SUFA and beyond.* Montreal: Institute for Research on Public Policy.

This book reminds us that the Social Union Framework Agreement (SUFA) and the much-touted health accords of 2000 and 2003 have not succeeded in establishing more constructive and co-operative intergovernmental relationships in Canadian social policy. Recommended particularly to Paul Martin.

Quarter, J., Mook, L. and Richmond, B.J. (2003). *What counts: Social accounting for nonprofits and cooperatives.* Upper Saddle River: Prentice Hall.

This is a groundbreaking contribution to the management of nonprofit and cooperative organizations. This book goes beyond traditional accounting and explains how performance can be measured with more accuracy. It is a must if you are on the board of a nonprofit organization providing human services and you would like to estimate the market value of the work done by the volunteers, or the contributions made by your organization to society.

Shragge, E. and Fontan, J.M. (2000). *Social economy: International debates and perspectives.* Montreal: Black Roses Books.

This book explains that the social economy is generally a local economy, and that local economic realities are worth paying attention to (in Canada and abroad) in an era of globalization. This is because social economy initiatives can help alleviate some negative impacts resulting from the downloading by government of their economic and social responsibilities.

## Related websites

Community-University Research Alliance (CURA) in Social Economy—www.aruc-es.uqam.ca

The *ARUC en économie sociale* is the largest group of researchers and community partners active in social economy research in Quebec. Based at UQAM, it is funded by the Social Sciences and Humanities Research Council of Canada.

Le Chantier de l'économie sociale—www.chantier.qc.ca/

The *Chantier* is the official voice of the social economy in Quebec. This site offers many good links to specific social economy initiatives, and also provides information on the state of the political debates surrounding the social economy in the province.

Social Policy Research Unit (University of Regina)—www.uregina.ca/spr

The interest for the social economy has already spilled over in English-Canada. At the University of Regina site you will find publications and some information about projects on the social economy in Saskatchewan.

Laboratoire de recherche sur les pratiques et les politiques sociales (LAREPPS), Université du Quebec à Montréal (UQAM)—www.travailsocial.uqam.ca

The LAREPPS is the social policy research unit of the School of Social Work at UQAM. Many researchers associated with the LAREPPS are conducting research projects on the social economy, often with collaborators from other Canadian provinces, European countries, or Latin America.

Centre de recherche sur les politiques et le développement social (Université de Montréal)—www.cpds.umontreal.ca.

The CRPD host an excellent website for those interested in the relationships between public policy and social development, not only in Quebec and in Canada, but also taking an international comparative perspective.

# Chapter Twenty-Two

———●———

# HEALTH, SOCIAL POLICY, SOCIAL ECONOMIES, AND THE VOLUNTARY SECTOR

## Pat Armstrong

## Introduction

The principles of solidarity, the democratic organization of work, and the participation of citizens in developing and delivering paid services through non-profit organizations that foster social cohesion and bonding are critical to health (Tremblay et al., 2002). And the importance of work, social support, participation, control, and services to health seem obvious. Such principles are central to what in Quebec is called a social economy approach, an approach that brings together various non-governmental agencies to undertake various forms of caring work. Other provinces rely on a less integrated voluntary sector to undertake similar work.

Undoubtedly, the social economy approach means some people are in better health and some receive better care. However, like all approaches, this one must be assessed in the context of our times and, in this case, with the determinants of health in mind. This chapter raises some questions about, and some areas for further reflection on, the social economy approach to improving the conditions for health. The issues are much the same for the voluntary sector in the rest of Canada but it is important to remember that the particular location matters. Thus, the implications in Quebec are necessarily somewhat different than in other parts of the country.

## First, what about women?

Health Canada recognizes gender as a determinant of health, yet a gendered analysis seems to have little place here. Health Canada recognizes gender and culture as two of the twelve determinants of health precisely because they are critical compo-nents in the structuring and impact of both health and care. All populations are gendered and in all populations gender makes a difference in terms of participation in, and the consequences of, health care. It also makes a difference in terms of the chances of being healthy and what health issues we face. Gender interacts with culture and racialized categories, as well as with economic and other locations, to shape both participation and consequence.

**Why is a gendered analysis critical?**
One major reason is that care work is women's work. Women account for over 80% of those providing paid care and a similar proportion of those providing direct personal care as unpaid providers. Work in the public sector, with its high rates of unionization, has meant relatively good jobs for women. Job security, decent wages and benefits, and even good working conditions characterized much of women's public sector employment until the end of the 1980s (Armstrong and Cornish, 1997).

---

**Box 22.1: Women's work in Canada**

**Current problem**
Better education and changing social attitudes have meant positive strides for many Canadian working women in the past two decades. At the same time, the economic changes associated with the globalized production of goods and services, free trade, privatization of services and resources, and de-regulation have brought increased inequalities for many. Recent labour market trends include involuntary part-time and home-based work, reduced training, decreased public sector employment (an important source of well-paid, relatively secure women's jobs), declining real wages, and reduced labour standard protections.

These conditions perpetuate long-standing inequalities. In 1998, the National Action Committee on the Status of Women reported that 40% of women had non-standard jobs (neither secure nor full-time) and women working full-time averaged 73% of men's pay. This pay gap was larger for female students, aboriginal women, women of colour, immigrants, women with disabilities, and older women. 61% of minimum wage earners were women. Unemployment rates were considerably higher for some groups of women (aboriginals, young women, women of colour) than is the national average for women and men.

Women perform 2/3 of unpaid work in Canada, worth up to $319 billion to the economy (Statistics Canada) and the equivalent of millions of full-time jobs (Genuine Progress Index Atlantic). Social service cutbacks are now shifting more responsibility to women and increasing their hours of unpaid work as they care for family members including the sick and frail elderly. Statistics Canada's 1998 General Social Survey found 38% of working mothers were severely time stressed, averaging 74 hours of paid and unpaid work weekly.

**The way forward**
To increase women's economic equality requires multiple strategies. It requires clear legislation and pro-active strategies for enforcing equal pay for work of equal value; a substantial minimum wage increase; strengthened rights to unionize; improved labour standards including those providing family leaves and coverage for migrant, domestic, and home workers; adequate social assistance and an end to workfare; and revitalized public services including quality child-care and homecare. Federal funding and legislation, not general tax cuts, are necessary to build the supports women need for their multiple roles in the new century.

---

Source: Swenarchuk, M. (2000). "Women's work," *Women's Global March 2000: Issue Sheet 9*. Ottawa: National Action Committee on the Status of Women, available at www.nac-cca.ca/march/infosht9_e.htm.

Social Determinants of Health

Reforms over the last decade have meant there are fewer hours of paid work for providers in the public sector who have been formally taught the required skills. At the same time, reforms have meant more hours of unpaid work in the household for those without formal training for the job or more hours in the often non-unionized third sector. Care and other support work in the third sector cannot be understood without understanding that it is women who do this work and that women's care is integrally linked to their unpaid caregiving (Armstrong and Armstrong, 2003).

While there is much talk about how people prefer to be cared for at home or in the community and have all services closer to home, there is much less talk about the preferences of those who must do the work. Six years before the 2002 Romanow Commission on the Future of Health Care, Prime Minister Chrétien appointed the National Forum on Health to make recommendations on the future of health care. Women told that group that they did not want to be "conscripted" into care work (see Charlottetown Declaration on the Right to Care, 2001). But this invisible conscription has only increased since then as more people are sent home quicker and sicker and fewer are allowed either admission into public institutions or publicly paid home care. Although this is often described as sending care back home or to the community, women are taking on tasks and responsibilities their grandmothers never dreamed about. They insert catheters and apply oxygen masks, handle breathing tubes and IVs. As a result, women giving and receiving care are often subject to violence and other risks, especially when the care is provided in isolated households. Without support or training and pushed to care, women providing care often end up in poor health and may provide poor care. Women

are rewarded by caregiving and many want to care. However, inadequate resources and lack of choice limit these rewards while making it harder to care. We have less research on other social services, but there is little reason to assume the impact is different there (Grant et al., 2003).

At the same time, the application of business practices to health and other social services combined with the cutbacks has contributed to deteriorating conditions for those who still have paid jobs. Women employed to provide these services are pushed to work harder and faster, with less control over the care and support they provide. Those organizations funded by the government are pressured to follow similar tactics. These developments are particularly obvious in health care. Increasingly, the women who cook, clean, do laundry, and serve food are defined as providing hotel services rather than care services (Cohen, 2001). This happens in spite of the fact that the women know they are care workers and the determinants of health literature tells us this is the case. Defining the work as ancillary or hotel services, as the Romanow report (Commission on the Future of Health Care, 2002, p. xxi) for example does, ignores both the evidence on their critical role in health care and the skills women bring to the work. So does sending care to be done in community organizations by women formerly on welfare and untrained for the job.

Women are not only the majority of providers, paid or not. They are also the majority of patients, and account for up to three-quarters of the institutionalized elderly. As the majority of the population and all of those giving birth, it is women who use care more. Moreover, women are more likely than men to have their care needs go unmet. It is also women who take children for care

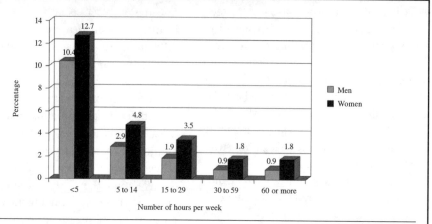

**Figure 22.1: Percentage of men and women aged 15 years and older spending varying amounts of time providing unpaid care or assistance to seniors, Canada, 2001**

Source: "Percentage of men and women aged 15 years and older spending varying amounts of time providing unpaid care or assistance to seniors, Canada, 2001," adapted from the Statistics Canada publication *The changing profile of Canada's labour force, 2001 Census* (Analysis series, 2001 Census), Catalogue 96F0030, February 11, 2003.

and who take responsibility for children's health (Grant et al., 2003).

Women are the majority of the poor as well. Women thus have fewer financial resources than men to assist them in getting or giving care. Their relative poverty also means that women are more dependent than men on other social services. And their responsibilities for children and households, combined with the barriers they face in the labour force, mean women have less access to labour-linked supports such as Employment Insurance. This means they are less likely than men to have benefit coverage through their paid job. This is particularly the case for women past retirement age, most of whom do not have pensions from their paid work. Indeed, women have fewer of the material resources that the health determinants literature tells us are important to health, and less of the power as well (Statistics Canada, 2000).

Cutbacks in health and social services hit women most because they rely on them

most. Equally important, reforms are increasingly based on notions of equity that define equity as same treatment. Those that fail to accommodate differences increase inequality among women. First Nations, Inuit, and Métis women face persistent and pervasive obstacles in giving and receiving care, in gaining and maintaining good health (Dion Stout et al., 2001). Like women from immigrant, refugee and visible minority communities, they often face racism, along with language and cultural barriers. And poor women find it harder not only to stay healthy and care for their children, but also to get the care they need.

Women are facing deteriorating conditions for health and care. However, the full implications of these conditions are often hidden by women's efforts to make up for the gaps in the social safety net and for the negative consequences of the reforms in the system, camouflaging just how far reforms have gone in increasing inequality. Indeed, women are expected to fill these gaps. They

Social Determinants of Health

feel responsible and are held responsible for communities and households. And this is mainly because they are women. Indeed, to talk of communities or households is to talk about women. Only a gendered analysis can reveal the forces at work in creating these conditions for health and care.

Nevertheless, a gender analysis is not central here. While it seems to be generally recognized that the Women's March on Poverty of 1996 was pivotal in initiating what is now called the social economy approach in Quebec, there is much less recognition of the consequences for women of this approach. The Quebec Women's Federation has been critical of these initiatives, arguing that inequality for women has continued to increase under the social economy regime (Salée, 2003). Certainly a social economy approach promotes job creation and paid, rather than volunteer work. This could be beneficial to women, given that women do most of the unpaid volunteer care and social work. However, the jobs created are often inferior to those otherwise provided in the public sector and either low paid or unpaid for at least some of the actual labour.

As Bernier and Dallaire (2002, p. 130) point out,

> In these organizations, which consist mostly of women, staff working conditions are deteriorating and volunteers are assuming more responsibilities for the population that is more and more distressed. Some agencies feel they have become the catch basin for the overflow that the public system can no longer absorb.

Boivin and Fortier (1999) go even farther, arguing that the social economy actually shifts women's good jobs in the public sector to poor jobs in the third sector. To quote Bernier and Dallaire (2002, p. 146) again, data on the social economy indicate

> that 9 out of 10 of the employees are women and that 40 per cent of them were receiving income security benefits before being hired. Though there are some notable exceptions among these enterprises, the hourly rate of their employees who provide direct services range from $6.80 to $8.30 an hour and close to half of these employees work only part-time.

Similar problems are evident in the voluntary sector throughout Canada. Jobs in the third sector can be more meaningful and healthy, allowing workers more control over their work and more obviously useful work to do. Nevertheless, there is a risk of the work becoming compulsory volunteerism for women. That is, women may be encouraged to take on the labour as part of their commitment to communities, with jobs underpaid and skills unrecognized, or even no pay at all for at least part of the work. When the workers are those formerly on welfare and pressured to take the job, the sense of control so critical to health may be lacking.

There are additional issues for women with the social economy approach and in the voluntary sector elsewhere in Canada. Four pillars are identified in the social economy. The market, the public sector, and the social economy account for three of them, and the household is quite appropriately included as the fourth. But this fourth pillar is too often identified in the social economy literature as an undifferentiated

**Women who work in some of the 90 women's centres in Montreal are witnessing rising poverty and the impacts of the attack on the public services which help these women.**

After massive cutbacks to Quebec's social services in the 90s, centres like the South Asian Women's Community Centre (SAWC) are seeing a drastic rise in demand for their services. "The load is getting bigger because public services are not doing their job ... so people get referred to us because we provide all our services for free," says Hitu Jugessur of SAWC. "And it is not just us. All women's centres are feeling the burden."

SAWC provides extensive services to immigrant and refugee women in seven different languages. Last year the SAWC received $30,000 in funding. After a long struggle, the amount now stands at $70,000. Yet, compared to centres such as the Africa-Feminin Women's Centre, which has worked with no funding whatsoever for the past 20 years, they are doing well.

**The roots of the crisis**

According to France Bourgeault of the Centre d'Action et d'Éducation des Femmes a discrepancy in salary between the genders, inadequate minimum wage, and social benefits, the housing crisis, lack of education about reinsertion into the job market, and mental health issues are among the primary factors contributing to the high rate of poverty for women in Quebec.

The housing crisis is of special concern to many centres. "There is no affordable housing available," says Jugessur. "We are dealing with people at the bottom of the social structure. We get many demands put on us whereas before there were housing banks around Montreal to help with finding accommodation. Those housing banks are not functioning because there are no houses available. So people call us directly."

As rents rise there are more and more evictions, people who can't pay their rent, and homelessness. "Since the beginning of the housing crisis last fall we see many new women who do not know what to do. They have always had work and a place to live. If for one month they can't pay their rent they get kicked out. They come to us extremely stressed out," says Suzanne Bourret of Herstreet, a day program for homeless women. "It is difficult to find and then pay for housing. For women who receive welfare, three-quarters of it has to go to rent. That leaves them with one week's worth of money to buy a month's worth of food. These factors lead to pan-handling, prostitution and of course being more prone to sexual and emotional abuse." Herstreet used to be open four days a week. However, in January—during the middle of the winter, traditionally their busiest time—they were forced to cut back to two days a week. Despite intense effort they have been unable to find funding.

More and more women are referred to women's centres because hospitals and CLSCs (community clinics) are unable to cope. "We are not clinicians, nor are we nurses or psychiatrists," says Jugessur. "But we are forced to deal with serious cases. We deal with it by trying to break isolation. Immigrant women particularly face a lot of isolation."

"In the public system they will prescribe anti-depressants as if that will solve everything—without looking at the woman's overall situation," says Jugessur. "She can be a refugee claimant, she's been raped or been witness to war and she comes here and there's no support system. They don't give importance to these things. It takes two minutes to write a prescription down on a piece of paper and send a woman home."

con't

con't

**Tax cuts**
The Quebec government promised massive tax cuts, to be implemented over three years, in the 2000 budget. The budget featured $4.5 billion in cuts for individuals and complete corporate exemptions to, among other things, health care services. "It is not a matter of lack of funds but of political will," says Jennifer Auchinleck of Project Genesis (a community drop-in centre). "There are no real debates over public services and people have it explained to them as 'We can't afford this anymore.' On a corporate level, the Quebec government has given extensive tax exemptions where public services, especially health care, are concerned. It is a clear policy decision. They are following an agenda of moving toward the privatisation of public services. There are groups that stand to benefit from the cuts."

Auchinleck is describing a trend that is common in other countries. Our governments have signed on to that agenda, and according to Auchinleck, it is not a direction that we in Quebec are willing to go in. "People do not want more cuts to public services."

"The key is being educated on the issues and taking action to have our voices heard," says Auchinleck. There have been victories in the recent past in housing and healthcare; the government has backed off from de-insuring dental and optometry services. As well, the fight for free medication for welfare recipients has been won. These have all been achieved through public pressure.

Women's groups as well have fought hard to gain more recognition. They are currently waging a campaign with the Régie régional de santé, the health and social services board, to ensure $165,000 in core funding for all women's centres in Montreal. This basic funding would not only enable them to maintain at-risk programs, while improving working conditions for employees, but also justly reward hard and increasingly necessary work.

Source: Kramer, T. (2002). *After the cutbacks.* May 4, 2002. Montreal: Alternatives for a Different World, online at www.alternatives.ca/article220.html.

household filled with "natural helpers" (Tremblay et al., 2002, p. 21). Such natural caregivers are too often assumed to be women. Study after study demonstrates that it is women who provide most of the unpaid personal care in the household (Morris, 2001). They are the ones who take up the slack left by the state when health care, education, and other social programmes are cut. They are the ones who are assumed to know naturally how to do the work. And they often do this work at the expense of their own economic futures and their health (Morris, 2001).

Equally important, there is little that is natural about the care they provide. To classify it as such is to ignore the skills required to do the work and to exert pressure on women to do the work as part of their genetic responsibility. Assumptions about natural caregiving "conscript" women into the work, as many of them told the National Forum on Health (1997, p. 19). Caring can be mutually rewarding, but only if there is a choice about doing the work and if the work is recognized. A workshop on women's caring in the home produced a summary of the principles required to develop homecare practices that work for all women.[1]

In addition, the power in these households is too frequently unequal. This inequality within households reflects those outside the household, each reinforcing the other. Women are paid less than men, and are more likely to be employed part-time or on a casual basis (Statistics Canada, 2000).

This inequality in the market in turn contributes to their responsibilities for domestic work. And their domestic responsibilities in turn contribute to their inequality in the labour force. Such inequality must not only be recognized as a starting point for a social economy approach devoted to the democratic organization of work but must also be addressed. Indeed, such an approach should positively promote equity by ensuring that the care work is both more equally rewarding and equally distributed. Given what we know about the determinants of health, such equity would necessarily contribute to the health of women.

## Second, what about power outside the household?

The for-profit sector has gained enormous power and has a significant interest in seeking profit in the areas of interest to the social economy and the voluntary sector more generally. Within this context, can there be collaboration through equal partnerships? Or will the practices of the for-profits prevail—especially during a period of neo-liberal governments that ally themselves so closely with such practices? Like marriages, these partnerships are located within wider contexts of inequality that make genuine partnerships difficult to develop or maintain. Research from the United Kingdom indicates that such partnerships are not about equality but rather mean absorption by the for-profit sector drivers (Knapp et al., 2001). Indeed, the transfer of care from public sector institutions to third sector ones may provide a cover, a camouflage, for a transfer of the more profitable aspects of care and other social services to for-profit and often international providers. This is what is happening in Ontario Community Care

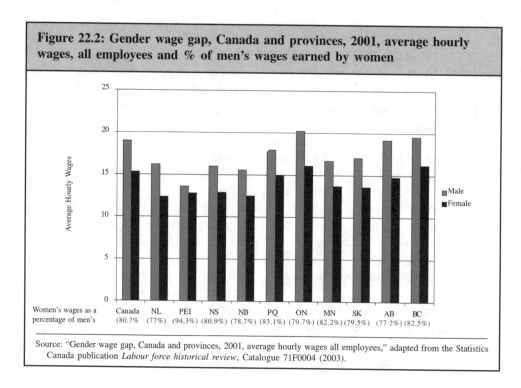

Figure 22.2: Gender wage gap, Canada and provinces, 2001, average hourly wages, all employees and % of men's wages earned by women

Source: "Gender wage gap, Canada and provinces, 2001, average hourly wages all employees," adapted from the Statistics Canada publication *Labour force historical review*, Catalogue 71F0004 (2003).

Social Determinants of Health

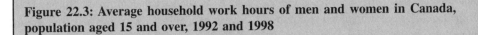

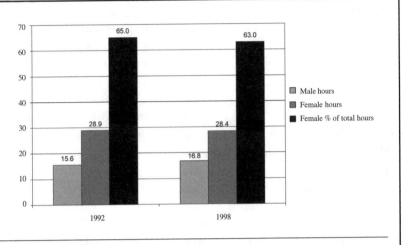

Access Centres and long-term care facilities as compulsory bidding pits for-profits against not-for-profits. The not-for-profits need to act like the for-profit ones in order to win the bid. The bulk of the service delivery gets shifted to for-profits in any case, with the less profitable and more burdensome work left to the not-for-profit sector. The result can be a legitimating of for-profit expansion, with the state still paying for care and other social services (Armstrong and Armstrong, 2002). In the process Canadians may either lose control to investors, many of whom are foreign, or be forced to act like them. As a result of this competitive model, the work for the mainly female labour force deteriorates along with their health.

## Third, does the social economy challenge the medical model?

My third question is also linked to power. The formal health care system now performs a narrower and narrower range of interventions, leaving social supports and care to the informal and third sector. Does this process not run the risk of reinforcing an hierarchical model of care dominated by a medical model at the core and complemented by different tasks undertaken by those defined as unskilled or significantly less skilled, mainly female helpers? And does it not leave the social determinants of health entirely outside the provision of care, rather than a central component in how we construct care? Instead of constructing care through organizations that combine social, economic and health services, such as was planned for the CLSCs (local community access centres) in Quebec, will the reliance on the third sector separate these health determinants? (Renaud, 1987).

This is evident in the Report from the Commission on the Future of Health Care in Canada (2002). Although there is mention of the factors that keep people well, there are no recommendations on the determinants of health. Instead, the focus is almost entirely on acute care services. Even when it comes to home care, it is recommended that public services be extended only to post-acute care and palliative care. Both are linked to health issues strictly though a medical model. Meanwhile, a distinct line is drawn between "direct health care services such as medical, diagnostic and surgical care; and ancillary services such as food preparation, cleaning and maintenance" (p. 6). Such a line distinguishes health care from other determinants, ignoring how determinants operate within the health care system, while reinforcing the dominance of a medical model for care.

## Fourth, what about tensions and contradictions within the social economy?

These two questions on power are in turn related to a fourth. The social economy combines conflicting goals and processes. Organizations may be promoting equal participation while acting as employers, for example. As employers, they need to keep costs down in order to remain as a supplier for the state or as a local service organization working with businesses. This can in turn mean social economy organizations seek to make people work harder and longer. Or what about the contradiction of encouraging participation even while women are already so overburdened they have no time to care? What about the tensions involved in seeking funding from either the private or public sector? Does the search for funding from private donors not involve appealing to neo-liberal perspectives? Moreover, does this not then mean that the decisions about funding get made by individuals and corporations rather than by Canadians as a whole, even though this means earnings forgone by the state? While social economy enterprises may prevent for-profit organizations from fulfilling this role, can they only do so by charging so little that women face inferior working conditions and by providing less skilled care? Does working with the private, for-profit sector mean that the need for commercial confidentiality limits the capacity of third sector organizations to share information with their members, and governments with their citizens, thus denying a central feature of democratic accountability? These are not necessarily inevitable consequences of a social economy approach or of a reliance on the voluntary sector. But they are issues that need to be addressed in assessing such an approach.

## Fifth, are local, non-profit organizations democratic?

My fifth question is about the range of organizations within the social economy and the extent to which they share power or act democratically in practice. Being local does not necessarily mean being democratic or responsive; nor does being non-profit necessarily mean either of these. Many religious organizations are non-profit without being democratic. Some are large, bureaucratic organizations based on hierarchies of power. And many nominally democratic organizations are far from based on equal participation. Some are based on cultural ties, with bonding fostered in a way that is exclusive. A significant proportion has a history of denying women equal access or participation. Even organizations nominally based on claims of social cohesion may give little priority to women's issues.

Research in Saskatchewan (Horne et al., 1999), for example, shows that the localization of decision-making combined with budget cuts meant women's issues were now defined as too expensive and too specialized for support.

According to a recent B.C. study (Benoit et al., 2002, p. 390–391) on maternity care,

> Control of decision-making may be closer to the community (i.e., at the regional level) but non-urban women in their communities have not had their voices heard by those in authority.

As a Quebec (Bernier and Dallaire, 2002, p. 150) report points out, localization may also be based on a false assumption that people have time to engage in democratic processes.

> Citizen involvement, which was supposed to facilitate reform by democratizing regional bodies and decision-making processes, has been frustrated by some of the effects of the reform itself. Women from community organizations are overburdened.

In other words, it is important to distinguish among organizations in the third sector and to scrutinize their organization and practices.

## Sixth, do the social economy and the voluntary sector more generally take the heat off the government while allowing it to act in ways that contradict the very principles of the social economy and some voluntary organizations?

Rekart (1993) has described how in B.C. the need for money forces organizations to adopt neo-liberal practices, providing services determined as necessary by the government and dropping their advocacy role in order to get funding. Similar issues have been raised in Quebec, with Doré for example (1991) arguing that community agencies are merely engaging in a form of contracting out that puts them in competition with other firms. Recent British research on homes for the aged "shows how local democracy, and talk about 'consulting' local opinion, are becoming increasingly meaningless under a government committed to imposing change from the centre" (McFadyean and Rowland, 2002, p. iv).

The promotion of the social economy or the voluntary sector may mean leaving the government unchanged and off the hook. This happened decades ago when it was argued that institutional care for the mentally ill was so bad that as many people as possible should be released and care should take place outside the institutions. The release was beneficial for some but those who remained in the institutions did not have the problems in their environment addressed and what went on in the institutions still had a profound impact on all those needing care. Local control may be primarily about shifting risks and responsibilities, without providing the resources required to do a good job.

It may also produce rather limited solidarity, with solidarity far too local and specific to lead to fundamental reforms. Indeed, it could undermine broader solidarities that lead to more equal distribution of resources of the sort provided by universal services.

Moreover, the technical focus that is condemned in the state is being replaced by a commitment to everything being evidence-based. This commitment may have the same effect as a technical focus, concentrating power in the hands of the experts in all four sectors. With so many actors, the tendency may be to rely on a rules-based approach. Such rules are too often based on general patterns that deny differences and individual participation or choice. Standardization rather than standards are the result, and citizens lose control in ways that are dangerous to their health.

So part of the last question, then, is: Can the social economy or the voluntary sector more generally change government practices? And what does this approach mean for the creation of solidarity and support through government?

## Finally, what about the international context and the free trade rules?

Does opening up services to the third sector risk opening them up to foreign providers? The Romanow Commission, and the studies prepared for it, make it clear that services are not necessarily protected from foreign intervention under free trade agreements (Jackson and Sanger, 2003). In shifting services out of the public sector, we may well be shifting them into the trade agreement regulations. This could mean that local control becomes less rather than more likely with a social economy approach.

## Conclusion

Raising these questions about the social economy and the voluntary sector does not mean denying the many benefits to health that such community organizations and collaborations have or may have in the future. Nor is it to contest the need for new paradigms of organization and care that put people and their concerns at the centre and that extend democratic control as a means of creating health.

However, it is to suggest that these approaches must be assessed within both an international context and within their specific political and historical locations. And this assessment must be made with the determinants of health in mind. Equally important, particular attention must be paid to gender and culture as determinants of health.

At the same time, it is necessary to develop ways of transforming the state in order to create the conditions for health. This has to be done in the context of a world where the pressure to make health and care products for sale is enormous, as is the pressure to make women in particular responsible for our health. If the social economy approach or the voluntary sector is to provide an alternative, it must also work to change the state at the same time as it is working towards a new local paradigm for service delivery and practices.

Health care services have created solidarity among citizens in Canada and Quebec, and could do so again. This requires a focus on developing public services directly linked to the health determinants, and on extending democratic practices in them. This does not mean abandoning a social economy approach and/or delivery by small, non-profit organizations. But it does mean that a social economy approach or the voluntary sector cannot be designed as the sole alternatives. This is a difficult, but not impossible, plan for health.

Social Determinants of Health

# Recommended readings

Armstrong, P. and Armstrong, H. (2003). "Thinking it through: Women work and caring in the new millennium," in Karen Grant et al. (Eds.) *Caring for/caring about.* Aurora: Garamond.
A careful analysis of the relation between gender, care and social policy.

Armstrong, P. et al. (2002). *Exposing privatization: Women and health reform in Canada.* Aurora: Garamond.
This book offers a summary of health reforms across Canada, paying particular attention to their impact on women. The chapter on Quebec is particularly useful in relation to the social economy approach.

Lee, K., Buse, K. and Fustukian, S. (Eds.). (2002). *Health policy in a globalizing world.* Cambridge: Cambridge University Press.
This book argues developments in the global political economy are influencing not only what are traditionally defined as health issues but are also changing who can influence health policy and priorities.

Sen, K. (Ed.). (2003). *Restructuring health services.* New York: St. Martin's Press.
A collection of articles written for an international meeting, this book presents health system change from the perspectives of policy-makers, researchers, and providers. "It shows how varied historical and socio-political circumstances are brought together by very similar mechanisms and processes of change."

# Related websites

Royal Commission on the Future of Health Care in Canada—www.healthcarecommission.ca
This website makes available all the research produced for the Royal Commission on the Future of Health Care in Canada (the Romanow Commission). It provides a rich bibliographic source on health issues and offers connections to other sources.

The Canadian Policy Research Network—www.cprn.ca
The Canadian Policy Research Network produces a variety of research studies relevant to the determinants of health.

The Canadian Women's Health Network—www.cwhn.ca
The Canadian Women's Health Network covers a broad range of issues related to health and health determinants. It connects to other useful websites and publications from the four Centres of Excellence for Women's Health can be downloaded from this website.

# Chapter Twenty-Three

## CONCLUSION: ADDRESSING AND SURMOUNTING THE POLITICAL AND SOCIAL BARRIERS TO HEALTH

### Dennis Raphael and Ann Curry-Stevens

## Introduction

The state of various social determinants of health and their effects upon the health of Canadians have been documented. There appears to be few grounds for optimism. Clearly, concerted actions are needed to raise Canadians' awareness of the importance of the social determinants of health and press policy-makers to undertake actions to improve their quality.

We consider three issues related to such an agenda. First, we consider the role ideology plays in whether a nation assigns a high priority to strengthening the social determinants of health. We examine the status of the Canadian welfare state and compare it to other nations. Second, we direct attention to various actions that can strengthen the social determinants of health in Canada. These involve actions at the community, municipal, provincial, and federal levels to implement policies and programs to strengthen the social determinants of health.

Finally, we provide an intensive analysis of some of the psychological, social, and political forces that lead to the social determinants of health being so low on the policy agenda. How does the public view health and its determinants? Why are social determinants of health so neglected by health-related professionals such as the health care, public health, and research communities? Are governments reluctant to raise the issues of the social determinants of health because of the role they are playing in weakening these health determinants?

## Health and the future of the welfare state

Numerous contributors to this volume have indicated that profound shifts in national social policy are behind the deterioration in the social determinants of health in Canada. Teeple (2000) sees increasing income and wealth inequalities and the weakening of infrastructure within Canada and elsewhere as resulting from the ascendance of concentrated monopoly capitalism and corporate globalization. Transnational corporations—many with home bases in the

U.S.—actively apply their increasing power to oppose reforms associated with the welfare state to reduce labour costs.

The forces that led to the development of the welfare state at the end of World War II were strong national identities, the need to rebuild Western economies, the strength of labour unions within national labour boundaries, the perceived threat of socialist alternatives, and a consensus for political compromise to avoid the boom-bust cycles of the economy. These led to policies that supported a more equitable distribution of income and wealth through social, economic, and political reforms such as progressive tax structures, social programs, and governmental structures that mitigated conflicts between business and labour, among others.

Since 1974, a fundamental change has occurred in the operation of national and global economics. The rise of transnational corporations that can easily shift investments across the globe serves to pressure nations into acceding to their demands for changes that reverse reforms associated with the welfare state. International trade agreements are one way to weaken both national identities and nationally based labour unions. Trade is now international, but unions continue to be nationally based. With such a power shift, business has less need to develop political compromises among themselves, labour, and governments.

To illustrate, nationally based labour unions have little influence when the economies of nations are increasingly globalized. Labour demands in one nation simply lead to companies moving elsewhere.

The decline of the Soviet Bloc, and its diffuse threat of supporting working class revolt, has also removed incentives for compromise by business with employees and labour in general. Finally, the overall slowing of economic growth has reduced resources available for the welfare state. Increased concentration of corporate and media ownership helps assure that justification for these changes, delivered in the form of neo-liberal ideology, is now the dominant discourse related to political and economic processes.

Recent scholarship places differences in the social determinants of health within explicitly political perspectives (Coburn, 2000; Navarro, 2002). Raphael and Bryant have compared the determinants of women's health in Canada with that seen in the U.K., U.S., Sweden, and Denmark (Raphael and Bryant, 2004). Jackson has compared Canada with the U.S. and Sweden (Jackson, 2002). These differences in national indicators have clear ideological and political antecedents (Navarro, 2000). The social democratic nations (e.g., Sweden, Norway, Finland) create the conditions necessary for health; liberal economies (e.g., U.S., U.K., Canada) less so (Navarro and Shi, 2001). These conditions include equitable distribution of wealth that create a large middle class, strong programs that support children, families, and women, and economies that support full employment (see Figure 23.1). Ideologies are malleable and national social policies can be changed. With this in mind we now consider means of moving such policy change along.

## Actions to strengthen the social determinants of health in Canada

Numerous contributors have described the forces driving the deterioration of a variety of social determinants of health in Canada. These changes are supported by a neo-liberal public discourse that involves a retreat from the welfare state—its equitable distribution

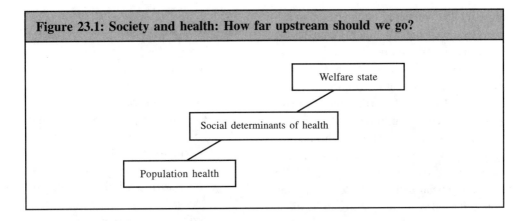

**Figure 23.1: Society and health: How far upstream should we go?**

Welfare state

Social determinants of health

Population health

of wealth, social programs, and life-span supports—that took Canadians so long to establish.

We provide a brief overview of policy recommendations to influence the social determinants of health. A recent and detailed exposition of these options is available (Raphael, 2003a). These concepts owe much to political economists who argue for a basic reorganization of the creation and distribution of societal resources. Practical ideas for action are drawn from the field of health promotion as outlined by the World Health Organization (World Health Organization, 1986).

**Targets for action: The political economy perspective**

Increasing income and wealth inequality and the weakening of social infrastructure result from the concentration of wealth and power within a nation with attendant weakening of civil society (Phillips, 2002; Raphael, 2003b). In response, there are calls for greater equity in political power (Zweig, 2000). This can be achieved by restoring programs and services and reintroducing more progressive income tax rates. Independent unions are a necessity as is legislation that strengthens the ability of workers to organize. Re-regulating many industries would reverse

current trends towards the concentration of power and wealth. Internationally, the development and enforcement of agreements to provide adequate working and living standards that would support and promote health and well-being across national barriers is essential. The provision of a social wage—government provided services that people need to live and develop their ability to work—is a way to restore the social infrastructure that has been so weakened in nations such as Canada and the U.S. Resistance to the privatization of public services is essential.

**Back to the basics: The Ottawa Charter for Health Promotion**

Many of the issues outlined within this volume are best addressed within the political sphere rather than through population and public health initiatives. But strong links exist between political economy and population health issues and health is an important intrinsic concern for Canadians. Yet, most Canadians remain focused on medical and lifestyle issues.

The *Ottawa Charter for Health Promotion* defines health promotion as the process of enabling people to increase control over, and to improve, their health (World Health Organization, 1986). In line with its predominantly structural approach to promoting health, the *Charter* outlines the basic prerequisites for health as being peace, shelter, education, food, income, a stable eco-system, sustainable resources, social justice and equity. It further outlines five pillars of action: building healthy public policy; creating supportive environments; strengthening community action; developing personal skills; and reorienting health services. Social justice and equity are the core values driving this approach. Nations that have seriously implemented health promotion approaches consistent with the *Charter* offer clear commitments to these principles (Mackenbach and Bakker, 2002).

## Working from the top: National policy options to promote health

Two examples of nations with commitments to improving the health of citizens through progressive public policy are Sweden and Finland (Burstrom et al., 2002; Lahelma et al., 2002). Both have a tradition of incorporating equity in governmental policies. The new *National Swedish Health Policy* outlines a number of policy recommendations to improve population health (Agren and Hedin, 2002). These activities are the responsibility of the National Institute of Public Health. Five strategies outlined are:

- *Increase social capital in the Swedish society.* This includes efforts to decrease social inequality and counteract discrimination of minority groups as well as the promotion of local democracy.
- *Promote better working conditions.* The most important issues are to decrease long-term negative stress, promote employees' influence at work and achieve more flexible working hours.

- *Improve conditions for children and young people.* Improve social support for families with children. Support and strengthen health-promoting schools.
- *Improve the physical environment.* Co-ordinate the work for sustainable environment with the struggle for improved health.
- *Provide good structural conditions for public health work at all societal levels.* Support to and co-ordination of research and education in public health science.

The Finnish government is committed to preventive public policy that includes supporting growth and development of children and young people, preventing exclusion, supporting personal initiative and involvement among the unemployed, and promoting basic security in housing (Ministry of Social Affairs and Health, 2001). Their means of achieving these goals clearly recognize the social determinants of health and include:

- Improving efficiency and co-operation among primary, specialized, and occupational health care providers.
- Providing support for the general functional capacity of people of differing ages.
- Promoting lifelong learning.
- Promoting well-being at work.
- Increasing gender equality, and social protection which provides an incentive to work.
- Giving priority to preventive policy, early intervention, and actions to interrupt long-term unemployment.
- Reducing regional welfare gaps.
- Promoting multiculturalism.

- Controlling substance abuse.
- Promoting active participation in international policymaking.
- Providing adequate income security as the key to building social cohesion.

Raphael draws upon various U.K. and Canadian documents to outline three general policy areas to reduce health inequalities and to improve the population health of Canadians (Raphael, 2002a). These concern the incidence of low income, reducing social exclusion, and restoring the social infrastructure, all social determinants of health identified as influencing health inequalities and population health.

### Policies to reduce the incidence of low income

The following steps would serve to reduce the number of Canadians living with low incomes, reduce economic inequality, and improve population health:

- Raise the minimum wage to a living wage.
- Improve pay equity.
- Restore and improve income supports for those unable to gain employment.
- Provide a guaranteed minimum income.

### Policies to reduce social exclusion

Numerous analyses have considered how social exclusion occurs and the role it plays in threatening population health (Atlantic Centre of Excellence for Women's Health, 2000; Shaw et al., 1999). The following steps—in addition to reducing low income— would reduce social exclusion in Canada:

- Enforce legislation that protects the rights of minority groups, particu-

larly concerning employment rights and anti-discrimination.
- Ensure that families have sufficient income to provide their children with the means of attaining healthy development.
- Reduce inequalities in income and wealth within the population, through progressive taxation of income and inherited wealth.
- Assure access to educational, training, and employment opportunities, especially for those such as the long-term unemployed.
- Remove barriers to health and social services which will involve understanding where and why such barriers exist.
- Provide adequate follow up support for those leaving institutional care.
- Create housing policies that provide enough affordable housing of reasonable standard.
- Institute employment policies that preserve and create jobs.
- Direct attention to the health needs of immigrants and to the unfavourable socioeconomic position of many groups, including the particular difficulties many New Canadians face in accessing health and other care services.

### Policies to restore and enhance Canada's social infrastructure

Canadian Federal program spending as a percentage of Gross Domestic product has been decreasing since 1987 such that current federal spending is at 1950 levels (Raphael, 2002b). Indeed, Hulchanski (2002) provides data that program spending is Canada is now lower than that seen in the U.S.!

These decreases have occurred in tandem with decreases in tax revenues

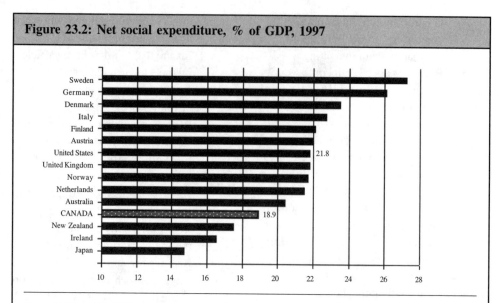

**Figure 23.2: Net social expenditure, % of GDP, 1997**

Sweden
Germany
Denmark
Italy
Finland
Austria
United States    21.8
United Kingdom
Norway
Netherlands
Australia
CANADA    18.9
New Zealand
Ireland
Japan

10  12  14  16  18  20  22  24  26  28

Source: Hulchanski, D. (2002). *Can Canada afford to help cities, provide social housing, and end homelessness? Why are provincial governments doing so little?* Toronto: Centre for Urban and Community Studies, University of Toronto. Online at www.tdrc.net/2rept29.htm.

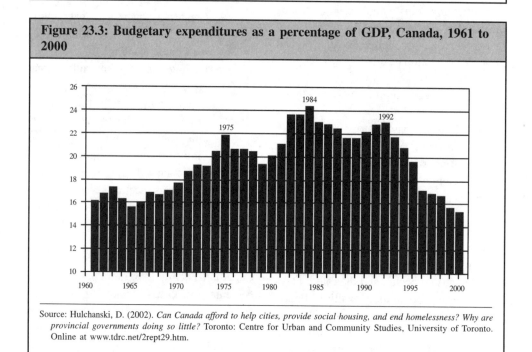

**Figure 23.3: Budgetary expenditures as a percentage of GDP, Canada, 1961 to 2000**

Source: Hulchanski, D. (2002). *Can Canada afford to help cities, provide social housing, and end homelessness? Why are provincial governments doing so little?* Toronto: Centre for Urban and Community Studies, University of Toronto. Online at www.tdrc.net/2rept29.htm.

resulting from modifications to the tax structure that favor the well-off. The concept of universality is an important cornerstone of policies designed to promote social inclusion. Programs that apply to all are more likely to engender political support from the public. The federal and provincial governments should:

- Restore health and service program spending to the average level of OECD nations.
- Develop a national housing strategy and allocate an additional 1% of federal spending for affordable housing.
- Provide a national day care program.
- Provide a national pharmacare program.
- Restore eligibility and level of employment benefits to previous levels.
- Require that provincial social assistance programs are accessible and funded at levels to assure health.
- Assure that supports are available to support Canadians through critical life transitions.

## Working from the middle: Municipal action to promote health

The most developed program of addressing health and its determinants at the municipal level is that of the *Healthy Cities Movement* (Ashton, 1992; Davies and Kelly, 1993). The movement originated in Toronto, Canada, but it was the European Office of the World Health Organization that turned it into a major political force.

Healthy Cities projects are committed to promoting health by influencing local structures and environments. They have a strong values base and consider health in a manner consistent with advanced ways of thinking about societal responsibilities towards their citizens. There are six key elements to the approach (World Health Organization Regional Office for Europe, 1997):

- *Commitment to health*: Projects are based upon a commitment to and definition of health as involving the interaction of physical, mental, social, and spiritual dimensions.
- *Political decision-making for health:* Since housing, environment, education, social services, and other city programs have a major effect on health in cities, strengthening these are important.
- *Intersectoral action*: Healthy Cities requires creating organizational mechanisms by which city departments and community members come together to contribute to health.
- *Community participation*: Projects promote active roles for people so they can have a direct influence on project decisions, the activities of city departments, and local life.
- *Innovation:* Projects recognize that promoting health and preventing disease requires a constant search for, and support for implementation of innovative ideas and methods.
- *Healthy public policy:* Projects achieve their goals by working to create policies that lead to healthier homes, schools, workplaces, and other parts of the urban environment.

The WHO Healthy Cities Office in Copenhagen has developed numerous guides for developing healthy cities projects (World Health Organization Regional Office for Europe, 2003).

## Working from the ground: Community action to promote health

The *Ottawa Charter for Health Promotion* identifies creating supportive environments and strengthening community action as key areas for health promotion action. Engaging local communities to identify and influence governmental and other institutional decisions that threaten health can promote health. The health promotion literature has identified numerous means by which these efforts can be carried out.

Projects can allow community members to identify their own health needs (Raphael et al., 2001b; Raphael et al., 2001a). Such approaches allow individuals and communities to increase control over the determinants of their health through strengthening communities and advocating for healthy public policy. They provide a direction for community-based health workers to take that is consistent with the main arguments concerning the social determinants of health contained within this volume (Popay and Williams, 1994; Williams and Popay, 1997). Health workers can support citizens in examination and discussions of the importance of the social determinants of health. Results can be fed back and form the basis for concerted community action. These sorts of undertakings combine the traditions of public health with those of civic involvement and participation to create effective action to improve the health of the population (Fischer, 2000). Yet there seems to be so little of these activities taking place. Why is this the case?

## Why are social determinants of health so low on the health policy and action agenda?

This book follows closely on the heels of a continuing major public debate about the health of Canadians related to the release of the Romanow *Commission on the future of health care in Canada* (Romanow, 2002). The terms of the debate remain largely fixed

on medical care and the services needed when illness strikes. While numerous submissions to the *Commission* spoke to the importance of social determinants of health for maintaining the sustainability of the health care system, these views did not emerge as a primary focus of the report. This is a rather common phenomena in Canadian health policy, health care, and public health discussions (Raphael, 2003c; Raphael, 2003d; Raphael et al., 2003).

Raphael has detailed some of the reasons why the health care, public health, and research communities eschew a focus on social determinants of health (Raphael, 2002c; Raphael, 2003e). Much of this involves a commitment to paradigms of health that stress biomedical determinants of health or individual responsibility for health and illness through "lifestyle choices." Such approaches are more determined by ideology than by evidence (Nettleton, 1997; Tesh, 1990). It also is very much driven by a perception that during periods of neo-liberal and increasingly conservative political environments raising these issues is—to put it bluntly—looking for trouble from those who hold the purse strings. Indeed, Raphael has suggested:

> Political pressure on federal, provincial, and local governments to conform to these shifting ideological sands blend well with the persistent bias of health workers in favour of individualistic, biomedical and lifestyle approaches to health. The media also prefers easy-to-understand biomedical and lifestyle headlines. The social-determinants-of-health approach is lost among such ideological imperatives. (Raphael, 2003e, p. 37)

Governments are loath to consider these issues as by any objective indicator polices of the past 20 years have served to weaken the social determinants of health. Indeed, government policy-making in Canada seems intent on weakening the social determinants of health. Federal program spending as a percentage of GDP is now at 1950s levels, and government policies have increased income and wealth inequalities, created crises in housing and food security, and increased the precariousness of employment (Raphael, 2001).

## Health and other service workers' priorities

There are pragmatic reasons for the image of health policy-makers, authorities, and advocates as ostriches digging their collective heads in the sand. Consider the everyday situation of those either responsible for formulating health policy or those working directly with vulnerable populations. In both cases, health assessments and solutions need to be offered. To appreciate fully the policy implications of the health issues identified in this volume is to come face-to-face with problems of vast proportions—poverty, inequality, poor access to food, workplace stress, inadequate housing, racism, and inadequate child care, among others.

What would it take to solve these monumental social and economic ills? In the Canada of 2004, it would require a profound reordering of political priorities and re-investment in social infrastructure and program spending. Such a reordering would not be revolutionary. It would simply represent adopting health policy directions consistent with many European nations and directions that, until recently, made Canada a world leader in developing and implementing healthy public policy. Without such commitment, it is unlikely that any

health promotion activities will make a dent in addressing emerging Canadian health issues.

Faced with such formidable policy options, many turn to community development as a means of improving health and well-being. Working on small-scale projects—frequently with limited resources—offers some workers enough hope for change. While this might resonate for some as a liberal model of change (Curry-Stevens, 2003), it is a location from which good work can be done. On a day-to-day basis, do you as a health or other worker choose to work directly with a community of people struggling for a better life or spend your days divorced from the vulnerable attempting to effect policy change by those who may never heed your call? For many, the choice of moving upstream to prevention looks less attractive, and perhaps futile.

## The general public

We can appreciate why health and other workers turn away from health paradigms based on the social determinants of health. Why then do vulnerable communities and individuals—those most affected by the conditions described in this volume—appear complacent in accepting the economic and social conditions under which they are required to live? Why are workers not pressing for fairer tax systems? Better wages? Fleeing low-income jobs? Demanding better minimum wage protection from their governments? Or insisting on expanding regulated childcare or assisted housing programs? In other words, where is the public outrage? A number of reasons may be responsible for this.

## On income and inequality issues, masked by debt

As incomes erode for a significant portion of the population, and they slide lower down the income ladder, why is there not greater outrage over declining standards of living? Especially as this is the case for numbers of Canadians that approach the majority?

Canadians are borrowing to compensate for this loss, with credit being made easier to secure and more abundantly provided. A study by the Vanier Institute of the Family (2002) explored the most recent data on the wealth of Canadians. Revealed are two trends on debt—one is that 30% of all households were now uncomfortable with their debt load and the second is that more families are failing to save for their retirement.

A study by Statistics Canada itself compared debt levels between 1984 and 1999. The findings confirm that Canadians are living with greater levels of debt, most likely to compensate for shortfalls in income. The debt figures are available as a percentage of assets. For every $100 of assets, Canadians now carry $18 of debt, rising from $14 in 1984. The highest burden is carried by those aged 25–34 years, and it is $40, more than double the debt load of others, and in comparison with 1984, up from $30 (Statistics Canada, 2001). The most compelling available data on this topic is that from the Canadian Labour Congress (2003) that indicates "the personal savings rate in the first half of 2003 was just 2.3%, well down from the already low level of 4.2% in 2002" (p. 2).

Credit remains unavailable to poor Canadians who lack the assets to secure loans. Such then is the trend towards deepening the psychological divide between the lower middle income groups and the working poor: those who are able to replace shrinking incomes with debt and those who suffer more directly.

## Hidden from view

The evidence provided by the various contributors to this volume is sometimes, but certainly not always, consistent with common sense. Or at least not the common sense being forwarded by our leading political parties, most of whom want the news about the economy to be seen as good news. This perception is important as our economy—the value of the Canadian dollar, the bond rating that foreign debtors place on the debts we owe, our interest rates and access to credit, the value of the stock market—is vulnerable to what can loosely be called "confidence." No mainstream political leader wants to expose how the market is failing the majority of its citizens and advancing the interests of a small proportion of the population. They would much rather hide this failing behind glowing reports of the rise in GDP or the increases in "average" incomes.

## Pointed in the wrong direction

It serves the economic elite for low and middle-income earners to point the blame for their social ills at other marginalized groups. These groups include immigrants "who steal our jobs," the welfare poor "who are just a drain on our resources," the beneficiaries of employment equity "who take the jobs we should have got," and even the unionized workers "who get much more that they deserve." One explaining factor is that competition increases as resources dry up, and that this competition generates hostility, particularly between those most alike. Any objective analysis of the current state of Canadian society quickly recognizes the role that uncaring corporations and those who wish to preserve their excessive income and wealth levels are playing in weakening the social determinants of health.

## Replaced by self-blame

Dominant culture in western civilization emphasizes individual achievement and personal agency. Embedded within our social and cultural norms is the myth of personal success, framing the individual as authors of our own lives. Such a notion of where agency originates redirects anger at the structural aspects of society that creates unhappiness towards the self. Those who do not achieve "view such failure in terms of personal inadequacy or the 'luck of the draw'" (McLaren, 2003, p. 77).

Through this process, we become agents in our own marginalization, a process identified by Gramsci as hegemony. Drawing from McLaren (2003), the prevailing image for our political system is a benevolent one, whereby the interests of the political and economic elite "supposedly represent the interests of all groups" (McLaren, 2003, p. 78). Canadians rarely confront their governments as to why they are not being firm with corporate giants or more generous to its citizens. While we are not coerced into such an analysis, we are conditioned to view the cause of our social ills as residing within us. The power of such analysis rests with the "common sense" of such beliefs, and it even seems to have been generated by that common sense.

Such beliefs manifest themselves in voting preferences and serve to profoundly disturb progressive Canadians as many struggling Canadians vote for right-wing political parties. While noting such a process in the U.S., Gore Vidal observes: "the genius of our system is that ordinary people go out and vote against their interests. The way our ruling class keeps out of sight is one of the greatest stunts in the political history of any country" (McLaren, 2003, p. 79). And, apparently, so too in Canada.

### Stuck in real human dilemmas

The mobility of workers stall as one gets poorer. Lacking money for first and last months' rent, a car to drive to distant locations, or even enough for public transit serves to keep many in dire poverty. Even information about wages is the privilege of higher income groups. The "money taboo" (Ehrenreich, 2001) keeps workers from sharing information that might fruitfully be used to even know where better paying jobs exist. All these dynamics serve to limit access to decent work.

Also at fault is the real drain that high housing costs place on our ability to make ends meet. The disappearance of cheap housing (safe or otherwise) leaves families in shelters, motels, trailers, and even cars. The withdrawal of the federal government and most provincial governments from public and cooperative housing (although signaled to reverse) deepens this crisis. If ever there was a market failure for the supply of a commodity in response to high demand, housing is truly that failure.

Another real dilemma is that pure exploitation of low-wage workers is rampant—both in terms of their wages and working conditions. Any non-unionized worker can be fired at whim. They are constantly watched by supervisors, treated as potential and likely thieves (with WalMart's notorious "time thief" accusations of workers who talk to others being an outrageous extension of this accusatory environment). Workers become likely to feel unworthy enough to actually believe they deserve such low wages (Ehrenreich, 2001).

### Feeling futile and disempowered ... distanced from our political leadership

Consider the political landscape today. Trust in government has been shrinking over the last 35 years (since such polling began). The EKOS survey, *Canadian and American national election studies,* uncovered the answer to the following question: "How much do you trust the government in Ottawa to do what is right?" The answer was resoundingly poor—falling from a high of 57% (answering "just about always/most of the time") in 1968 to a level of just 27% in May 2002. And the ever-popular Ipsos-Reid *Canada Trust Survey* was repeated in 2003, revealing that the trust[1] Canadians place in the federal politicians ranks last of a list of 26 professions—even car salespeople rank one position higher at 25th. Local politicians score no better, as they take the 24th spot. Those who score higher include pharmacists (1st), doctors (2nd), teachers (4th), the police (5th), charitable organizations (9th), religious institutions (14th), lawyers (18th), journalists (19th), trade unions (21st), and CEOs (22nd). Emerging is a growing crisis in the reputation of our political leadership.

Further evidence of this dramatic change is revealed in the EKOS survey, as it articulates the shrinking importance of the public interest. The following question was posed: "When the federal government makes decisions, whose interests do you think are given the greatest importance?" From 1998 to 2002, the public interest shrank from 18% of the population to 16%, while the combined importance of "the interest of politicians and their friends" and "the interest of big business" rose from 60% to 67% in just four years.

There is clear evidence of growing distrust in politicians and rising concern with the interests and activities of big business. In tandem, these trends displace the importance of the public interest. As a decision-making body, today's political leaders show themselves to be seriously out-of-step with the majority of the population. To explore the causes of this destabilizing dynamic, we need to turn to theory drawn from the study of privilege. Hobgood (2000) asserts that there is a natural process in play

for the privileged whereby their separation (socially and economically) from the majority population leads to an ignorance that stems from their lack of contact with the lived realities of the average and more vulnerable citizens. This ignorance, in time, leads to an arrogance that stems from assuming that the world works for the majority in much the same way that it works for the privileged.

Asserting this to be a natural process of alienation, Hobgood thus calls on us to problematize the world of privilege. It is they who are out-of-touch and suffering the effects of social exclusion (Curry-Stevens, 2004), not the majority world that lies below them. The gravely serious arrogance that is bred unfolds as follows: the privileged person looks at the lived reality of the less privileged and assumes that the world works for others the way it works for themselves. The reality is, in fact, contrary to this logic. They assume that if they lived their lives as a poor, blue-collar, racialized, immigrant or as woman, that they would achieve largely the same accomplishments as they have as white, male and upper class. What they do not realize is that nothing would be the same. They would not have gotten off home plate. As encapsulated by Hatfield (2002), when discussing George Bush Junior, "He's one of those guys who was born on third base and thinks he hit a triple" (p. 53).

## And finally, duped by the hope (and sometimes the promise) that we too can be rich

Let's start at the beginning—our statistics reveal that only 15% of Canadian families earn more than $100,000/year. Yet the myth of income mobility is held out in front of us like a carrot, intertwined by the promise that hard work will get us ahead. Social commentators such as Michael Moore

(2003) claim that in the United States, citizens are afraid to hold corporations accountable as they bought the lie "that we too could some day become rich. So we don't want to do anything that could harm us on that day we end up millionaires" (p. 140). In calculations done for Moore's book, he asserts that the chance of the average American at middle income levels becoming rich to be about one in a million. Similarly, too, we imagine this statistic for Canadians.

Having scanned these various social and economic impediments to change, there remains the need to debunk the rhetoric of the status quo—and their political project towards lower labour costs, lower taxes, smaller governments, and an enhanced role for corporate voices in the governing decisions of the country. These pressures have served to reconfigure social policy as we know it, but from our view, their position is weak—becoming exposed as self-interested, with cracks beginning to show.

## Challenging the assertion: "We can't afford this"

The costs of resolving all our social ills may appear to be prohibitive. One answer would be "We cannot afford not to effect such spending" as the costs of attending later to the problems of poverty and homelessness as two examples escalate later down the line, as more lives are damaged. Yet time frames in politics do not stretch far. They are limited to 5-year time horizons, or less if the next election looms.

So what arguments exist today in defense of enhanced social spending? Beginning with the basics of economic growth, we can illustrate that enhanced spending is not simply an expenditure item. Any spending that serves to employ someone has a ripple effect. First, employment returns income taxes to the government, reducing the net outlay of the expenditure. Second, employment removes someone from the roles of unemployment insurance or social assistance and puts them into the workforce. Thirdly, that income in turn is spent on goods and services that generate economic activity and the cycle of earnings and spending. It is only when those dollars are removed from the system through expenditures outside of the country or through savings that the ripple effects stop.

Consider whether government spending creates more ripple effects if placed in the hands of the rich or the poor. When placed in the hands of the rich, it is more likely to end up as savings or spent outside of the country. This is the reason that deductions in capital gains taxes or reduced income taxes do not serve our economy. Yet direct social spending strongly serves economic growth, particularly if it is placed in the pockets of those who spend it locally. Hundreds of businesses went bankrupt in the Toronto area when social assistance rates were cut and purchase of goods and services were reduced. Cuts in employment insurance serve the same function—reducing the quality of life in our neighbourhoods as the spending power of Canadians shrinks.

What has been deemed in the corporate interest has been assessed to be in the interests of small businesses. Survey after survey of the various independent business associations reveals an interpretation that taxes serve to strangle their business, thus contributing to small and mid-sized businesses acting as allies in cuts to social programs and a regimen of lower taxes. But what if the question were posed differently? What if we asked them if they wanted greater disposable income in the hands of people in their neighbourhood? And would they be likely to increase sales if that were true? And would they rather increase sales or have lower taxes?

# Conclusion

Developments in Europe indicate that concerted public health and community efforts can profoundly influence the development of policies that determine the extent of health inequalities and the overall state of population health within a nation. The policy directions being undertaken by nations such as Sweden and Finland are two such examples. Similarly, the success of the WHO European Office Healthy Cities initiative is another example of the power of cities and communities to influence health policy. Canada has a rich history of concerted public pressure that can lead to positive policy change.

*The Toronto charter on the social determinants of health*—see Appendix—is based on the content of this volume. Toronto and Ottawa City Councils have endorsed the Charter and it is going before additional municipal councils across Canada for endorsement. This Charter itself is a tool for promoting health and social justice, both within and outside of Canada. It can be an impetus for change, notably by municipal council endorsement followed by political action.

The social determinants of health concept can help make the links between government policy, the market, and the health and well-being of Canadians. For those working in the health sector, it can serve as motivation for working for change. The interests of their clients, patients or consumers are served by speaking out against poverty, social exclusion, inequality, and inadequate services. There are potent barriers however, to such actions. We hope that this volume will assist in these efforts.

# Notes

1. This survey also inquired about the behaviors and attitudes that are most valued components of trust. These include honesty, integrity, and reliability.

# Recommended readings

Raphael, D. (2003). "Towards the future: Policy and community actions to promote population health," in R. Hofrichter (Ed.) *Health and social justice: A reader on politics, ideology, and inequity in the distribution of disease*, pp. 453–468. San Francisco: Jossey Bass/Wiley .

   This chapter provides means by which health public policy can be developed to influence the social determinants of health. Examples of successful initiatives are provided from Canada and elsewhere.

Raphael, D. (2002). *Social justice is good for our hearts: Why societal factors—not lifestyles—are major causes of heart disease in Canada and elsewhere*. Toronto: CSJ Foundation for Research and Education. Online at www.socialjustice.org.

   This monograph is an example of how a social determinants of health analysis can inform analysis of the causes of major diseases in Canada and elsewhere. While compelling evidence of the importance of social determinants of health is present, action to address these issues is frequently limited.

Mackenbach, J. and Bakker, M. (Eds.). (2002). *Reducing inequalities in health: A European perspective*. London: Routledge.

   Social determinants of health approaches to health policy are much more prevalent in Europe than North America. This volume provides numerous case studies of efforts to address social determinants of health that provides examples for Canadian policy-makers to follow.

Social Determinants of Health

Rebick, J. (2000) *Imagine democracy*. Toronto: Stoddart.

When considering change, very quickly our analysis turns to our system of democracy, with its associated faults of corporate influence, first-past-the-post electoral decisions, representative instead of participatory democracy and the trust deficit that these (and other) factors engender. Rebick assesses our Canadian system and develops an argument for her model of effective citizenship.

Navarro, V. (Ed.). (2002). *The political economy of social inequalities: Consequences for health and quality of life*. Amityville: Baywood Press.

This is a collection of papers that explicitly considers how ideology and politics influence the social determinants of health. The importance of the welfare state for health is clearly demonstrated.

## Related websites

National Institute of Public Health. (2002). Sweden's New Public-Health Policy—www.fhi.se/pdf/roll_eng.pdf

This document provides an excellent example of a social determinants of health approach to national health policy. The website www.fhi.se/english/eng_summaries.asp provides other examples of Swedish health policy.

World Health Organization, European Office. (2003). Healthy cities and urban governance—www.who.dk/healthy-cities

This website provides resources for developing healthy cities based on 15 years of European experience. The Healthy Cities movement originated in Toronto, but has seen its successful implementation in Europe.

Social Determinants of Health Listserv at York University, Canada

To subscribe, send the message "subscribe SDOH *yourname*" in the text area to listserv@yorku.ca

This international listserv was established to (a) provide the latest information on scholarship on social determinants of health; (b) explore the implications of these conditions for the health of citizens; and (c) provide support for those attempting to strengthen these social determinants of health in their local jurisdictions.

Canadian Health Coalition—www.healthcoalition.ca

This is the site of the Canadian Health Coalition—the major activist-oriented site on health issues. It has an excellent list of resources in their archives of current issues within health care. Although focused on medical care, it also provides information about food and food safety, genetically-modified foods, privatization of health care, and the pharmaceutical industry. It positions itself as a watchdog on the Canadian health system.

Rabble.ca—www.rabble.ca

Any set of resources is incomplete without a site that is dedicated to keeping us up-to-date on what is happening in Canada and around the world. Rabble.ca is an online news source that draws from Canada's best progressive journalists (both well known and lesser known) and provides commentary on current political issues.

# Appendix

---

## STRENGTHENING THE SOCIAL DETERMINANTS OF HEALTH: THE TORONTO CHARTER FOR A HEALTHY CANADA

From November 29 to December 1, 2002, a conference of over 400 Canadian social and health policy experts, community representatives, and health researchers met at York University in Toronto, Canada to: (a) consider the state of ten key social or societal determinants of health across Canada; (b) explore the implications of these conditions for the health of Canadians; and (c) outline policy directions to improve the health of Canadians by influencing the quality of these determinants of health. The conference took place at a time when Canadian social and health policies were undergoing profound changes related to shifting political, economic, and social conditions.

Ten social determinants of health—early life, education, employment and working conditions, food security, health services, housing, income and income distribution, social exclusion, the social safety net, and unemployment and job insecurity were chosen on the basis of their prominence in Health Canada and World Health Organization policy statements and documents.

The conference was a response to accumulating evidence that growing social and economic inequalities among Canadians are contributing to higher health care costs and other social burdens. Indeed, the Kirby Report on the *Federal role in health care* points out that 75% of our health is determined by physical, social, and economic environments. Evidence was also accumulating that a high level of poverty—an outcome of the growing gap between rich and poor—has profound societal effects as poor children are at higher risk for health and learning problems in childhood, adolescence, and later life, and are less likely to achieve their full potential as contributors to Canadian society.

The *Social determinants of health across the life-span* conference coincided with the release of the Romanow Report on the *Future of health care in Canada* that called for strengthening the Canadian health care system by expanding its coverage, resisting privatization, and increasing financial investment. The report also discusses the importance of economic and social determinants of health. The evidence heard at the conference reinforced the view that immediate and long-term improvements in the health of Canadians depend upon investments that address the sources of health and disease.

**The participants at the *Social determinants of health across the life-span conference* therefore resolve:**

*Whereas* the evidence is overwhelming that the health of Canadians is profoundly affected by the social and economic determinants of health, including—but not restricted to—early life, education, employment and working conditions, food security, health care services, housing, income and its distribution, social exclusion, the social safety net, and unemployment and employment security; and

*Whereas* the evidence presented at the conference clearly indicates that the state and quality of these key determinants of health are linked to Canada's political, economic and social environments and that many governments across Canada have not responded adequately to the growing threats to the health of Canadians in general, and the most vulnerable in particular; and

*Whereas* these social determinants of health are also human rights as defined in the *Universal Declaration of Human Rights* and the *International Covenant on Economic, Social and Cultural Rights*, which Canada is obliged to protect and promote; and

*Whereas* the evidence presented indicates that investments in the basic social determinants of health will profoundly improve the health of Canadians most exposed to health threatening conditions—the poor, the marginalized, and those Canadians excluded from participation in aspects of Canadian society by virtue of their living conditions—therefore providing health benefits for all Canadians; and

*Whereas* the evidence presented to us has indicated the following to be the case:

1.  **Early childhood development** is threatened by the lack of affordable licensed childcare and continuing high levels of family poverty. It has been demonstrated that licensed quality childcare improves developmental and health outcomes of Canadian children in general, and children-at-risk in particular. Yet, while a national childcare program has been promised, 90% of Canadian families with children lack access to such care.
2.  **Education** as delivered through public education systems has helped to make Canada a world leader in educational outcomes but our education systems are now at risk due to funding instability and poorly developed curriculum in many provinces. These conditions may weaken the trend toward greater number of students graduating despite evidence that those who do so show significantly better health and family functioning than non-graduates.
3.  **Employment and working conditions** are deteriorating for some groups— especially young families—with potential attendant health risks. One in three adult jobs are now either peripheral or precarious as a result of increasing contracting out of core jobs and privatization of public employment. These jobs are often temporary, with low pay and high stress. Precarious working situations are directly

related to the weakening of labour legislation in many jurisdictions. These changes threaten the gains made by workers in the past, jeopardizing their health and well-being.

4.  **Food security** among Canadians and their families is declining as a result of policies that reduce income and other resources available to low-income Canadians. In Canada, food insecurity exists among 10.2% of Canadian households representing 3 million people. Monthly food bank use is 747,665 or 2.4% of the total Canadian population, which is double the 1989 figure; 41% of the food bank users or 305,000 are children under the age of 18.

5.  **Health care services** can become a social determinant of health by being reorganized to support health. Many examples of effective—but all-too-rarely implemented—means of preventing deterioration among the ill through chronic disease management and rehabilitation are available. Screening that has been carefully assessed for its effectiveness can support health. Preventing disease in the first place by promoting the social and living conditions that support healthy lifestyles has also been neglected. While the Romanow Report reaffirmed the principles of the Canada Health Act, missing were strong statements about the important roles public health, health promotion, and long-term care play in supporting health.

6.  **Housing shortages** are creating a crisis of homelessness and housing insecurity in Canada. Lack of affordable housing is weakening other social determinants of health as many Canadians are spending more of their income on shelter. More than 18% of Canadians live in unacceptable housing situations and one in every five renter households spent 50% or more of their income on housing in 1996, an increase of 43% since 1991.

7.  **Income and its equitable distribution** have deteriorated during the past decade. Despite a 7-year stretch of unprecedented economic growth, almost half of Canadian families have seen little benefit as their wages have stagnated. Governments at all levels have let the after-tax-and-transfer income gap between rich and poor grow from 4.8:1 in 1989 to 5.3:1 in 2000. The growing vulnerability of lower-income Canadians threatens early childhood, education, food security, housing, social inclusion, and ultimately, health. Low-income Canadians are twice as likely to report poor health as compared to high-income Canadians.

8.  **Social exclusion** is becoming increasingly common among many Canadians. Social exclusion is the process by which Canadians are denied opportunities to participate in many aspects of cultural, economic, social, and political life. It is especially prevalent among those who are poor, Aboriginal people, New Canadians, and members of racialized—or non-white—groups. As our racialized composition grows, it is unacceptable that these groups earn 30% less than whites and are twice as likely to be poor. These trends contribute to social and political instability in our society.

9.  **Social safety nets** are changing in character as a result of shifting federal and provincial priorities. The 1990s have seen a weakening of these nets that constitute threats to both the health and well-being of the vulnerable. The social economy

may provide opportunities for community organizations to provide services in more democratic, transparent and community-sensitive ways. It may be, however, unable to meet emerging needs without further burdening caregivers in the community, many of whom are women, or inadequately compensating them.

10. **Unemployment** continues at high levels and **employment security** is weakening due to the growth of precarious, unstable, and non-advancing jobs. Higher stress, increasing hours of work, and increasing numbers of low-income jobs are the mechanisms that link employment insecurity and unemployment to poor health outcomes. Unionized jobs are the most likely to help avoid these health-threatening conditions.

11. **Canadian women, Aboriginal people, Canadians of colour, and New Canadians** are especially vulnerable to the health-threatening effects of these deteriorating conditions. This is most clear regarding income and its distribution, employment and working conditions, housing affordability, and the state of the social safety net.

It is therefore resolved that:

*Governments at all levels* should review their current economic, social, and service policies to consider the impacts of their policies upon these social determinants of health. Areas of special importance are the provision of adequate income and social assistance levels, provision of affordable housing, development of quality childcare arrangements, and enforcement of anti-discrimination laws and human rights codes. It is also important to increase support for the social infrastructure including public education, social and health services, and improvement of job security and working conditions;

*Public health and health care associations and agencies* should educate their members and staff about the impacts of governmental decisions upon the social determinants of health and advocate for the creation of positive health promoting conditions. Particularly important is these associations and agencies joining current debates about Canadian health and social policy decisions and their impacts upon population health;

*The media* should begin to seriously cover the rapidly expanding findings concerning the importance of the social determinants of health and their impacts upon the health of Canadians. This would strike a balance between the predominant coverage of health from a biomedical and lifestyle perspective. It would also help educate the Canadian public about the potential health impacts of various governmental decisions and improve the potential for public involvement in public policymaking; and that

### Immediate Action

As a means of moving this agenda forward, the conference recommends that Canada's federal and provincial/territorial governments immediately address the sources of health and the root causes of illness by matching the $1.5 billion targeted for diagnostic services in the

Romanow *Report on the future of health care in Canada* and allocating this amount towards two essential determinants of health for children and families: 1) affordable, safe housing; and 2) a universal system of high quality educational childcare; and

## Long-Term Action

Similar to governmental actions in response to the *Acheson inquiry into health inequalities in the United Kingdom*, the federal government should establish a *Social Determinants of Health Task Force* to consider these findings and work to address the issues raised at this conference. The *Task Force* would operate to identify and advocate for policies by all levels of government to support population health. The federal and provincial governments would respond to these recommendations in a formal manner through annual reports on the status of these social determinants of health.

**So Resolved, this December 1, 2002, in Toronto, Canada, and Ratified, February 10, 2003**

# References

## Chapter 1

Blane, D. (1999). "The life course, the social gradiant and health," in Marmot, M.G. and Wilkinson, R.G. (Eds.). *Social determinants of health*. Oxford: Oxford University Press.

Blane, D., Brunner, E. and Wilkinson, R. (Eds.). (1996). *Health and social organization: Towards a health policy for the twenty-first century*. New York: Routledge.

Brunner, E. and Marmot, M.G. (1999). "Social organization, stress, and health," in Marmot, M.G. and Wilkinson, R.G. (Eds.), *Social determinants of health*. Oxford: Oxford University Press.

Canadian Institute on Children's Health. (2000). *The health of Canada's children: A CICH profile, 3rd edition*. Ottawa: Canadian Institute on Children's Health.

Canadian Population Health Initiative. (2002). *Canadian population health initiative brief to the Commission on the Future of Health Care in Canada*. CPHI. Online at cihi.ca.

Canadian Public Health Association. (2003). *CPHA policy statements*. Canadian Public Health Association (CPHA). Online at www.cpha.ca/english/policy/pstatem/polstate.htm.

Davey Smith, G. (Ed.). (2003). *Inequalities in health: Life course perspectives*. Bristol: Policy Press.

Donaldson, L. (1999). *Ten tips for better health*. London: Stationary Office. Online at www.archive.official-documents.co.uk/document/cm43/4386/4386–tp.htm.

Engels, F. (1845/1987). *The condition of the working class in England*. New York: Penguin Classics.

Epp, J. (1986). *Achieving health for all: A framework for health promotion*, for Health and Welfare Canada. Online at www.frcentre.net/library/AchievingHealthForAll.pdf.

Gordon, D. (1999). Message posted July 21 on the Spirit of 1848 Electronic Listserve. David Gordon is a professor at the University of Bristol in Bristol, UK.

Health Canada. (1998). "Taking action on population health: A position paper for health promotion and programs branch staff" (Health and Welfare Canada). Online at www.hc–sc.gc.ca/hppb/phdd/pdf/tad_e.pdf.

Jarvis, M.J. and Wardle, J. (1999). "Social patterning of individual health behaviours: The case of cigarette smoking," in Marmot, M.G. and Wilkinson, R.G (Eds.), *Social determinants of health*. Oxford: Oxford University Press.

Kawachi, I. and Kennedy, B. (2002). *The health of nations: Why inequality is harmful to your health*. New York: New Press.

Kuh, D. and Ben-Shilmo, Y. (Eds.). (1997). *A life course approach to chronic disease epidemiology*. Oxford: Oxford University Press.

Lalonde, M. (1974). *A new perspective on the health of Canadians: A working document*. (Health and Welfare Canada). Online at www.hc-sc.gc.ca/hppb/phdd/pube/perintrod.htm.

Lynch, J.W., Davey Smith, G., Kaplan, G.A. and House, J.S. (2000). "Income inequality and mortality: Importance to health of individual income, psychosocial environment, or material conditions," *British medical journal* 320, 1220–1224.

McKinlay, J. and McKinlay, S.M. (1987). "Medical measures and the decline of mortality," in Schwartz, H.D. (Ed.), *Dominant issues in medical sociology*. New York: Random House.

Raphael, D. (2001). "From increasing poverty to societal disintegration: How economic inequality affects the health of individuals and communities," in Armstrong, P., Armstrong, H. and Coburn, D. (Eds.), *Unhealthy times: The political economy of health and care in Canada*. Toronto: Oxford University Press.

Raphael, D. (2003), "A society in decline: The social, economic, and political determinants of health inequalities in the USA," in Hofrichter, R. (Ed.), *Health and social justice: A reader on politics, ideology, and inequity in the distribution of disease*. San Francisco: Jossey-Bass/Wiley.

Raphael, D. (2002). *Social justice is good for our hearts: Why societal factors—not lifestyles—are major causes of heart disease in Canada and elsewhere*. Centre for Social Justice Foundation for Research and Education (CSJ). Online at www.socialjustice.org/pubs/justiceHearts.pdf.

Raphael, D., Anstice, S., Raine, K. and McGannon, K. (2003). "The social determinants of the incidence and management of Type 2 Diabetes Mellitus: Are we prepared to rethink our questions and redirect our research activities?" *Leadership in health services* 16, 10–20.

Raphael, D. and Farrell, E.S. (2002). "Beyond medicine and lifestyle: Addressing the societal determinants of cardiovascular disease in North America," *Leadership in health services* 15, 1–5.

Ross, N., Wolfson, M., Dunn, J., Berthelot, J.M., Kaplan, G. and Lynch, J. (2000). "Relation between income inequality and mortality in Canada and in the United States: Cross sectional assessment using census data and vital statistics," *British medical journal* 320 (7239), 898–902.

Shaw, M., Dorling, D., Gordon, D. and Davey Smith, G. (1999). *The widening gap: Health inequalities and policy in Britain*. Bristol: Policy.

Shields, M. and Tremblay, S. (2002). "The health of Canada's communities," *Health reports (Statistics Canada), Supplement* 13 (July).

Tarlov, A. (1996). "Social determinants of health: The sociobiological translation," in Blane, D., Brunner, E. and Wilkinson, R. (Eds.), *Health and social organization: Towards a health policy for the 21st Century*. London: Routledge.

Teeple, G. (2000). *Globalization and the decline of social reform*. Aurora: Garamond.

Townsend, P., Davidson, N. and Whitehead, M. (Eds.). (1992). *Inequalities in health: The Black report and the health divide*. New York: Penguin.

Virchow, R. (1848/1985). *Collected essays on public health and epidemiology*. Cambridge: Science History Publications.

Wilkins, R., Berthelot, J.-M. and Ng, E. (2002). "Trends in mortality by neighbourhood income in urban Canada from 1971 to 1996," *Health reports (Stats Can), Supplement* 13, 1–28.

Wilkinson, R. and Marmot, M. (2003). *Social determinants of health: The solid facts*. Copenhagen: World Health Organization, Europe Office. Online at www.dk/document/e81381.pdf.

World Health Organization. (1986). *Ottawa charter for health promotion*. World Health Organization, Europe Office. Online at www.hc-sc.gc.ca/hppb/phdd/docs/charter/.

# Chapter 2

Abella, R. (1984). *Equality in employment: The report of the Commission on Equality in Employment*. Ottawa: Supply and Services Canada.

Anderson, J. and Curry-Stevens, A. (2000). *The growing wealth divide*. Toronto: CSJ Foundation for Research and Education.

Canada Employment and Immigration Advisory Council. (1992). *Last in, first out: Racism in employment*. Ottawa: Government of Canada.

Canadian Council for Refugees. (2000). *Report on systemic racism and discrimination in Canadian refugee and immigration policies*. Montreal: Canadian Council for Refugees.

Canadian Labour Congress. (Fall 2003). *Economy: Economic review and outlook* 14 (2).

Canadian Race Relations Foundation. (1999). "Unequal access: A Canadian profile of racial differences," in *Education, employment and income*. Toronto: Canadian Race Relations Foundation.

Commission on Systemic Racism in the Ontario Criminal Justice System. (1994). *Report of the Commission on Systemic Racism in the Ontario Criminal Justice System*. Toronto: Queen's Printer for Ontario.

Curry-Stevens, A. (June 2003). "Arrogant capitalism: Changing futures, changing lives," *Canadian review of social policy* 51, 137–142.

Curry-Stevens, A. (2001). *When markets fail people: Exploring the widening gap between rich and poor in Canada*. Toronto: CSJ Foundation for Research and Education.

Frenette, M. and Morisette, R. (2003). *Will they ever converge? Earnings of immigrant and Canadian-born workers over the last two decades*. Ottawa: Statistics Canada.

Galabuzi, G.-E. (2001). *Canada's creeping economic apartheid*. Toronto: CSJ Foundation for Research and Education.

Lewis, S. (1992). *Stephen Lewis report on race relations in Ontario*. Submitted to Premier Bob Rae. Online at www.geocities.com/CapitolHill/6174/lewis.html.

Ornstein, M. (1999). *The differential effect of income criteria on access to rental accommodation on the basis of age and race: 1996 Census Results*. Toronto: Centre for Equality Rights in Accommodation.

Ornstein, M. (1994). *Income and rent: Equality seeking groups and access to rental accommodation restricted by income criteria*. Toronto: Institute for Social Research.

Sauve, R. (2002). *The dreams and the reality: Assets, debts and net worth of Canadian households*. Ottawa: Vanier Institute on the Family.

Scott, K. (2002). "A lost decade: Income inequality and the health of Canadians," presentation to the Social Determinants of Health Across the Life-span Conference (Toronto, November 2002).

Statistics Canada. (2001b). *The assets and debts of Canadians: An overview of the results of the survey of financial security*. Ottawa: Statistics Canada.

Statistics Canada. (2001a). *2001 Census of Canada*. Ottawa: Statistics Canada.

Task Force on the Participation of Visible Minorities in the Federal Public Service. (2000). *Embracing change in the federal public service*. Ottawa: Treasury Board of Canada.

Yalnizyan, A. (2000). *Canada's great divide: The politics of the growing gap between rich and poor in the 1990s*. Toronto: Centre for Social Justice.

Yalnizyan, A. (1998). *The growing gap: A report on growing inequality between the rich and poor in Canada*. Toronto: Centre for Social Justice.

## Chapter 3

Barrett, C., Bussière, L., Darby, P., Lafleur, B., MacDuff, D. and Vail, S. (2003). *Performance and potential 2003–04: Defining the Canadian advantage*. Online at www.conferenceboard.ca.

Bill 112. *An Act to combat poverty and social exclusion* (2002, chapter 61). National Assembly, second session, 36th legislature. Quebec Official Publisher.

Choinière, R., Lafontaine, P. and Edwards A.C. (2000). "Distribution of cardiovascular risk factors by socioeconomic status among Canadian adults," *Canadian Medical Association journal* 162 (9, Supplement), S13–S24.

Choinière R., M.J. and Paradis C. (2003). *Le portrait statistique de la santé des Montréalais*. Montreal: Direction de Santé Publique, Régie régionale de la Santé et des Services sociaux de Montréal-Centre.

Epp, J. (1986). *Achieving health for all: A framework for health promotion*. Health and Welfare Canada. Online at www.hc-sc.gc.ca/hppb/phdd/approach/linked.html.

Ferland, M. (2003). *Variation des écarts de l'état de santé en fonction du revenu au Québec de 1987 à 1998*. Ottawa: Institut de la statistique du Québec.

Gaumer, B., Desrosiers, G. and Keel, O. (2002). *Histoire du Service de Santé de la ville de Montréal 1865–1975*. Quebec City: Institut québecois de recherche sur la culture, Les presses de l'Université Laval.

Human Resources Development Canada. (May 2003). *Understanding the 2000 low income statistics based on the market basket measure* (Applied Research Bulletin, Strategic Policy). Online at www.hrdc-drhc.gc.ca/sp-ps/arb-dgra/publications/research/2003docs/SP-569-03/e/SP-569-03_E_toc.shtml.

Kawachi, I. "Income inequality and health," in Berkman, L. and Kawachi, I. (Eds.), *Social epidemiology*. Oxford: Oxford University Press, 2000.

Kawachi, I. and Kennedy, B. (1997). "The relationship of income inequality to mortality: Does the choice of indicator matter?" *Soc Sci Med* 45 (7), 1121–1128.

Kawachi, I., Kennedy, B., Lochner, K. and Prothrow-Stith, D. (1997). "Social capital, income inequality, and mortality," *Am J Public Health* 87 (9), 1491–1498.

Kidder, K., Stein, J., and Fraser, J. (2000). *The health of Canada's children: A CICH profile, 3rd edition*. Ottawa: Canadian Institute on Children's Health (CICH).

Lalonde, M. (1974). *A new perspective on the health of Canadians: A working document* (Health and Welfare Canada). Online at www.hc–sc.gc.ca/hppb/phdd/pube/perintrod.htm

Lessard, R., Roy, D., Choinière, R., Bujold, R. et. al. (1998). *Social inequalities in health: Annual report of the health of the population*. Montreal: Direction de la Santé Publique. Online at www.santepub–mtl.qc.ca/Publication/autres/rapport1998.html#english.

Lessard, R., Roy, D., Choinière, R., Lévesque, J.F. and Perron, S. (2002). *Urban health: A vital factor in Montreal's development*. Montreal: Direction de Santé Publique. Online at www.santepub–mtl.qc.ca/Publication/autres/annualreport2002.html.

Lynch, J.W., Smith, G.D., Kaplan, G.A. and House, J.S. (2000). "Income inequality and mortality: Importance to health of individual income, psychosocial environment, or material conditions," *British medical journal* 320, 1200–1204.

Mackenbach, J.P.(2002). "Income inequality and population health," *British medical journal* 324, 1–2.

Massé, R. and Gilbert, L. (2003). *Programme national de santé publique 2003—2012*. Quebec: Ministère de la Santé et des Services Sociaux.

Ministère de la Santé et des Services sociaux. (1992). *La politique de la santé et du bien-être*. Québec.

Nöel, A. (December 2002). *A law against poverty: Quebec's new approach to combating poverty and social exclusion* (Background Paper: Family Network). Canadian Policy Research Networks. Online at www.cpds.umontreal.ca/fichier/cahiercpds03–01.pdf.

Phipps, S. (2003). *The impact of poverty on health: A scan of research literature*. Canadian Institute for Health Information. Online at cihi.ca.

Ross, D. and Roberts, P. (1999). *Income and child well-being: A new perspective on the poverty debate*. Canadian Council on Social Development.

Ross, N., Wolfson, M., Dunn, J., Berthelot, J.M., Kaplan G. and Lynch, J. (2000). "Relation between income inequality and mortality in Canada and in the United States: Cross sectional assessment using census data and vital statistics," *British medical journal* 320, 898–902.

Séguin, L. et al. (2001). "Standard of living, health and development, Part I: Poverty, health, conditions at birth and infant health," *Longitudinal study of child development in Québec (ÉLDEQ 1998–2002)* 1 (3), Quebec: Institut de la statistique du Québec. Online at www.omiss.ca/english/reference/bibliography/childhood.html.

United Nations Human Development Report. (2003). "Millennium Development Goals: A compact among nations to end human poverty." Oxford: United Nations Development Programme, Oxford University Press. Online at www.undp.org/hdr2003/.

Webber, M. (1998). "Measuring low income and poverty in Canada: An update," *Income and labour dynamic working paper series*. Ottawa: Statistics Canada.

Wilkins, R., Berthelot, J.-M. and Ng, E. (2002). "Trends in mortality by neighbourhood income in urban Canada from 1971 to 1996," *Health reports (Stats Can), Supplement* 13, 1–28.

# Chapter 4

Arthur, M.B. and Rousseau, D.M. (Eds.). (1996). *The boundaryless career: A new employment principle for a new organizational era*. New York: Oxford University Press.

Cadin, L., Bender, A.F., Saint-Giniez, V. and Pringle, J. (2000). *Carrières nomades et contextes nationaux: Revue de gestion des ressources humaines*. Paris: AGRH.

Chapon, S. and Euzéby, C. (2002). "Vers une convergence des modèles sociaux européens?" *Revue internationale de sécurité sociale* 55 (2), 49–71.

Dasgupta, S. (2001). *Employment security: Conceptual and statistical issues.* Geneva: International Labour Office.

Esping-Andersen, G. (1985). *Politics against markets: The social democratic road to power.* Princeton: Princeton University Press.

Freyssinet, J. (2003). "Les trois inflexions des politiques de l'emploi," *Alternatives économiques* 210, 38–45.

Le Boterf, G. (1998). *L'ingénierie des compétences.* Paris: Les Editions d'Organisation.

Lowe, G., Schellenberg, G. and Davidman, K. (1999). *Re-thinking employment relationships.* CPRN Discussion Paper no. W-5.

Organization for Economic Cooperation and Development. (1996). *L'économie fondée sur le savoir.* Paris: OECD.

Paugam, S. (1998). "Le revenu minimum d'insertion en France après six ans; un bilan contrasté," *Interventions économiques, Montreal* 28, 21–45. Online at www.teluq.uquebec.ca/interventionseconomiques.

Standing, G. (1999). *Global labour flexibility: Seeking distributive justice.* London: Palgrave.

Tremblay, D.-G. (2004). *Virtual communities of practice: What impacts for individuals and organizations?* Forthcoming in the National Business and Economics Society 2004 Conference Proceedings, NBES, USA.

Tremblay, D.-G. (2003a). "New types of careers in the knowledge economy? Networks and boundaryless jobs as a career strategy in the ICT and multimedia sector," *Communications & strategies.* Montpellier-Manchester: IDATE.

Tremblay, D.-G. (2003b). "Telework: A new mode of gendered segmentation? Results from a study in Canada," *Canadian journal of communication* 28 (4), 461–478.

Tremblay, D.-G. (2003c). "Youth Employment situation and employment policies in Canada," in Roulleau-Berger, Laurence (Ed.), *Youth and work in the post-industrial city of North America and Europe.* Boston: Brill Editor.

Tremblay, D.-G. (2003d). *Innovation, management et économie: Comment la théorie économique rend-elle compte de l'innovation?* Note de recherche de la Chaire du Canada sur les enjeux socio-organisationnels de l'économie du savoir. No 2003, 21. Online at www.teluq.uquebec.ca/chaireecosavoir.

Tremblay, D.-G. (2002a). "Les économistes institutionnalistes: les apports des institutionnalistes à la pensée économique hétérodoxe," *Interventions économiques* 28. Online at www.teluq.uquebec.ca/interventionseconomiques.

Tremblay, D.-G. (2002b). "Informal learning communities in the knowledge economy," *Proceedings of the 2002 World Computer Congress.* International Federation for Information Processing, August 27–29, 2002. Montreal: Elsevier Press.

Tremblay, D.-G. (2002c). "Balancing work and family with telework? Organizational issues and challenges for women and managers," *Women in management* 17 (3/4).

Tremblay, D.-G. (1997). *Économie du travail: les réalités et les approches théoriques.* Montreal: Editions St-Martin.

Tremblay, D.-G. (1990). *L'emploi en devenir.* Quebec City: Institut québécois de recherche sur la culture.

Tremblay, D.-G. and Chevrier, C. (2002a). "Portrait du marché du travail au Canada et au Québec: Une analyse statistique différenciée selon le genre," *Direction de la recherche.* Online at www.teluq.uquebec.ca/chaireecosavoir.

Tremblay, D.-G. and Chevrier, C. (2002b). "Les motifs de recours au travail autonome par les entreprises et les avantages et inconvénients qu'y voient les travailleurs autonomes," *Direction de la recherche.* Online at www.teluq.uquebec.ca/chaireecosavoir.

Tremblay, D.-G. and Fontan, J.-M. (1994). *Le développement économique local: La théorie, les pratique, les expériences.* Quebec City: Presses de l'Université du Québec.

Tremblay, D.-G. and Rolland, D. (2000). "Labour regime and industrialisation in the knowledge economy: The Japanese model and its possible hybridisation in other countries," *Labour and management in development journal* 7. Online at www.ncdsnet.anu.edu.au.

References

Tremblay, D.-G. and Rolland, D. (1998). *Modèles de gestion de main-d'oeuvre: Typologies et comparaisons internationales*. Quebec City: Presses de l'université du Québec.

Tremblay, D.-G. and Villeneuve, D. (1998). *Aménagement et réduction du temps de travail: Les enjeux, les approches, les méthodes*. Montreal: Editions St-Martin.

## Chapter 5

Ackerman, B. and Alstott, A. (1999). *The stakeholder democracy*. New Haven: Yale University Press.

Ala-Mursula, L., Vahtera, J., et al. (2002). "Employee control over working time: Associations with subjective health and sickness absences," *Journal of epidemiology and community health* 56, 272–278.

Appelbaum, E., Bailey, T., Berg, P. and Kalleberg, A. (2000). *Manufacturing advantage: Why high-performance work systems pay off*. Ithaca: ILR.

Appelbaum, S., Lavigne-Schmidt, S., Peytchev, M., and Shapiro, B. (1999). "Downsizing: Measuring the costs of failure," *Journal of management development* 18 (5).

Beach, C., Finnie, R., et al. (2002). "Earnings over time," *Perspectives on labour and income* 3 (11).

Belanger, J. (2000). "The influence of employee involvement on productivity: A review of research," Applied Research Branch Discussion Paper R-00-4E, Human Resource Development Canada.

Betcherman, G. and Chaykowski, R. (1996). "The changing workplace: Challenges for public policy," Applied Research Branch Discussion Paper, R-96-13E. Ottawa: Human Resources Development Canada.

Betcherman, G. and Lowe, G.S. (1997). *The future of work in Canada: A synthesis report*. Ottawa: Canadian Policy Research Network.

Burke, M., and Shields, J. (1999). The job-poor recovery: Social cohesion and the Canadian labour market. Toronto: Ryerson Polytechnic University.

Burrell, D. (2001). "Weekend woes: Working hard can be hazardous to your holidays," *Psychology today* 34 (20), 20.

Carter, T. (1999), *The aftermath of reengineering: Downsizing and corporate performance*. New York: Haworth.

CFO Forum. (1995). "Downsizing downsized," *Institutional investor* 29 (12), 28.

Cohen, M. (1997). "Downsizing and disability go together," *Business and health* 15 (1), 10.

Cranford, C.J., Vosko, L.F., et al. (2003). "Precarious employment in the Canadian labour market: A statistical portrait," *Just labour* 3 (Fall), 6–22.

Davis-Blake, A., Broschak, J. and George, E. (2003). "Happy together? How using nonstandard workers affects exit, voice, and loyalty among standard employees," *The academy of management journal* 46 (4), 475–485.

Dooley, D. (2003). "Unemployment, underemployment and mental health: Conceptualizing employment status as a continuum," *American journal of community psychology* 32, 9–20.

Duxbury, L. and Higgins, C. (2001). *Work-life balance in the new millenium: Where are we? Where do we go from here?* Ottawa: Canadian Policy Research Networks.

Duxbury, L.E., Higgins, C.A. and Lee, C. (1994). "Work–family conflict: A comparison by gender, family type and perceived control," *Journal of family issues* 15 (3), 449–466.

Elmuti, D. and Kathawala, Y. (2000). "Business reengineering: Revolutionary management tool, or fading fraud?" *Business forum* 25 (1/2), 29–36.

Ertel, M., Pech, E. and Ullsperger, P. (2000). "Telework in perspective: New challenges to occupational health and safety," in Isaksson, K., Hogstedt, C., Eriksson, C. and Theorell, T. (Eds.), *Health effects of the new labour market*. New York: Kluwer Academic.

Fagan, C. (2003). *Working-time preferences and work–life balance in the EU: Some policy considerations for enhancing quality of life*. Dublin: European Foundation for the Improvement of Working and Living Conditions.

Fagan, C. and Burchell, B. (2002). *Gender, jobs and working conditions in the European Union*. Dublin: European Foundation for the Improvement of Working and Living Conditions.

Fairris, D. and Tohyama, H. (2002). "Productive efficiency and the lean production system in Japan and the United States," *Economic and industrial democracy* 23 (4), 529–554.

Farias, G. and Varma, A. (1998). "Research update: High performance work systems: What we know and what we need to know," *HR human resource planning* 21 (2) 50–54.

Ferber, M.A. and O'Farrell, B. (1991). *Work and family: Policies for a changing workforce.* Washington: National Academy Press.

Ferrie, J.E. (2001). "Is job insecurity harmful to health?" *Journal of the Royal Society of Medicine* 94, 71–76.

Franks, S. (1999). *Having none of it: Women, men and the future of work.* London: Granta Books.

Frone, M., Russell, M. and Cooper, L. (1997). "Relation of work–family conflict to health outcomes: A four-year longitudinal study of employed parents," *Journal of occupational and organizational psychology* 70 (4), 325–335.

Gore, S. (1978). "The effect of social support in moderating the health consequences of unemployment," *Journal of health and social behaviour* 19 (June), 157–165.

Green, F. (2002). "Work intensification, discretion and the decline of well-being at work," Paris: Conference on Work Intensification.

Hammer, M. and Champy, J. (1993). *Reengineering the corporation: A manifesto for business revolution.* New York: HarperCollins.

Heery, E. and Salmon, J. (2000). "The insecurity thesis," in Heery, E. and Salmon, J. (Eds.), *The insecure workforce.* London: Routledge.

Heisz, A., Jackson, A., et al. (2002). *Winners and losers in the labour market of the 1990s.* Ottawa: Statistics Canada.

Herzenberg, S.A., Alic, J.A., et al. (1998). *New rules for a new economy: Employment and opportunity in post-industrial America.* Ithaca and London: ILR.

Jahoda, M. (1982). *Employment and unemployment: A social psychological analysis.* Cambridge: Cambridge University Press.

Kasl, S.V. (1998). "Measuring job stressors and studying the health impact of the work environment: An epidemiologic commentary," *Journal of occupational health psychology* 3 (4), 390–401.

Kivimaki, M., Vahtera, J., Pentti, J. and Ferrie, J. (2000). "Factors underlying the effect of organisational downsizing on health of employees: Longitudinal cohort study," *British medical journal* 320 (7240), 971–985.

Lewchuk, W., de Wolff, A., King, A. and Polanyi, M.F. (2003). "From job strain to employment strain: Health effects of precarious employment," *Just labour* 3 (Fall), 23–35.

Lewchuk, W., de Wolff, A., King, A. and Polanyi, M.F. (2003). "Beyond job strain: Employment strain and the health effects of precarious employment," unpublished paper.

Martens, M.F.J., Nijhuis, F.J.N., et al. (1999). "Flexible work schedules and mental and physical health: A study of a working population with non-traditional hours," *Journal of organizational behavior* 20, 35–46.

Marshall, K. (1996). "A job to die for," *Perspectives on labour and income* (Summer), 26–31.

Maxwell, J. (2002). *Smart social policy: "Making work pay."* Ottawa: Canadian Policy Research Networks.

Mehmet, O., Mendes, E., et al. (1999). *Towards a fair global labour market: Avoiding a new slave trade.* London: Routledge.

Mohr, G. B. (2000). "The changing significance of different stressors after the announcement of bankruptcy: A longitudinal investigation with special emphasis on job insecurity," *Journal of organizational behavior* 2, 337–359.

Morris J.K., Cook, D.G. and Shaper, A.G. (1992). "Non-employment and changes in smoking, drinking and body weight," *British medical journal* 304, 536–541.

Morissette, R. and Rosa, J. (2003). "Alternative work practices and quit rates: Methodological issues and empirical evidence for Canada," *Statistics Canada Research Paper*, No. 11F0019 #199.

Mustard, C.A., Cole, D.C., Shannon, H.S., Pole, J., Sullivan, T.J., Allingham, R. and Sinclar, S.J. (2001). "Does the decline in Worker's compensation claims (1990–1999) in Ontario correspond to a decline in workplace injuries?" Working Paper #168. Toronto: Institute for Work and Health.

Nolan, J. (2002). "The intensification of everyday life," in Burchell, B. and Wilkinson, F. (Eds.), *Job insecurity and work intensification.* London: Routledge.

Osberg, L. and Sharpe, A. (2003). "An index of labour market well-being for OECD countries," *CSLS research report 2003–05*, 1–37. Ottawa: Centre for the Study of Living Standards.

Polanyi, M.F. and Tompa, E. (2002). "Rethinking the health implications of work in the new global economy" (Working Paper, Comparative Program on Health and Society). Toronto: Munk Centre for International Studies, University of Toronto. Online at www.utoronto.ca/mcis.

Price, R.H., Choi, J.N., et al. (2002). "Links in the chain of adversity following job loss: How financial strain and loss of personal control lead to depression, impaired functioning, and poor health," *Journal of occupational health psychology* 7 (4), 302–312.

Probst, T.M. and Brubaker, T.L. (2001). "The effects of job insecurity on employee safety outcomes: Cross-sectional and longitudinal explorations," *Journal of occupational health psychology* 6 (2), 139–159.

Ramsay, H., Scholarios, D. and Harley, B. (2000). "Employees and high-performance work systems: Testing inside the black box," *British journal of industrial relations* 18 (4), 501–531.

Raphael, D. (2001). "From increasing poverty to social disintegration: how economic inequality affects the health of individuals and communities," in Armstrong, P., Armstrong, H. and Coburn, D. (Eds.), *Unhealthy times: The political economy of health and care in Canada*. Toronto: Oxford University Press.

Schor, J.B. (2002). *The overworked American: The unexpected decline of leisure*. New York: Basic Books.

Shields, M. (1999). "Long working hours and health," *Health reports* 11 (2), 33–48.

Smith, V. (1997). "New forms of work organization," *Annual review of sociology* 23, 315–339.

Sparks, K., Faragher, B., et al. (2001). "Well-being and occupational health in the 21$^{st}$ century workplace," *Journal of occupational and organizational psychology* 74 (4), 489–509.

Sparks, K., Cooper, C., Fried, Y. and Shirom, A. (1997). "The effects of hours of work on health: A meta-analytic review," *Journal of occupational and organizational psychology* 70 (4), 391–408.

Sverke, M., Hellgren J., et al. (2002). "No security: A meta-analysis and review of job insecurity and its consequences," *Journal of occupational health psychology* 7 (3), 242–264.

Tremblay, D.-G. (2002). "New ways of working and new types of work? What developments lie ahead?" *Report for the Futures Forum: "Places of Work."* Ottawa: Policy Research Initiative.

Tremblay, D.-G. (2003e). *New types of careers in the knowledge economy: Networks and boundaryless jobs as a career strategy in the ict and multimedia sector*. Research Note of the Canada Research Chair on the Knowledge Economy No 2003-12A. Online at www.teluq.uquebec.ca/chaireecosavoir

Tremblay, D.-G. (2003f). *The new division of labour and women's jobs: Results from a study conducted in Canada from a gendered perspective*. Research Note of the Canada Research Chair on the Knowledge Economy No 2003-19A. Online at www.teluq.uquebec.ca/chaireecosavoir.

Tremblay, D.-G. (2003g). *Working time and work-family balancing; A Canadian perspective*. Research Note of the Canada Research Chair on the Knowledge Economy No 2003-18. Online at www.teluq.uquebec.ca/chaireecosavoir.

Tremblay, D.-G. and Rolland, D. (2003). *The Japanese model and its possible hybridization in other countries*. Research Note of the Canada Research Chair on the Knowledge Economy No 2003-20A. Online at www.teluq.uquebec.ca/chaireecosavoir.

Tremblay, D.-G., Davel, E. and Rolland, D. (2003). *New management forms for the knowledge economy: HRM in the context of teamwork and participaton*. Research Note of the Canada Research Chair on the Knowledge Economy No 2003-14A. Online at www.teluq.uquebec.ca/chaireecosavoir.

Townson, M. (2003). *Women in non-standard jobs: The public policy challenge*. Ottawa: Status of Women Canada.

Turner, J.B. (1995). "Economic context and the health effects of unemployment," *Journal of health and social behaviour* 36 (3), 213–229.

Varma, A., Beatty, R., Schneier, C. and Ulrich, D. (1999). "High performance work systems: Exciting discovery or passing fad?" *Human resource planning* 22 (1), 26–37.

Wagar, T. (1998). "Exploring the consequences of workforce reduction," *Canadian journal of administrative sciences* 15 (4), 300–309.

Warr, P.B. (1987). *Work, unemployment and mental health*. Oxford: Clarendon Press.

Wilkinson, R.G. (1996). *Unhealthy societies: The afflictions of inequality*. London: Routledge.

Wood, S. (1999). "Human resource management and performance," *International journal of management reviews* 1 (4), 367–413.

Yates, C., Lewchuk, W. and Stewart, P. (2001). "Empowerment as a Trojan horse: New systems of work organization in the North American automobile industry," *Economic and industrial democracy* 22, 517–541.

## Chapter 6

Applebaum, Eileen. (1997). *The impact of new forms of work organization on workers*. Washington: Economic Policy Institute.

Betcherman, G., McMullen, K. and Davidman, K. (1998). *Training for the new economy: A synthesis report*. Ottawa: Canadian Policy Research Networks.

Drolet, M., and Morrissette, R. (1998). "The upward mobility of low-paid Canadians, 1993–1995," Statistics Canada *SLID Working Paper 98-07*.

Duxbury, L. and Higgins, C. (2002). *The 2001 national work–life conflict study* (Health and Welfare Canada). Online.

Esping-Andersen, G. (1999). *Social foundations of postindustrial economies*. Oxford: Oxford University Press.

European Industrial Relations Observatory (EIRO) (2001). a) *Working time developments: Annual update*; b) *Non-permanent employment, quality of work and industrial relations*; c) *Working time developments and the quality of work*. Online at www.eiro.eurofound.eu.int.

Finnie, Ross. (2000). *The dynamics of poverty in Canada*. Ottawa: C.D. Howe Institute.

Human Resource Development Canada Labour Program. (2000). *Statistical analysis of occupational injuries and fatalities*. Ottawa: Government of Canada.

Jackson, A. (2002). "The unhealthy Canadian workplace: Research Paper #19." Ottawa: Canadian Labour Congress. Online at www.action.web.ca/home/clcpolcy/attach/The%20Unhealthy%20Canadian%20Workplace1.pdf.

Jackson, A. (2000). *Why we don't have to choose between social justice and economic growth: The myth of the equity-efficiency trade-off*. Canadian Council on Social Development. Online at www.ccsd.ca/pubs/2000/equity.

Jackson, A. and Kumar, P. (1998). *Measuring and monitoring the quality of jobs and the work environment in Canada*. Online at www.csls.ca/events/oct98/jacks.pdf.

Jencks, C., Perlman, L. and Rainwater, L. (1988). "What is a good job? A new measure of labour market success," *American journal of sociology* 93 (May), 1322–1357.

Karasek, R. and Theorell, T. (1990). *Healthy work: Stress, productivity and the reconstruction of working life*. New York: Basic Books.

Lewchuk, W. and Robertson, D. (1996). "Working conditions under lean production: A worker-based benchmarking study," *Asia Pacific business review* (Summer).

Livingstone, D.W. (2002). *Working and learning in the information age: A profile of Canadians*. Ottawa: Canadian Policy Research Networks.

Lowe, G. (2000). *The quality of work: A people centred agenda*. Oxford: Oxford University Press.

Statistics Canada. (2001). *Health Indicators*. Cat. 82-221-XIE. Online.

Statistics Canada. (2001). *Learning a living. A report on adult education and training in Canada*. Cat. 81-586-XIE. Online.

Sullivan, T. (Ed.). (2000). *Injury and the new world of work*. Vancouver and Toronto: UBC Press.

Survey of Labour and Income Dynamics (Ongoing). Ottawa: Statistics Canada.

Sussman, D. (2002). "Barriers to job-related training," *Perspectives on labour and income*. Ottawa: Statistics Canada. Online.

Wilkins, K. and Beaudet, M.P. (1998). "Work stress and health," *Health reports* 10.3 (Winter), 47–62.

World Health Organization. (1999). *Labour market changes and job insecurity*. WHO Regional Publications/European Series, No. 81.

Advisory Committee on the Changing Workplace. (1997). *Collective reflection on the changing workplace: Report of the Advisory Committee on the Changing Workplace.* Ottawa: Public Works and Government Services Canada.

The Atkinson Charitable Foundation. (1999)."Are Canadians working too many hours? Part 2." Online at www.atkinsonfoundation.ca/publications/work2.pdf/view.

Aronowitz, S., Esposito, D., DiFazio, W. and Yard, M. (1998). "The post-work manifesto," in Aronowitz, S. and Cutler, J. (Eds.), *Post-work: The wages of cybernation.* New York: Routledge.

Betcherman, G., and Lowe, G.S. (1995). "Inside the black box: Human resource management and the labour market," in Adams, R.J., Betcherman, G. and Bilson, B. (Eds.), *Good jobs, bad jobs, no jobs: Tough choices for Canadian labour law.* Toronto: CD Howe Institute.

Bluestone, B. and Harrison, B. (2000). *Growing prosperity. The battle for growth with equity in the twenty-first century.* Boston: Houghton Mifflin.

Broad, D. (2000). *Hollow work, hollow society? Globalization and the causal labour problem in Canada.* Halifax: Fernwood.

Brooker, A.-S. and Eakin, J.M. (2001). "Gender, class, work-related stress and health: Toward a power-centred approach," *Journal of community and applied social psychology* 11, 97–109.

Brown, P. and Lauder, H. (2001). *Capitalism and social progress: The future of society in a global economy.* London: Palgrave.

Cooperrider, D.L. and Srivastva, S. (1987). "Appreciative inquiry in organizational life," in Pasmore, W. and Woodman, R. (Eds.), *Research in organizational change and development: Vol. 1.* Greenwich, CT: JAI Press.

Dagg, A. (1997). "Worker representation and protection in the 'New Economy,'" in *Collective reflection on the changing workplace: Report of the Advisory Committee on the Changing Workplace.* Ottawa: Government of Canada.

Das Gupta, T. (1996). *Racism and paid work.* Toronto: Garamond.

Duxbury, L. and Higgins, C. (1998). *Work–life balance in Saskatchewan: Realities and challenges.* Regina: Government of Saskatchewan. Online.

Duxbury, L. and Higgins, C. (2001). *Work–life balance in the new millennium: Where are we? Where do we go from here?* CPRN Discussion Paper W-12. Ottawa: Canadian Policy Research Networks.

Duxbury, L.E., Higgins, C.A. and Lee, C. (1994). "Work–family conflict: A comparison by gender, family type and perceived control," *Journal of family issues* 15 (3), 449–466.

Ertel, M., Pech, E. and Helsperger, P. (2000). "Telework in perspective: New challenges to occupational health and safety," in Isaksson, K., Hogskdt, C., Eriksson, C. and Theorell, T. (Eds.), *Health effects of the new labour market.* New York: Kluwer Academic.

European Commission. (1997). *Green paper: Partnership for a new organization of work.* European Commission [2002, 11/20/2002].

European Foundation for the Improvement of Living and Working Conditions. (2002a). *Quality of work and employment in Europe: Issues and challenges* (Foundation Paper). Dublin, Ireland: EFILWC (European Foundation for the Improvement of Living and Working Conditions). Online at www.eurofound.eu.int/publications/files/EF0212EN.pdf.

European Foundation for the Improvement of Living and Working Conditions. (2002b). *Interactions between the labour market and social protection: Seminar report.* Brussels: European Foundation for the Improvement of Working and Living Conditions.

Ferrie, J.E. (2001). "Is job insecurity harmful to health?" *Journal of the Royal Society of Medicine* 94, 71–76.

Ferrie, J.E., Shipley, M.J., Marmot, M.G., Stansfeld, S. and Smith, G.D. (1998). "The health effects of major organisational change and job insecurity," *Social science and medicine* 46 (2), 243–254.

Frone, M.R. (2000). "Work–family conflict and employee psychiatric disorders: The national comorbidity study," *Journal of applied psychology* 85, 888–895.

Goldberg, M. and Green, D. (1999). *Raising the floor: The social and economic benefits of minimum wages in Canada.* Vancouver: Canadian Centre for Policy Alternatives.

Gorz, A. (1999). *Reclaiming work: Beyond the wage-based society*, translated by C. Turner. Cambridge: Polity.

Herzenberg, S.A., Alic, J.A. and Wial, H. (1998). *New rules for a new economy: Employment and opportunity in postindustrial America*. Ithaca and London: ILR.

Human Resources and Development Canada. (1994). *Report of the advisory group on working time and distribution of work*. Ottawa: Government of Canada.

Johnson, J. and Hall, E. (1988). "Job strain, workplace social support and cardiovascular disease: A cross-sectional study of a random sample of the Swedish working population," *American journal of public health* 78, 1336–1342.

Johnson, J.V. and Hall, E.M. (1999). "Class, work and health," in Amick, B. (Ed.), *Society and health*. New York: Oxford University Press.

Jones, F., Bright, J.E.H., Searle, B. and Cooper, L. (1998). "Modelling occupational stress and health: The impact of the demand-control model on academic research and on workplace practice," *Stress medicine* 14, 231–236.

Karasak, R. (1985). *Job content instrument: Questionnaire and user's guide (Revision 1.1 ed.): Job/Heart Project*. New York: Columbia University Press.

King, C.T., McPherson, R.E. and Long, D.W. (2000). "Public labor market policies for the twenty-first century," in Marshall, R. (Ed.), *Back to shared prosperity: The growing inequality of wealth and income in America*. Armonk, NY: M.E. Sharpe.

Kristensen, T. (1995). "The demand-control-support model: Methodological challenges for future research," *Stress medicine* 11, 17–26.

Landsbergis, P. et al. (2003). "Research findings linking workplace factors to CVD outcomes," in Schnall, P. et al. (Eds.). *Occupational medicine: State of the art reviews: The workplace and cardiovascular disease*. Philadelphia: Hanley & Belfus.

Lavis, J.N. and Farrant, M.S.R. (1998). *Unemployment, job insecurity and health: From understanding to action*. Toronto: Report submitted to the Population Health Fund, Health Canada, unpublished.

Lerner, S., Clark, C.M.A. and Needham, W.R. (1999). *Basic income: Economic security for all Canadians*. Toronto: Between the Lines.

MacIntyre, S. (2003). "Evidence based policy making," *British medical journal* 326, 5–6.

Marshall, K. (2001). "Part-time by choice," *Perspectives* (Spring 2001), 20–27.

Mason, R. and Mitroff, I. (1981). *Challenging strategic planning assumptions: Theory, cases and techniques*. New York, Chichester, Brisbane, Toronto: John Wiley and Sons.

Maxwell, J. (2002). *Smart social policy: "Making work pay."* Ottawa: Canadian Policy Research Networks.

Pocock, B., van Wanrooy, B., Strazzari, S. and Bridge, K. (2001). *Fifty families: What unreasonable hours are doing to Australians, their families and their communities*. Melbourne: Australian Council of Trade Unions.

Polanyi, M.F. and Cole, D.C. (2003). "Stakeholder engagement on repetitive strain injuries: Lessons from Ontario," in Sullivan, T.J. and Frank, J.W. (Eds.), *Preventing and managing work-related disability*. London: Taylor and Francis.

Polanyi, M., Frank, J.W., Shannon, H.S., Sullivan, T.J. and Lavis, J. (2000). "Promoting the determinants of good health in the workplace," in Poland, B.D., Green, L.W. and Rootman, I. (Eds.), *Settings for health promotion: Linking theory and practice*. Thousand Oaks: Sage.

Polanyi, M. and Tompa, E. (2002). *Rethinking the health implications of work in the new global economy (Working Paper)*. Toronto: Munk Centre for International Studies, Comparative Program on Health and Society, University of Toronto. Online at www.utoronto.ca/cphs/WorkingPapers.shtml.

Reskin, B. and Padavic, I. (1994). *Women and men at work*. Thousand Oaks: Sage.

Schor, J.B. (2002). *The overworked American: The unexpected decline of leisure*. New York: Basic Books.

Schnall, P.S., Landsbergis, P.A. and Baker, D. (1994). "Job strain and cardiovascular disease," *Annual review of public health* 15, 381–411.

Shotter, J. and Gustavsen, B. (1999). *The role of "dialogue conferences" in the development of "learning regions": Doing "from within" our lives together what we cannot do apart*. Stockholm: Center for Advanced Studies in Leadership, Stockholm School of Economics.

Siegrist, J. (2001). "A theory of occupational stress," in Dunham, J. (Ed.), *Stress in the workplace: Past, present, future*. London: WHURR.

Siegrist, J. (1996). "Adverse health effects of high-effort/low-reward conditions," *Journal of occupational health psychology* 1 (1), 27–41.

Siegrist, J. and Peter, R. (1998). *Measuring effort-reward imbalance: Guidelines*. Dusseldorf: University of Dusseldorf.

Skocpol, T. (2000). *The missing middle*. New York, London: Norton.

Sparks, K., Cooper, C., Fried, Y. and Shirom, A. (1997). "The effects of hours of work on health: A meta-analytic review," *Journal of occupational and organizational psychology* 70 (4), 391–408.

Spurgeon, A., Harrington, J.M., and Cooper, C.L. (1997). "Health and safety problems associated with long working hours: A review of the current position," *Occupational and environmental medicine* 54, 367–375.

Theorell, T. (2001). "Stress and health: From a work perspective," in Dunham, J. (Ed.), *Stress in the workplace: Past, present, future*. London: WHURR.

Vail, J., Wheelock, J. and Hill, M. (1999). *Insecure times: Living with insecurity in contemporary society*. London: Routledge.

Van Der Doef, M. and Maes, M. (1999). "The job demand–control (–support) model and psychological well-being," *Work & stress* 13, 87–114.

Weisbord, M.R. and Janoff, S. (1995). *Future search: An action guide to finding common ground in organizations and communities*. San Francisco: Berrett-Koehler.

Wichert, I. (2002). "Job security and work intensification," in Burchell, B. and Wilkinson, F. (Eds.), *Job insecurity and work intensification*. London: Routledge.

# Chapter 8

Andersson, B.E. (1992). "Effects of day care on cognitive and socioemotional competence of thirteen year old Swedish school children," *Child development* 63, 20–36.

Beach, J., Bertrand, J. and Cleveland, G. (1998). *Our child care workforce: From recognition to remuneration—more than a labour of love: Main report*. Ottawa: Child Care Human Resources Steering Committee.

Cleveland, G., Colley, S., Friendly, M. and Lero, D. (2003). *The state of Canadian ECEC data*. Toronto: Childcare Resource and Research Unit, University of Toronto.

Doherty, G., Friendly, M. and Forer, B. (2002). *By default or design? An analysis of quality in for profit and non-profit child care centres using the You Bet I Care! data sets, occasional paper #18*. Toronto: Childcare Resource and Research Unit, University of Toronto.

Doherty, G., Lero, D., Goelman, H., LaGrange, A. and Tougas, J. (2000). *You bet I care! A Canada-wide study on wages, working conditions and practices in child care centers*. Guelph, Ontario: Centre for Families, Work and Well-Being, University of Guelph.

Environics Research Group. (1998). *Child care issues and the child care workforce: A survey of Canadian public opinion*. Toronto: Environics Research Group.

European Commission Network on Childcare. (1996). *Quality targets in services for young children: Proposals for a ten year action plan*. London: Thomas Coram Research Unit, University of London.

Federal/Provincial/Territorial Ministers Responsible for Social Services (March 13, 2003). *Press release*. "Supporting Canada's children and families." Toronto: Multilateral Framework on Early Learning and Child Care.

Friendly, M. (2001). *Is this as good as it gets? Child care as a test case for assessing the Social Union Framework Agreement*. Ottawa: Canadian review of social policy. Online at www.childcarecanada.org/pubs/ bn/isthisasgoodasitgets.html.

Friendly, M., Beach, J. and Turiano, M. (2002). *Early childhood education and care in Canada 2001*. Toronto: Childcare Resource and Research Unit, University of Toronto.

Gallagher, J.J., Rooney, R. and Campbell, S. (1999). "Child care licensing regulations and child care quality in four states," *Early childhood research quarterly* 14 (3), 313–333. Washington: National Association for the Education of Young Children and Elsevier Science, Inc.

Goelman, H., Doherty, G., Lero, D., LaGrange, A. and Tougas, J. (2000). *You bet I care! Caring and learning environments: Quality in child care centres across Canada.* Guelph, ON: Centre for Families, Work and Well-Being, University of Guelph.

Masse, L.N. and Barnett, S. (2002*). Benefit-cost analysis of the Abecedarian Early Childhood Intervention.* New Brunswick, N.J.: National Institute for Early Education Research, Rutgers University.

Meyers, M.K. and Gornick, J.C. (2000). *Early childhood education and care (ECEC): Cross-national variation in service organization.* New York: Institute for Child and Family Policy, Columbia University School of Social Work. Organization for Economic Co-operation and Development.

Organization for Economic Co-operation and Development (OECD). (2001). *Starting strong: Early childhood education and care.* Paris: OECD.

Schweinhart, L.J. and Weikart, D.P. (1993). "Changed lives, significant benefits: The High Scope Perry Preschool Project to date," *High scope resource* 1 (Summer), 10–14. Ypsilanti, MN: High Scope Press.

Shonkoff, J. and Phillips, D. (2000). *From Neurons to neighbourhoods: The science of early childhood development.* Washington: National Academies Press.

Social Policy Committee, Federal Liberal Caucus. (2002). Getting the architecture right now. Ottawa: Social Policy Committee, Federal Liberal Caucus.

United Nations Children's Fund. (2001). *The state of the world's children 2001.* New York: United Nations.

White, L. (2002). "The child care agenda and the social union," in Skogstad, G. and Bakvis, H. (Eds.), *Federalism in the new millennium.* Toronto: Oxford University Press.

Whitebook, M., Howes, C. and Phillips, D. (1990). *Who cares? Child care teachers and the quality of care in America: Final report of the national staffing study.* Oakland, CA: Child Care Employee Project.

## Chapter 9

Anderson, J.C., Williams, S., McGee, R. and Silva, P. A. (1987). "DSM-III disorders in preadolescent children: Prevalence in a large sample from the general population," *Arch. gen. psychiatry* 44, 69–76.

Applied Research Branch Strategic Policy, H.R.D.C. (1998). *Readiness to learn, child development and learning outcomes: Background* (Rep. No. T–98–4E.a). Ottawa: Human Resources Development Canada.

Bennett, K.J. and Offord, D.R. (1998). "Schools, mental health and life quality," in National Forum on Health (Ed.), *Determinants of health: Settings and issues* 3, 47–86.

Bouchard, C. (1999). "The community as a participative learning environment: The case of centraide of Greater Montreal 1,2,3 Go! Project," in Keating, D.P. and Hertzman, C. (Eds.), *Developmental health and the wealth of nations: Social, biological, and educational dynamics.* New York: Guilford.

Boyle, M.H. and Lipman, E.L. (2002). "Do places matter? Socioeconomic disadvantage and behavioral problems of children in Canada," *J consult clin. psychol.* 70, 378–389.

Boyle, M.H. and Offord, D.R. (1987a). *Ontario child health study.* Hamilton: Child Epidemiology Unit, Department of Psychiatry, McMaster University.

Boyle, M.H., Offord, D.R., Hofmann, H.G., Catlin, G.P., Byles, J.A., Cadman, D.T., Crawford, J.W., Links, P.S., Rae-Grant, N.I. and Szatmari, P. (1987b). "Ontario Child Health Study. I. Methodology," *Arch. gen. psychiatry* 44, 826–831.

Briggs-Gowan, M.J., Horwitz, S.M., Schwab-Stone, M.E., Leventhal, J.M. and Leaf, P.J. (2000). "Mental health in paediatric settings: Distribution of disorders and factors related to service use," *J. Am. acad. child adolesc. psychiatry* 39, 841–849.

Browne, G., Byrne, C., Roberts, J., Gafni, A., Majumdar, B. and Kertyzia, J. (2001a). *"Sewing the Seams": Effective and efficient human services for school-aged children.* System-Linked Research Unit, McMaster University 3N46: Report for Integrated Services for Children Division, Government of Ontario.

Browne, G., Byrne, C., Roberts, J., Gafni, A., Watt, S., Haldane, S., Thomas, I., Ewart, B., Schuster, M., Underwood, J., Kingston, S.F. and Rennick, K. (1999a). "Benefitting all the beneficiaries of social assistance: The 2-year effects and expense of subsidized versus nonsubsidized quality child care and recreation," *National academies of practice forum* 1 (2), 131–142.

Browne, G., Byrne, C., Roberts, J., Gafni, A. and Whittaker, S. (2001a). "When the bough breaks: Provider-initiated comprehensive care is more effective and less expensive for sole support parents on social assistance," *Social science and medicine* 53, 1697–1710.

Browne, G., Roberts, J., Byrne, C., Gafni, A., Weir, R. and Majumdar, B. (2001b). "The costs and effects of addressing the needs of vulnerable populations: Results of 10 years of research," *Can j nurs. res.* 33, 65–76.

Browne, G., Roberts, J., Gafni, A., Byrne, C., Kertyzia, J. and Loney, P. (2003). "Conceptualizing and validating a measure of human service integration," unpublished.

Browne, G., Roberts, J., Gafni, A., Byrne, C., Weir, R., Majumdar, B. and Watt, S. (1999). "Economic evaluations of community-based care: Lessons from twelve studies in Ontario," *Journal of evaluation in clinical practice* 5 (3), 191–209.

Browne, G., Roberts, J., Gafni, A., Weir, R., Watt, S. and Byrne, C. (1995). "More effective and less expensive: Lessons from five studies examining community approaches to care," *Health policy* 34, 95–112.

Browne, G., Roulston, J., Ewart, B., Schuster, M., Edwardh, J. and Boily, L. (2000). "Investments in comprehensive programming: services for children and single-parent mothers on welfare pay for themselves within one year," in Cleveland, G. (Ed.), *Our children's future: Child care policy in Canada.* Toronto: University of Toronto Press.

Browne, G., Byrne, C., Roberts, J., Gafni, A., Majumdar, B. and Kertyzia, J. (2002). "Convergence: Why Ontario should develop community-based models of integrated service for school-aged children," *System-linked research unit working paper series #01—02.* Hamilton: McMaster University.Online at www.fhs.mcmaster.ca/slru.

Byrne, C., Browne, G., Roberts, J., Gafni, A., Bell, B., Chalklin, L., Kraemer, J., Mills, M. and Wallik, D. (2003). "Adolescent emotional/behavioural problems and risk behaviour in Ontario primary care: Comorbidities and costs," *Clinical excellence for nurse practitioners* (forthcoming).

Catalano, R.F. and Berrglund, M.L. (1999). "Positive youth development in the US: research findings on evaluation of positive youth development programs." Online at www.aspe.hhs.gov/hsp/PositiveYouthDev99.

Durlak, J.A. and Wells, A.M. (1997). "Primary prevention mental health programs for children and adolescents: A meta-analytic review," *American journal of community psychology* 25 (2), 115–152.

Fonagy, P. (2000). "Evidence based child mental health: the findings of a comprehensive review." Paper presented at Child mental health interventions: What works for whom? Centre for Child and Adolescent Psychiatry. Oslo, Norway, 29 May 2000.

Greenberg, M.T., Domitrovich, C. and Bumbarger, B. (1999). Preventing mental disorders in school-age children: A review of the effectiveness of prevention programs. State College PA: Prevention Research Center for the Promotion of Human Development.

College of Health and Human Development Pennsylvania State University. Online at www.prevention.psu.edu/pubs/docs/CMHS.pdf

Growing Together Short-Term Evaluation. (2001). Findings from research on the effectiveness of early intervention and their relevance for the Growing Together program. Toronto and Halifax: Growing Together Short-Term Evaluation.

Health Canada (2000). Better Beginnings Better Futures, 2000. Website with materials online at bbbf.queensu.ca/pub.html.

Mustard, J.F. and McCain, M.M. (1999). "Response to Corcoran Editorial: In defence of childhood spending," *Financial post* (December 7).

Offord, D.R., Boyle, M.H., Szatmari, P., Rae-Grant, N.I., Links, P.S., Cadman, D.T., Byrne, J.A., Crawford, J.W., Munroe Blum, H., Byrne, C., Thomas, H. and Woodward, C.A. (1987). "Ontario child health study: II: Six month prevalence of disorder and rates of service utilization," *Archives of general psychiatry* 44, 832–36.

Offord, D.R., Kraemer, H.C., Kazdin, A.E., Jensen, P.S., Harrington, R. and Gardner, J.S. (1999). "Lowering the burden of suffering: monitoring the benefits of clinical, targeted, and universal approaches," in Keating, D.P. and Hertzman, C. (Eds.), *Developmental health and the wealth of nations: Social, biological, and educational dynamics.* New York: Guilford.

Ontario Association of Children's Mental Health Centres. (2001). *Children's mental health issues: Children's mental health—an urgent priority for Ontario*. Online at www.cmho.org/pdf_files/cmhopprioritynews1b.pdf.

Human Resources Development Canada/Statistics Canada. (2000). *Growing up in Canada: National longitudinal survey of children and youth*, Rep. No. Statistics Canada catalogue 89-550. Ottawa: Statistics Canada.

Schorr, L. (1988). *Within our reach: Breaking the cycle of disadvantage*. New York: Doubleday.

Volpe, R., Batra, A. and Bomio, S. (1999). "Third generation school-linked services for at risk children," *Institute of child study*. Toronto: OISE, University of Toronto.

Williams, J.D. (Ed.). (2002). *Vulnerable children: Findings from Canadian's National Longitudinal Survey of Children and Youth*. Edmonton: University of Alberta Press/Human Resources Development Canada.

## Chapter 10

Adams, M. (December 29, 2001). "We're hiding from the future," Globe and mail, A13.

Bohatyretz, S. and Lipps, G. (1999). "Diversity in the classroom: Characteristics of elementary students receiving special education," *Education quarterly review* 6 (2) 7–19.

Bowlby, J.W. and McMullen, K. (2002). *At a crossroads: First results for the 18 to 20 year old cohort of the youth in transition survey*. Canada: Human Resources Development Canada. Online at www.hrdc-drhc.gc.ca/sp-ps/arb-dgra/publications/research/2002docs/YITS/yits-encov.pdf.

Bricker, D. and Greenspon, E. (2001). *Searching for certainty: Inside the new Canadian mindset*. Toronto: Doubleday.

Canadian Education Statistics Council. (2000). *Education indicators in Canada: Report of the pan-Canadian education indicators program 1999*. Ottawa: Statistics Canada. Online at www.statcan.ca/english/freepub/81–582–XIE/81–582–XIE.pdf.

Chandler, M. and Lalonde, C. (1998). "Cultural continuity as a hedge against suicide in Canada's first nations," *Transcultural psychiatry* 35 (2), 193–211.

Compas/National Post (2001). Special report on the state of education: Quarterly report, Don Mills, Ontario: National Post.

Corak, M. (1999). *Death and divorce: The long-term consequences of parental loss on adolescents*. Family and Labour Studies, Statistics Canada. Online at www.ideas.repec.org/p/wpd/statca/11f0019mie19991-35.html.

Council of Ministers of Education Canada, Statistics Canada, and Human Resources Development Canada. (2001). *Measuring up: The performance of Canada's youth in reading, mathematics and science (OECD PISA Study—First Results for Canadians aged 15)*. Ottawa: Statistics Canada.

Department of Indian Affairs and Northern Development. (2002). *Basic departmental data*. Minister of Public Works and Government Services. Online at www.ainc–inac.gc.ca/pr/sts/bdd02/bdd02_e.html.

Guppy, N. and Davies, S. (1999). "Understanding Canadians' declining confidence in public education," *Canadian journal of education* 24 (3), 265–280.

Kerr, D. and Beaujot, R. (May 2001). "Family relations, low income and child outcomes: A comparison of children in intact, lone, and step families," London, ON: University of Western Ontario, Population Studies Centre, Discussion paper 01-8. Online at www.ssc.uwo.ca/sociology/popstudies/dp/dp01–8.pdf.

Lipps, G. and Yiptong-Avila, J. (1999). *From home to school: How Canadian children cope: Initial analyses using data from the second cycle of the school component of the national longitudinal survey of children and youth*. Canada: Culture, Tourism and the Centre for Education Statistics. Online at www.statcan.ca/english/indepth/81–003/feature/eqar1999006002s4a04.pdf.

Lochhead, C. (Autumn 2000). "The trend toward delayed for childbirth: health and social implications," *ISUMA* 1 (2). Online at www.isuma.net/v01n02/lochhead/lochhead_e.pdf.

McCall, D. (1998). *Transitions within elementary and secondary levels: Third national forum on education*. St. Johns, NF: Council of Ministers of Education Canada. Online at www.cmec.ca/nafored/english/cap.pdf.

National Centre for Education Statistics. (1999). *Third International Mathematics and Science Study*. Washington: National Centre for Education Statistics. Online at www.nces.ed.gov/timss/results.asp.

Organization for Economic Cooperation and Development (2000). *Health data*. Online at www.library.mun.ca/hsl/guides/oecd.php.

Pepler, D.J. and Craig, W.M. (1997). "Bullying: Research and interventions," *Youth Update*. Oakville: Institute for the Study of Antisocial Youth.

Ravanera, Z.R. (July 2000). "Family tranformation and social cohesion: Project overview and integrative framework," a revised version of Ravanera, Z.R. and Rajulton, F., "Multiple levels of analysis: prospects and challenges for the family transformation and social cohesion project," a paper presented at the annual meeting of the Canadian Population Society in Edmonton, Alberta, May 28–30, 2000.

Ross, D. and Roberts, P. (1999). "Income and child well being: New perspectives on the poverty debate." Canadian Council on Social Development. Online at www.ccsd.ca/pubs/inckids/index.htm.

Ross, D., Roberts, P. and Scott, K. (2000). "Family income and child well-being," *ISUMA* 1 (2) 51–54.

Ryan, B.A. and Adams, G.R. (1999) "How do families affect children's success in school," *Education quarterly review* 6 (1).

Schachter, H. (2002). *Memos to the Prime Minister: What Canada could be in the 21$^{st}$ century*. Toronto: Wiley.

School Achievement Indicators Program. (2002). *Writing II*. Toronto: Council of Ministers of Education Canada. Online at www.cmec.ca/saip/scribe3/indexe.stm.

School Achievement Indicators Program. (2001). *Mathematics learning: The Canadian context*. Toronto: Council of Ministers of Education Canada. Online at www.cmec.ca/saip/math2001/public/context.en.pdf.

School Achievement Indicators Program. (1999). *Science II*. Toronto: Council of Ministers of Education Canada. Online at www.cmec.ca/saip/science2/index.en.stm.

School Achievement Indicators Program. (1998). *Reading and writing II*. Toronto: Council of Ministers of Education Canada. Online at www.cmec.ca/saip/rw98le/pages/tablee.stm.

School Achievement Indicators Program. (1997). *Report on mathematics assessment*. Toronto: Council of Ministers of Education Canada. Online at www.cmec.ca/saip/math97/index.en.stm.

School Achievement Indicators Program. (1996). *Science*. Toronto: Council of Ministers of Education Canada. Online at www.cmec.ca/saip/sci96/index.htm.

Statistics Canada. (2000). "Rural youth: Stayers, leavers and return migrants," *The daily*. Online at www.statcan.ca/Daily/English/000905/d000905b.htm.

Statistics Canada. (2000). "Education indicators in Canada: Report of the pan-Canadian education indicators program 1999," *The daily*. Online at www.statcan.ca/english/freepub/81–582–XIE/free.htm.

Statistics Canada. (2002). "Youth in Transition Survey, 2000," *The daily*. Online at www.statcan.ca/Daily/English/020123/d020123a.htm.

Statistics Canada. (1998). "1996 Census: Education, mobility, and migration," *The daily*. Online at www.statcan.ca/Daily/English/980414/d980414.htm#1996%20Census.

Statistics Canada. (2001)."Top 10 places of birth for total immigrants, immigrants arriving before 1961 and recent immigrants for Canada, 1996 census: 20% sample data." Online at www.statcan.ca/english/census96/nov4/table1.htm.

Statistics Canada. (1994). "Languages in Canada, catalogue No. 96-313 E Table 3.4 and 1996 Census Nation Tables."

Tremblay, R.E. (2000). "The origins of youth violence," *ISUMA* 1 (2). Online at www.isuma.net/v01n02/tremblay/tremblay_e.pdf.

# Chapter 11

American Medical Association Ad Hoc Committee on Health Literacy. (1999). "Health literacy: Report of the council on scientific affairs," *JAMA* 281 (6), 553–557.

Anderson, A. (2003). *Better health, better schools, better futures*. Toronto: OISE/UT.

Antone, E.M. (2003). "Aboriginal peoples: Literacy and learning," *Literacies* 1 (Spring), 9–12.

Baker, D.W., Parker, R.M., Williams, M.V., Clark, W.S., and Nurss, J. (1997). "The relationship of patient reading ability to self-reported health and use of health services," *American journal of public health* 87 (6),1027–1030.

Baker, D.W., Gazmararian, J.A., Williams, M.V., Scott, T., Parker, R.M., Green, D., Ren, J., Peel, J. (2002). "Functional health literacy and the risk of hospital admission among Medicare managed care enrolees," *American journal of public health* 92 (8),1278–83.

Begley, S. (1996). "Your child's brain," *Newsweek* (February 19).

Boyd, M. (1991). "Gender, nativity and literacy: Proficiency and training issues," *Adult literacy in Canada: Results of national study*. Ottawa: Statistics Canada, 86–94.

Breen, M.J. (1998). "Promoting literacy, improving health," *Canada health action: Building on the legacy: V2 Adults and Seniors*. Ottawa: National Forum on Health.

Calamai, P. (2000). *The three L's: Literacy and life-long learning. An address to the Westnet 2000 conference* (Calgary, November 2, 2000). Online at www.nald.ca/fulltext/3ls.

Calamai, P. (1999) *Literacy Matters Report*, Toronto, ABC CANADA Literacy Foundation. Online at www.abc–canada.org/public_awareness/literacy_matters_report.asp.

Calamai, P. (1987). *Broken words: Why five million Canadians are illiterate: A special Southam survey.* Online at www.nald.ca/fulltext/Brokword/cover.htm.

Canadian Business Task Force on Literacy. (1987). *The cost of illiteracy to Canadian business*. Toronto: Westmount Research Consultants.

Canadian Public Health Association. (2003). *Literacy and health research workshop: Setting priorities in Canada.* Online at www.nlhp.cpha.ca/clhrp/index_e.htm#workshop.

Canadian Public Health Association. (2000). *What the HEALTH! A Literacy and Health Resource for Youth.* Ottawa: Canadian Public Health Association. Online at www.worlded.org/us/health/docs/culture/materials/curricula_009.html.

Charette, M.F. and Meng, R. (August 1998). "The determinants of literacy and numeracy and the effect of literacy and numeracy on our market outcomes," *Canadian journal of economics/revue canadienne d'economique* 13 (3). Online at www.nald.ca/fulltext/pat/Charette/page1.htm.

Daniels, S., Kennedy, B. and Kawachi, I. (2000). "Justice is good for our health: How greater economic equality would promote public health," *Boston review* February/March 2000. Online at www.bostonreview.net/BR25.1/daniels.html.

Darville, R. (1992). *Adult literacy work in Canada*. Toronto: Canadian Association for Adult Education.

Davies, R. (1995). *Men for change*. Halifax: Private correspondence.

Davis, T.C., Meldrum, H., Tippy, P.K.P., et al. (1996). "How poor literacy leads to poor health care," *Patient care* 30 (16), 94–124.

DeWit, D.J., Akst, L., Braun, K., Jelley, J., Lefebver, L, McKee, C., et al. (2002). *Sense of school membership: A mediating mechanism linking student perceptions of school culture with academic and behavioural functioning: Baseline data report of the school culture project*. Toronto: Centre for Addiction and Mental Health.

Edwards, C. (1995). "Due diligence: The challenge of language and literacy," *Accident prevention* 42 (6),18–21.

Education Quality and Accountability Office. (2003). *Ontario secondary school literacy test report of provincial results*. Online at www.eqao.com.

Federal, Provincial and Territorial Advisory Committee on Population Health. (1999). *Toward a healthy future*. Ottawa: Health Canada.

Friedland, R. (1998). "New estimates of the high costs of inadequate health literacy," *Promoting health literacy: A call to action,* Proceedings of Pfizer Conference (October 7–8, 1998), 6–10.Washington: Pfizer Inc.

Frontier College. (1989). *Learning in the workplace*. Toronto: Frontier College. Online at www.frontiercollege.ca/english/programs/wkplace.htm.

Gazmararian, J.A., Baker, D.W., Williams, M.V., Parker, R.M., Scott, T.L., Green, D.C., Fehrenbach, S.N., Ren, J. and Koplan, J.P. (1999). "Health literacy among Medicare enrollees in a managed care organization," comment in *JAMA* 282 (6), 527.

Grossman, M., and Kaestner, R. (1997). "The effects of education on health," in Behermann R., Stacey, N. (Eds.), *The social benefits of education*. Ann Arbor: University of Michigan Press.

Grotsky, R. (1989). *Workplace literacy and health and safety: A research report*, prepared for the Industrial Accident Prevention Association by Learning Communications Inc.

Guerra, C.E. and Shea, J.A. (2003). "Functional health literacy: Comorbidity and health status," *Journal of general internal medicine* 18 (1), 174.

Hawthorne, G. (1997). "Preteenage drug use in Austrialia: Key predictors and school-based drug education," *Journal of adolescent health* 20 (5), 384–395.

Health Canada. (2003). "How does literacy affect the health of Canadians?" Online at www.hc–sc.gc.ca/hppb/phdd/literacy/literacy.html.

Jadad, A.R. (1999). "Promoting partnerships: Challenges for the internet age," *British medical journal* 318 (September 18), 761–764.

Kalichman, S.C., Ramachandran, B., and Catz, S. (1999). "Adherence to combination antiretroviral therapies in HIV patients of low literacy," *J. gen internal medicine* 5, 267–273.

Kirsch, I.S., Jungeblut, A., Jenkins, L., and Kolstad, A. (1993). *Adult literacy in America: A first look at the results of the National Adult Literacy Survey (NALS)*. Washington: National Center for Educational Statistics, U.S. Department of Education.

Mustard, F. and McCain, M.N. (1999). *Early years study*. Toronto: Queen's Printer for Ontario.

OECD and Statistics Canada. (2000). *Literacy in the information age: Final report of the international adult literacy survey*. Online at www.statcan.ca/english/freepub/89-588-XIE/about.htm.

Parker, R.M., Ratzan, S.C., and Lurie, N. (2003). "Health literacy: A policy challenge for advancing high quality health care," *Health affairs* 22 (4), 147.

Parkland Regional College. (1998). *Reaching the rainbow: Aboriginal literacy in Canada*. Melville SK: Parkland Regional College.

Perrin, B. (1989). *Literacy and health: Making the connection: The research report of the literacy and health project phase one: Making the world healthier and safer for people who can't read*. Ontario Public Health Association and Frontier College. Online at www.opha.on.ca/resources/literacy1research.pdf.

Puchner, L.D. (1993). *Early childhood, family, and health issues in literacy: International perspectives*. Philadelphia, PA: NCAL International Paper IP93–2.

Roberts, P. and Fawcett, G. (1998). *At risk: A socio-economic analysis of health and literacy among seniors*. Statistics Canada Cat. No. 89–552–MPE, no. 5.

Rootman, I. (1991). "Literacy and health in Canada: Contribution of the LSUDA survey," in Statistics Canada, *Adult literacy in Canada: Results of a national study*. Ottawa: Minister of Industry, Science and Technology.

Rootman, I., Gordon-El-Bihbety, D., Frankish, J., Hemming, H., Kaszap, M., Langille, L., Quantz, D. and Ronson, B. (2003). *National literacy and health research program, needs assessment and environmental scan*. Online at www.nlhp.cpha.ca/clhrp/index_e.htm.

Rootman, I. and Ronson, B. (2003). "Literacy and health research in Canada: Where have we been and where should we go?" Research paper. Ottawa: International Think Tank on Reducing Health Disparities and Promoting Equity for Vulnerable Populations.

Rudd, R. E., Moeykens, B. A. and Colton, T. (1999). "Health and literacy: A review of medical and public health literature," NCSALL: *The annual review of adult learning and literacy*, Volume 1, Chapter 5.

Sarginson, R. J. (1997). *Literacy and health: A Manitoba perspective*. Winnipeg: Literacy Partners of Manitoba. Online at www.mb.literacy.ca/publications/lithealth/ack.htm.

Schillinger, D., Grumbach, K., Piette, J., Wang, F., Osmond, D., Daher, C., Palacios, J., Sullivan, G. D. and Bindman, A.B. (2002). "Association of health literacy with diabetes outcomes," *Journal of the American Medical Association* 288 (4), 475–82.

Schweinhart, L. J., Barnes, H. V., Weikart, D. P., Barnett, W. S. and Epstein, A. S. (1993). *Significant benefits: The High/Scope Perry preschool study through age 27*. Ypsilanti, MI: High/Scope Press.

Scott, T. L., Gazmararian, J. A., Williams, M. V., Baker, and D. W. (2002). "Health literacy and preventive health care use among Medicare enrollees in a managed care organization," *Medical care* 40 (5), 395–404.

Shohet, L. (1997). "Canadian budget shines spotlight on family literacy." Online at www.nald.ca/naldnews/97spring/budget.htm.

Statistics Canada. (1996). *Reading the future: A portrait of literacy in Canada.* Online at www.nald.ca/nls/ials/ialsreps/high1.htm.

Totten, M. and Quigley, P. (2003). *Bullying, school exclusion and literacy*, unpublished discussion paper sponsored by the Canadian Public Health Association.

Weiss, B. D., Blanchard, J. S., McGee, D. L., Hart, G., Warren, B., Burgoon, M. and Smith, K. J. (1994). "Illiteracy among Medicaid recipients and its relationship to health care costs," *Journal of health care for the poor and underserved* 5 (2), 99–111.

Weiss, B. D. (2001). "Health literacy: An important issue for communicating health information to patients," *Chinese medical journal* 64 (11), 603–8.

WHO. (2003). *The World Health Organization's health promoting school: Creating an environment for emotional and social well-being.* Geneva: Information Series on School Health, Document 10.

WHO, UNESCO, World Bank and UNICEF. (2000). *Focusing resources on effective school health: A FRESH start to enhancing the quality and equity of education.* World Education Forum 2000, Final Report. Online at www.freshschools.org/whatisfresh.htm.

Young, D. E. and Smith, L. L. (1992). *The involvement of Canadian native communities in their health care programs: A review of the literature since the 1970's.* Edmonton: Canadian Circumpolar Institute and Centre for the Cross-Cultural Study of Health and Healing.

# Chapter 12

Che, J., and Chen, J. (2001). "Food insecurity in Canadian households," *Health reports* 12, 11–22.

Hamilton, W. L., Cook, J. T., Thompson, W. W., Buron, L., Frongillo, E., Olson, C., et al. (1997). *Household food security in the United States in 1995: Summary report of the Food Security Measurement Project.* Washington: United States Department of Agriculture Food and Consumer Service.

Kendall, A., Olson, C. M. and Frongillo, E. A. (1995). "Validation of the Radimer/Cornell measures of hunger and food insecurity," *Journal of nutrition* 125, 2793–2801.

McIntyre, L., Connor, S. K., and Warren, J. (2000). "Child hunger in Canada: Results of the 1994 National Longitudinal Survey of Children and Youth," *Canadian Medical Association journal* 163, 961–965.

McIntyre, L., Glanville, N. T., Officer, S., Anderson, B., Raine, K. D., and Dayle, J. B. (2002). "Food insecurity of low-income lone mothers and their children in Atlantic Canada," *Canadian journal of public health* 93, 411–415.

McIntyre, L., Glanville, N. T., Raine, K. D., Dayle, J. B., Anderson, B., and Battaglia, N. (2003). "Low-income lone mothers compromise their nutrition to feed their children," *Canadian Medical Association journal* 168, 686–691.

McIntyre, L., Walsh, G. and Connor, S. K. (2001). *A follow-up study of child hunger in Canada.* Working Paper W–01–1–2E. Ottawa: Human Resources Development Canada.

Olson, C. M. (1999). "Nutrition and health outcomes associated with food insecurity and hunger," *Journal of nutrition* 129, 521S–524S.

Rainville, B. and Brink, S. (2001). *Food insecurity in Canada, 1998–1999.* Research paper R–01–2E. Ottawa: Human Resources Development Canada.

Riches, G. (1997). "Hunger, food security and welfare policies: Issues and debates in First World societies," *Proceedings of the Nutrition Society* 56, 63–74.

Rose, D. and Oliveira, V. (1997a). *Validation of a self-reported measure of household food insufficiency with nutrient intake data.* Washington: United States Department of Agriculture.

Rose, D. and Oliveira, V. (1997b). "Nutrient intakes of individuals from food–insufficient households in the United States," *American journal of public health* 87, 1956–61.

Sarlo, C. (1996). *Poverty in Canada, 2nd edition.* Vancouver: Fraser Institute.

Tarasuk, V. (2001). "Household food insecurity with hunger is associated with women's food intakes, health and household circumstances," *Journal of nutrition* 131, 2670–2676.

Tarasuk, V. S. and Beaton, G. H. (1999). "Household food insecurity and hunger among families using food banks," *Canadian journal of public health* 90, 109–113.

Tarasuk, V. and Reynolds, R. (1999). "A qualitative study of community kitchens as a response to income-related food insecurity," *Canadian journal of dietetic practice and research* 60, 11–16.

Townsend, M. S., Peerson, J., Love, B., Achetberg, C. and Murphy, S. P. (2001). "Food insecurity is positively related to overweight in women," *Journal of nutrition* 131, 1738–1745.

United Nations Food and Agriculture Organization (FAO). (2002). *The state of food insecurity in the world.* Washington: FAO.

Wehler, C. A., Scott, R. I. and Anderson, J. J. (1996). *The community childhood hunger identification project: A survey of childhood hunger in the United States.* Washington: Food Research and Action Center.

Wilson, B. and Tsoa, E. (2002). *HungerCount 2002. Eating their words: Government failure on food security.* Toronto: Canadian Association of Food Banks.

## Chapter 13

Alaimo, K., Olson, C. M. and Frongillo, E. A. (2001a). "Food insufficiency and American school-aged children's cognitive, academic, and psychosocial development," *Pediatrics* 108, 44–53.

Alaimo, K., Olson, C. M. and Frongillo, E. A. (2001b). "Low family income and food insufficiency in relation to overweight in US children: Is there a paradox?" *Archives of pediatrics and adolescent medicine* 155, 1161–1167.

Alaimo, K., Olson, C. M. and Frongillo, E. A. (2002). "Family food insufficiency, but not low family income, is positively associated with dysthymia and suicide symptoms in adolescents," *Journal of nutrition* 132, 719–725.

Alaimo, K., Olson, C. M., Frongillo, E. A. and Briefel, R. (2001c). "Food insufficiency, family income, and health of US preschool and school-aged children," *American journal of public health* 91, 781–786.

Badun, C., Evers, S. and Hooper, M. (1995). "Food security and nutritional concerns of parents in an economically disadvantaged community," *J Can Diet Assoc* 56, 75–80

Basiotis, P. P. and Lino, M. (2002). *Food insufficiency and prevalence of overweight among adult women.* Alexandria VA: USDA Center for Nutrition Policy and Promotion.

Bull, N. L. (1991). "The distribution of energy and nutrient intakes within households," *Journal of human nutrition and dietetics* 4, 421–425.

Campbell, C. C. and Desjardins, E. (1989). "A model and research approach for studying the management of limited food resources by low income families," *Journal of nutrition education* 21, 162–171

Campbell, C., Katamay, S. and Connolly, C. (1988). "The role of nutrition professionals in the hunger debate," *Journal of the Canadian Dietetic Association* 49, 230–235.

Che, J. and Chen, J. (2001). "Food insecurity in Canadian households," *Health reports* 12, 11–22.

Cristofar, S. P. and Basiotis, P. P. (1992). "Dietary intakes and selected characteristics of women ages 19–50 years and their children ages 1–5 years by reported perception of food sufficiency," *Journal of nutrition education* 24, 53–58.

Davis, B., Katamay, S., Desjardins, E., Sterken, E. and Patillo, M. (1991). "Nutrition and food security: A role for the Canadian Dietetic Association," *Journal of the Canadian Dietetic Association* 52, 141–145.

Dowler, E. and Leather, S. (2000). "'Spare some change for a bite to eat?' From primary poverty to social exclusion: the role of nutrition and food," in Bradshaw, J. and Sainsbury, R. (Eds.), *Experiencing poverty.* Aldershot: Ashgate.

Dowler, E. and Calvert, C. (1995). *Nutrition and diet in lone-parent families in London.* London: Family Policy Studies Centre.

Emes, J. and Kreptul, A. (1999). *The adequacy of welfare benefits in Canada.* Vancouver: The Fraser Institute. Online at www.fraserinstitute.ca/publications/.

Enns, C. W. (1987). "Comparison of nutrient intakes by male vs. female heads of households," *Journal of the American Dietetic Association* 87, 1551–1553.

Fitchen, J. M. (1988). "Hunger, malnutrition, and poverty in the contemporary United States: Some observations on their social and cultural context," *Food and foodways* 2, 309–333.

Social Determinants of Health

Gunderson, C. and Gruber, J. (2001). "The dynamic determinants of food insufficiency," in *Second food security measurement and research conference, vol. II: Papers*. Washington: U.S. Department of Agriculture.

Hamelin, A. M., Beaudry, M. and Habicht, J.-P. (2002). "Characterization of household food insecurity in Quebec: food and feelings," *Social science and medicine* 54, 119–132.

Health Canada. (1997). *Canada's food guide to healthy eating*. Ottawa: Health Canada.

Joint Steering Committee. (1996). *Nutrition for health: An agenda for action*. Ottawa: Health Canada.

Kendall, A., Olson, C. M. and Frongillo, E. A. (1996). "Relationship of hunger and food insecurity to food availability and consumption," *Journal of the American Dietetic Association* 96, 1019–1024.

Kirkpatrick, S. and Tarasuk, V. (2003). "Income and household food expenditure in Canada," *Public health nutrition* 6, 589–597.

Kleinman, R. E., Murphy, J. M., Little, M., Pagano, M., Wehler, C. A., Regal, K. and Jellinek, M. S. (1998). "Hunger in children in the United States: Potential behavioral and emotional correlates," *Pediatrics* 101, 1–6.

Klesges, L. M., Pahor, M., Shorr, R. I. and Wan, J. Y. (2001). "Financial difficulty in acquiring food among elderly disabled women: Results from the Women's Health and Aging Study," *American journal of public health* 91, 68–75.

Lang, T. (1997). "Dividing up the cake: Food as social exclusion," in Walker, A. and Walker, C. (Eds.), *Britain divided*. London: CPAG.

Leather, S. (1996). *The making of modern malnutrition*. London: The Caroline Walker Trust.

Lee, P. (1990). "Nutrient intakes in socially disadvantaged groups in Ireland," *Proceedings of the Nutrition Society* 49, 307–321.

Louk, K. R., Schafer, E., Schafer, R. B. and Keith, P. (1999). "Comparison of dietary intakes of husbands and wives," *Journal of nutrition education* 31, 145–152.

McIntyre, L., Connor, S. K. and Warren, J. (2000). "Child hunger in Canada: Results of the 1994 National Longitudinal Survey of Children and Youth," *Canadian Medical Association journal* 163, 961–965.

McIntyre, L., Glanville, T., Officer, S., Anderson, B., Raine, K. D. and Dayle, J. B. (2002). "Food insecurity of low-income lone mothers and their children in Atlantic Canada," *Canadian journal of public health* 93, 411–415.

McIntyre, L., Glanville, T., Raine, K. D., Anderson, B. and Battaglia, N. (2003). "Do low-income lone mothers compromise their nutrition to feed their children?" *Canadian Medical Association journal* 168, 686–691.

McLaughlin C., Tarasuk, V. and Kreiger N. (2003). "An examination of at-home food preparation activity among low-income, food-insecure women," *Journal of the American Dietetic Association* 103, 1506–1512.

Murphy, J. M., Wehler, C. A., Pagano, M. E., Little, M., Kleinman, R. E., and Jellinek, M. S. (1998). "Relationship between hunger and psychosocial functioning in low-income American children," *Journal of the American Academy of Child and Adolescent Psychiatry* 37, 163–170.

National Council of Welfare. (1990). *Women and poverty revisited*. Ottawa: Minister of Supply and Services Canada. Online.

National Council of Welfare. (2002). *Welfare incomes, 2000 and 2001*. Ottawa: Minister of Public Works and Government Services Canada. Online at www.ncwchbes.net.

Nelson, K., Brown, M. E. and Lurie, N. (1998). "Hunger in an adult patient population," *Journal of the American Medical Association* 279, 1211–1214.

Nelson, K., Cunningham, W., Andersen, R., Harrison, G. and Gelberg, L. (2001). "Is food insufficiency associated with health status and health care utilization among adults with diabetes?" *Journal of general internal medicine* 16, 404–411.

Nelson, M. (1986). "The distribution of nutrient intake within families," *British journal of nutrition* 55, 267–277.

Olson, C. M. (1999). "Nutrition and health outcomes associated with food insecurity and hunger," *Journal of nutrition* 129, 521S–524S.

Radimer, K. L., Allsopp, R., Harvey, P. W. J., Firman, D. W. and Watson, E. K. (1997). "Food insufficiency in Queensland," *Australian and New Zealand journal of public health* 21, 303–310.

Radimer, K. L., Olson, C. M. and Campbell, C. C. (1990). "Development of indicators to assess hunger," *Journal of nutrition* 120, 1544–1548.

Radimer, K. L., Olson, C. M., Greene, J. C., Campbell, C. C. and Habicht, J.-P. (1992). "Understanding hunger and developing indicators to assess it in women and children," *Journal of nutrition education* 24, 36S–45S.

Riches, G. (2002). "Food banks and food security: Welfare reform, human rights and social policy: Lessons from Canada?" *Social policy and administration* 36, 648–663.

Riches, G. (1997). "Hunger in Canada: Abandoning the right to food," in *First World hunger, food security and welfare politics*. London: Macmillan.

Rose, D. (1999). "Economic determinants and dietary consequences of food insecurity in the United States," *Journal of nutrition* 129, 517S–520S.

Rose, D. and Oliveira, V. (1997a). "Nutrient intakes of individuals from food-insufficient households in the United States," *American journal of public health* 87, 1956–1961.

Rose, D. and Oliveira, V. (1997b). *Validation of a self-reported measure of household food insufficiency with nutrient intake data*. Washington: Department of Agriculture.

Sarlio-Lahteenkorva, S. and Lahelma, E. (2001). "Food insecurity is associated with past and present economic disadvantage and body mass index," *Journal of nutrition* 131, 2880–2884.

Tarasuk, V. (2001a). "A critical examination of community-based responses to household food insecurity in Canada," *Health education and behavior* 28, 487–499.

Tarasuk, V. S. and Beaton, G. H. (1999). "Women's dietary intakes in the context of household food insecurity," *Journal of nutrition* 129, 672–679.

Tarasuk, V. and Maclean, H. (1990). "The food problems of low-income single mothers: An ethnographic study," *Canadian home economics journal* 40, 76–82.

Tarasuk, V. S. (2001b). "Household food insecurity with hunger is associated with women's food intakes, health, and household circumstances," *Journal of nutrition* 131, 2670–2676.

The Canadian Dietetic Association. (1991). "Hunger and food security in Canada: Official position of the Canadian Dietetic Association," *Journal of the Canadian Dietetic Association* 52, 139–139.

Townsend, M. S., Peerson, J., Love, B., Achterberg, C. and Murphy, S. P. (2001). "Food insecurity is positively related to overweight in women," *Journal of nutrition* 131, 1738–1745.

Travers, K. D. (1995). "'Do you teach them how to budget?': Professional discourse in the construction of nutritional inequities," in Maurer, D. and Sobal, J. (Eds.), *Eating agendas: Food and nutrition as social problems*. Hawthorne NY: Aldine DeGruyter.

Travers, K. D. (1996). "The social organization of nutritional inequities," *Social science and medicine* 43, 543–553.

Travers, K. D., Cogdon, A., McDonald, W., Wright, C., Anderson, B. and MacLean, D. R. (1997). "Availability and cost of heart healthy dietary changes in Nova Scotia," *Journal of the Canadian Dietetic Association* 58, 176–183.

Travers, K. D. (1997). "Reducing inequities through participatory research and community empowerment," *Health education and behavior* 24, 344–356.

Vozoris, N., Davis, B. and Tarasuk, V. (2002). "The affordability of a nutritious diet for households on welfare in Toronto," *Canadian journal of public health* 93, 36–40.

Vozoris, N. and Tarasuk, V. (2003). "Household food insufficiency is associated with poorer health," *Journal of nutrition* 133, 120–126.

Wehler, C. A., Scott, R. I. and Anderson, J. J. (1992). "The community childhood hunger identification project: A model of domestic hunger: Demonstration project in Seattle, Washington," *Journal of nutrition education* 24, 29S–35S.

# Chapter 14

Canadian Housing and Renewal Association. (2003). *Expiry of operating agreements: Findings on the big picture* (Quebec/Ontarion regional meeting document, June 11, 2003).

Social Determinants of Health

Canada Mortgage and Housing Corporation. (2002). *Opening doors* (Annual Report 2002).

Carter, T. (2000). *Canadian housing policy: Is the glass half empty or half full?* (Canadian Housing and Renewal Association Research Paper, April 2000).

Cooper, M. (2001). *Housing affordability: A children's issue* (Research report). Canadian Policy Research Networks, March 2001.

Federation of Canadian Municipalities. (2002). "Is this really an affordable rental housing program?" (Affordability assessment, November 2002.) Ottawa: Federation of Canadian Municipalities.

Hulchanski, D. (2001). "A tale of two Canadas: Homeowners getting richer, renters getting poorer" (Research Bulletin #2). Toronto: Centre for Urban and Community Studies, August, 2001.

Mahoney, Hon. S. (2003). "Letter to National Housing and Homelessness Network with Update on Spending Commitments under the Affordable Housing Program," Ottawa, December 5, 2003.

Martin, P. (1990). "Finding room." National Liberal Task Force on Housing. Online at www.housingagain.web.net/pmartin.html

National Housing and Homelessness Network. (2002). "Housing for all Canadians: More federal money required, more federal leadership required." (Pre-Budget Submission to the House of Commons Standing Committee on Finance, September 3, 2003).

National Housing and Homelessness Network.(2003). "NHHN housing report card" (November 14, 2003). Online at www.povnet.org/downloads/nhhnreportcardnov2003.pdf.

National Housing and Homelessness Network. (2001). "State of the crisis 2001: A report on housing and homelessness in Canada." Online at www.tdrc.net/2report3.htm.

Ontario Housing Supply Working Group. (2001). *Affordable rental housing supply: The dynamics of the market and recommendations for encouraging new supply* (May 2001). Online at www.mah.gov.on.ca/userfiles/HTML/nts_1_3369_1.html.

Reitsma-Street, M., Schofield, J., Lund, B. and Kasting, C. (2001). *Housing policy options for women living in urban poverty: An action research project in three Canadian cities* (February, 2001). Online at www.swc-cfc.gc.ca/pubs/0660613417/index_e.html.

TD Economics (2003). *Affordable housing in Canada: In search of a new paradigm* (2003). Online at www.action.web.ca/home/housing/alerts.shtml.

Toronto Disaster Relief Committee. (1998). *State of emergency declaration: An urgent call for emergency humanitarian relief and prevention measures.* Toronto: Toronto Disaster Relief Committee (October 1998).

Toronto Disaster Relief Committee. (2000). *State of the Crisis.* Toronto: Toronto Disaster Relief Committee

# Chapter 15

Ambrosio E., Baker D., Crowe C. and Hardill, K. (1992). *The street health report: A study of the health status and barriers to health care of homeless women an men in the City of Toronto.* Toronto: Street Health.

Bines, W. (1994). *The health of single homeless people.* York University: Centre for Health Policy.

Bryant, T. (in press). "The role of political ideology in rental housing policy in Ontario, Canada," *Housing Studies.*

Bryant, T. (2002). "The role of knowledge in progressive social policy development and implementation," *Canadian review of social policy* 49/50, 5–24.

Bryant, T. (2003). "A critical examination of the hospital restructuring process in Ontario, Canada," *Health policy* 64, 193–205.

Brunner, E. and Marmot, M. (1999). "Social organization, stress, and health," in Marmot, M. and Wilkinson, R. (Eds.), *Social determinants of health.* Oxford: Oxford University Press.

Canada Mortgage and Housing Corporation. (2001). *Welfare income versus current average market rent, Toronto CMA.* Ottawa: Canada Mortgage and Housing Corporation.

Canada Mortgage and Housing Corporation. (2000). *Housing market survey: Statistics Canada small area data: Special tabulations calculations.* Ottawa: The Advocate Institute.

City of Calgary. (2002). "The 2002 count of homeless persons, 2002 May 15." Calgary: City of Calgary Planning and Policy Department.

Coburn, D. (2000). "Income inequality, lowered social cohesion and the poorer health status of populations: The role of neo-liberalism," *Social science and medicine* 51, 135–146.

Coleman, W.D., Skogstad, G.D. and Atkinson, M.M. (1997). "Paradigm shifts and policy networks: Cumulative change in agriculture," *Journal of public policy* 16:3, 273–301.

Daily Bread Food Bank. (2002). *Fact Sheet: Turning our backs on our children: Hunger + decrepit housing = unhealthy, unsafe children.* Toronto: Daily Bread Food Bank.

Davey Smith, G. (2003). *Inequalities in health.* Bristol: Policy Press.

Dedman, D. J., Gunnell, D., Davey Smith, G. and Frankel, S. (2001). "Childhood housing conditions and later mortality in the Boyd Orr cohort," *Journal of epidemiology and community health* 55:10–15.

Dunn, J. R. (2002). *A population health approach to housing: A framework for research.* Ottawa: National Housing Research Committee and CMHC. Online at www.hpclearinghouse.ca/hcn/download/A_Population_Health_Approach_to_Housing_FINAL.pdf.

Dunn, J.R. (2000). "Housing and health inequalities: Review and prospects for research," *Housing Studies* 15:3, 341–366.

Howlett, M. and Ramesh, M. (1995). *Studying public policy: Policy cycles and policy subsystems.* Toronto: Oxford University Press.

Hulchanski, J.D. (2001). *A tale of two Canadas: Homeowners getting richer, renters getting poorer.* Toronto: Centre for Urban and Community Studies, University of Toronto.

Hulchanski, J.D. (2002). *Housing policy for tomorrow's cities. Discussion Paper F/27 Family Network.* Ottawa: Canadian Policy Research Networks.

Hwang, S. (2001). "Homelessness and health," *Canadian Medical Association journal* 164: 2, 229–233.

Hwang, S., Fuller-Thomson, E., Hulchanski, J. D., Bryant, T., Habib, Y. and Regoeczi, W. (1999). *Housing and population health: A review of the literature.* Toronto: Faculty of Social Work, University of Toronto.

Jenkins, R. (1982). *Hightown rules: Growing up in a Belfast housing estate.* Leicester: National Youth Bureau.

Kirby, M. (2002). *The study of the state of the health care system in Canada.* Ottawa: Senate of Canada. Online at www.albertadoctors.org/advocacy/sustainability.

Kushner, C. (1998). *Better access, better care: A research paper on health services and homelessness in Toronto.* Toronto: Toronto Mayor's Homelessness Action Task Force.

Layton, J. (2000). *Homelessness: The making and unmaking of a crisis.* Toronto: Penguin.

Marmot, M. and Wilkinson, R. (Eds.). (1999). *Social determinants of health.* Oxford: Oxford University Press.

Marsh, A., Gordon, D., Pantazis, C. and Heslop, P. (1999). *Home sweet home?: The impact of poor housing on health.* Bristol: Policy.

Martin, P. and Fontana, J. (1990). *Finding room: Housing solutions for the future.* Ottawa: Liberal Party of Canada.

Mazankowski, D. (2001). *A framework for reform.* Edmonton: Premier's Advisory Council on Health. Online at www.albertadoctors.org/advocacy/sustainability/.

National Housing and Homelessness Network. (2002). "More than half provinces betray commitments: NHHN 'report card' on anniversary of Affordable Housing Framework Agreement." Online at www.tdrc.net/2replst.htm.

Platt, S., Martin, C., Hunt, S. and Lewis, C. (1989). "Damp housing, mould growth and symptomatic health state," *British medical journal* 298, 1673–8.

Romanow, R. (2002). *Building on values: The future of health care in Canada. Final report.* Saskatoon: Commission on the Future of Health Care in Canada.

Sandeman G., Lyon, C., Lyons, G., Jackson. M., McKeen, M., Murray, J. and Robinson, K. (2002). *Community plan to address homelessness and housing insecurity in Peterborough City and County.* Peterborough: City of Peterborough.

Social Determinants of Health

Savage, A. (1988). *Warmth in winter: Evaluation of an information pack for elderly people*. Cardiff: University of Wales College of Medicine Research Team for the Care of the Elderly.

Shaw, M. (2001). "Health and housing: A lasting relationship," *Journal of epidemiology and community health* 55, 291.

Shaw, M., Dorling, D. and Davey Smith, G. (1999). "Social exclusion," in Marmot, M. and Wilkinson, R. (eds.), *Social determinants of health*. New York: Oxford University Press.

Shaw, M., Dorling, D., Gordon, D. and Davey Smith, G. (1999). *The widening gap: Health inequalities and policy in Britain*. Bristol: Policy.

Standing Senate Committee on Social Affairs, Science and Technology. (2002). *The health of Canadians: The federal role*. Ottawa: Senate of Canada.

Statistics Canada. (2004). "Owner households and tenant households by major payments and gross rent as a percentage of 2000 household income, provinces and territories." Online at www.statcan.ca/english/Pgdb/famil65a.htm.

Statistics Canada. (1984, 1999). *Survey of financial security*. Ottawa: Statistics Canada.

Strachan, D. (1988). "Damp housing and childhood asthma: Validation of reporting of symptoms," *British medical journal* 297, 1223–6.

Toronto Disaster Relief Committee. (1998). *The one per cent solution*. Toronto: TDRC. Online at www.tdrc.ca.

Watt, J. (2003). *Adequate and affordable housing: A child health issue*. Ottawa: Child and Youth Health Network for Eastern Ontario.

Wilkinson, D. (1999). "Poor housing and ill health: A summary of research evidence." Edinburgh: The Scottish Office. Online.

World Health Organization. (1986). *Ottawa charter on health promotion*. Geneva: WHO.

# Chapter 16

Adams, D. (1995). *Health issues of women of colour: A cultural diversity perspective*. Thousand Oaks: Sage.

Anderson, J. M. (2000). "Gender, race, poverty, health and discourses of health reform in the context of globalization: A post-colonial feminist perspective in policy research," *Nursing inquiry* 7 (4), 220–229.

Anderson, J. and Kirkham, R. (1998). "Constructing nation: The gendering and racializing of the Canada health care system," in Strong-Boag, V. and Grace, S. (Eds.), *Painting the maple: Essays on race, gender, and the construction of Canada*. Vancouver: UBC Press.

Anderson, J., Blue, C., Holbrook, A. and Ng, M. (1993). "On Chronic illness: Immigrant women in Canada's workforce: A feminist perspective," *Canadian journal of nursing research* 25/2.

Agnew, V. (2002). *Gender, migration and citizenship resources project: Part II: A literature review and bibliography on health*. Toronto: Centre for Feminist Research, York University.

Alliance for South Asian AIDS Prevention (ASAP). (1999). *Discrimination & HIV/AIDS in South Asian communities: Legal, ethical and human rights challenges: An ethnocultural perspective*. Toronto: ASAP/Health Canada.

Beiser, M. (1998). *After the door has been opened: Mental health issues affecting immigrants and refugees in Canada: Report of the Canadian Taskforce on mental health issues affecting immigrants and refugees*. Ottawa: Health and Welfare Canada.

Bloom, M. and Grant, M. (2001). *Brain gain: The economic benefits of recognizing learning and learning credentials in Canada*. Ottawa: Conference Board of Canada.

Bolaria, B. and Bolaria, R. (Eds.). (1994). *Immigrant status and health status: Women and racial minority immigrant workers in racial minorities, medicine and health*. Halifax: Fernwood.

Byrne, D. (1999). *Social exclusion*. Buckingham: Open University Press.

Chard, J., Badets, J. and Howatson-Lee, L. (2000). "Immigrant women," in *Women in Canada, 2000: A gender-based statistical report*. Ottawa: Statistics Canada.

Chen, J., Wilkins, R. and Ng, E. (1996). "Life expectancy of Canada's immigrants from 1986 to 1991," *Health reports* 8/3 (1996), 29–38.

Cross Boundaries. (1999). *Healing journey: Mental health of people of colour project.* Toronto: Across Boundaries.

De Wolff, A. (2000). *Breaking the myth of flexible work.* Toronto: Contingent Workers Project.

Dossa, P. (1999). *The narrative representation of mental health: Iranian women in Canada.* Vancouver: RIIM.

Dunn, J. and Dyck, I. (1998). *Social determinants of health in Canada's immigrant population: Results from the National Population Health Survey.* Working paper series #98-20. Vancouver: Vancouver Centre of Excellence, Research on Immigration and Integration in the Metropolis.

Fernando, S. (1991). *Mental health, race and culture.* London Macmillan/Mind.

Galabuzi, G. (2001). *Canada's creeping economic apartheid: The economic segregation and social marginisation of racialised groups.* Toronto: CJS Foundation for Research & Education.

Globerman, S. (1998). *Immigration and health care: Utilization patterns in Canada.* Vancouver: RIIM.

Guidford, J. (2000). *Making the case for economic and social inclusion.* Ottawa: Health Canada.

Health Canada. (1998). *Metropolis health domain seminar: Final report.* Ottawa: Health Canada.

Henry, F. and Tator, C. (2000). "The theory and practice of democratic racism in Canada," in Kalbach, M. A. and Kalbach, W. E. (Eds.), *Perspectives on ethnicity in Canada.* Toronto: Harcourt.

Human Resources Development Canada (HRDC). (2002). *Knowledge matters: Skills and learning for Canadians: Canada's Innovation Strategy.* Ottawa: HRDC. Online at www.hrdc–drhc.gc.ca/sp–ps/sl–ca/doc/summary.shtml.

Human Resources Development Canada (HRDC). (2001). "Recent immigrants have experienced unusual economic difficulties," *Applied research bulletin* 7 (1), Winter/Spring.

Hutchinson, J. (2000). "Urban policy and social exclusion, " in J. Percy-Smith (Ed.), *Policy responses to social exclusion: Toward inclusion?* Buckingham, U.K.: Open University Presss.

Jackson, A. (2001). "Poverty and immigration," *Perception* 24(4), Spring.

Jenson, J. (2002). *Citizenship: Its relationship to the Canadian diversity model.* Canadian Policy Research Networks (CPRN). Online at www.cprn.org.

Jenson. J. and Papillon, M. (2001). *The changing boundaries of citizenship: A review and a research agenda.* Canadian Policy Research Networks (CPRN). Online at www.cprn.org.

Kawachi, I. R. and Kennedy, B. (2002). *The health of nations: Why inequality is harmful to your health.* New York: New Press.

Kawachi, I., Wilkinson, R. and Kennedy, B. (1999). "Introduction," in Kawachi, I., Kennedy, B. and Wilkinson, R. (Eds.), *The society and population health reader: Volume I: Income inequality and health.* New York: New Press.

Kazemipur, A. and Halli, S. (1997). "Plight of immigrants: The spatial concentration of poverty in Canada," *Canadian journal of regional sciences* (special issue), XX 1/ 2 Spring–Summer 1997, 11–28.

Kazemipur, A. and Halli, S. (2000). *The new poverty in Canada.* Toronto: Thompson Educational Publishing.

Kilbride, K.M, Anisef, P., Baichman-Anisef, E. and Khattar, R. (2000). *Between two worlds: The experiences and concerns of immigrant youth in Ontario.* Toronto: CERIS and CIC–OASIS. Online at www.settlement.org.

Kunz, J. L., Milan. A. and Schetagne, S.. (2001). *Unequal access: A Canadian profile of racial differences in education, employment, and income.* Toronto: Canadian Race Relations Foundation.

Kymlicka, W. and Norman, W. (1995). "Return of the citizen: A survey of recent work on citizenship theory," in Beiner, Ronald (Ed.), *Theorizing citizenship.* Albany: SUNY Press.

Lee, Y. (1999). "Social cohesion in Canada: The role of the immigrant service sector," *OCASI Newsletter* 73, Summer/Autumn 1999.

Lynch, J. (2000). "Income inequality and health: Expanding the debate," *Social science and medicine* 51, 1001–1005.

Madanipour, A. (1998). "Social exclusion and space," in Madanipour, A., Cars G. and Allen, J. (Eds.), *Social exclusion in European cities.* London: Jessica Kingsley.

Marmot, M.(1993). *Explaining socioeconomic differences in sickness absence: The Whitehall II Study.* Toronto: Canadian Institute for Advanced Research.

Marmot, M. and Wilkinson, R. (Eds.). (1999). *Social determinants of health.* Oxford: Oxford University Press.

Marx, K. (1977). *Capital: A critique of political economy, volume one.* New York: Vintage Press.

Noh, S., Beiser, M., Kaspar, V., Hou, F. and Rummens, J. (1999). "Perceived racial discrimination, discrimination, and coping: A study of Southeast Asian refugees in Canada," *Journal of health and social behaviour* 40, 193–207.

Ontario Advisory Council on Women's Issues. (1990). *Women and mental health in Ontario: Immigrant and visible minority women.* Ottawa: Ministry of Health.

Ornstein, M. (2000). *Ethno-racial inequality in the City of Toronto: An analysis of the 1996 Census.* Toronto: City of Toronto. Online at www.ceris.metropolis.net.

Pendakur, R. (2000). *Immigrants and the labour force: Policy, regulation and impact.* Montreal: McGill-Queen's University Press.

Pon, Gordon (2000). "Beamers, cells, malls and cantopop: Thinking through the geographies of Chineseness," in C.E. James (Ed.), *Experiencing difference.* Halifax: Fernwood.

Preston, V. and Man, G. (1999). "Employment experiences of Chinese immigrant women: An exploration of diversity," *Canadian women's studies* 19, 115–122.

Quinn, J. (2002). "Food bank clients often well-educated immigrants," *The Toronto Star*, March 31, 2002, A12.

Raphael, D. (1999). "Health effects on economic inequality," *Canadian review of social policy* 44, 25–40.

Raphael, D. (2001). "From increasing poverty to societal disintegration: How economic inequality affects the health of individuals and communities," in Armstrong, P., Armstrong, H. and Coburn, D. (Eds.), *Unhealthy times: The political economy of health and care in Canada.* Toronto: Oxford University Press.

Reitz, J. G. (2001). "Immigrant skill utilization in the Canadian labour market: Implications of human capital research," *Journal of international migration and integration* 2/3, Summer 2001.

Room, G. (1995). "Conclusions," in Room, G. (Ed.), *Beyond the threshold: The measurement and analysis of social exclusion.* Bristol: Policy.

Saloojee, A. (2002). *Social inclusion, citizenship and diversity: Moving beyond the limits of multiculturalism.* Toronto: Laidlaw Foundation.

Shaw, M., Dorling, D. and Smith, G. D. (1999). "Poverty, social exclusion, and minorities," in Marmot, M. and Wilkinson, R. (Eds.), *Social determinants of health.* Oxford: Oxford University Press.

Shields, J. (2002). "No safe haven: Markets, welfare and migrants" (paper presented to the Canadian Sociology and Anthropology Association, Congress of the Social Sciences and Humanities), Toronto ON, June 1, 2002).

Siemiatycki, M. and Isin, E. (1997). "Immigration, ethno-racial diversity and urban citizenship in Toronto," *Canadian journal of regional sciences* (special issue) XX: 1, 2, Spring–Summer 1997, 73–102.

Wilkinson, R. (1996). *Unhealthy societies: The afflictions of inequality.* New York: Routledge.

Wilkinson, R. and Marmot, M. (2003). *Social determinants of health: The solid facts.* Copenhagen: World Health Organization. Online at www.who.dk/document/e81384.pdf.

Wilson, W. J. (1987). *The truly disadvantaged: Inner city, the underclass and public policy.* Chicago: University of Chicago Press.

Yanz, L., Jeffcoat, B., Ladd, D. and Atlin, J. (1999). *Policy options to improve standards for women garment workers in Canada and internationally.* Toronto: Maquila Solidarity Network/Status of Women Canada.

Yepez Del Costello, I. (1994). "A comparative approach to social exclusion: Lessons from France and Belgium," *International labour review* 133/5–6, 613–633.

# Chapter 17

Bach, M. (2002). *Social inclusion as solidarity: Rethinking the child rights agenda.* Toronto: Laidlaw Foundation.

Barata, P. (2000). *Social exclusion in Europe: Survey of literature.* Toronto: Laidlaw Foundation (unpublished mimeo).

Bloor, M. and McIntosh, J. (1990). "Surveillance and concealment," in Cunningham-Burley, S. L. and

McKeganey, N. L. (Eds.), *Readings in medical sociology.* New York: Tavistock/Routledge.

Dahrendorf, R. (1959). *Class and class conflict in industrial society.* Stanford: Stanford University Press.

Durning, A. (1989). "Mobilizing at the grassroots," in Brown, L., et al. (Eds.), *State of the world 1989.* New York: Norton.

Foucault, M. (1979). *Discipline and punish: The birth of the prison.* Middlesex: Peregrine Books.

Foucault, M. (1980). *Power/knowledge: Selected interviews and other writings.* Gordon, C. (Ed.). New York: Pantheon.

Friedmann, J. (1992). *Empowerment: The politics of alternative development.* Oxford: Blackwell.

Galeano, E. (1973). *Open veins of Latin America: Five centuries of the pillage of a continent.* New York: Monthly Review Press.

Guildford, J. (2000). *Making the case for social and economic inclusion.* Halifax: Health Canada, Population and Public Health Branch, Atlantic Region.

Gyebi, J., Brykczynska, G. and Lister, G. (2002). *Globalisation: Economics and women's health.* London: U.K. Global Health Forum. Online at www.ukglobalhealth.org.

Hochschild, A.R. (2000) "Global care chains and emotional surplus value," in Hutton, W. and Giddens, A. (Eds.), *Global capitalism.* New York: New Press.

Hunter, A. and Staggenborg, S. (1988). "Local communities and organized action," in Milofsky, C. (Ed.), *Community organization: Studies in resource mobilization and exchange.* Oxford: Oxford University Press.

Kelsey, J. (2002). *At the crossroads: Three essays.* Wellington: Bridget Williams Books.

Labonte R., Edwards, R., Green, C., Hershfield, L., Thompson, P., Sushnigg, C. and Sykes, R. (1994). *Equity in action: Analyses of 33 locality equity projects.* Toronto: Ontario Premier's Council on Health, Wellbeing and Social Justice.

Labonte, R. (1999) "Social capital and community development: Practitioner emptor," *Australian and New Zealand journal of public health* 23 (4), 93–96.

Labonte, R. (2003) "Globalization, trade and health: Unpacking the linkages, defining the healthy public policy options," in Hofrichter, R. (Ed.), *Health and social justice: Politics, ideology and inequity in the distribution of disease.* San Francisco: Jossey-Bass.

Lister, R. (2000). *Strategies for social inclusion: Promoting social inclusion or social justice?* New York: St. Martin's Press.

Sen, A. (2000). *Development as freedom.* New York: Knopf.

Taylor, S. and Ashworth, C. (1987). "Durkheim and social realism: An approach to health and illness," in Scambler, G. (Ed.), *Sociological theory and medical sociology.* New York: Methuen.

Unsworth, B. (1993). *A sacred hunger.* New York: Norton.

# Chapter 18

Aboriginal Nurses Association of Canada. (1996). *HIV/AIDS and the impact on aboriginal women in Canada.* Ottawa: Aboriginal Nurses Association of Canada.

D'Cunha, C. (1999). *Diabetes: Strategies for prevention.* Toronto: Ontario Ministry of Health and Long-Term Care.

Diabetes Division Bureau of Cardio-Respiratory Diseases and Diabetes. (1999). *Diabetes in Canada.* Ottawa: Laboratory Center for Disease Control, Health Canada.

Diverty, B. and Perez, C. (1998). "The health of northern residents," *Health reports* 9 (4), 49–55.

Federal Provincial and Territorial Advisory Committee on Population Health. (1999). *Statistical report on the health of Canadians.* Ottawa: Federal Provincial and Territorial Advisory Committee on Population Health.

First Nations and Inuit Health Branch, and Health Canada. (1999). *A Second diagnostic on the health of First Nations and Inuit people in Canada* December 2002. Ottawa: First Nations and Inuit Health Branch, Health Canada. Online at www.hc.sc.gc.ca/fnihb/cp/publications/second_diagnostic_fni.pdf.

Social Determinants of Health

First Nations and Inuit Regional Health Survey National Steering Committee. (1999). *First Nations and Inuit regional health survey: National Report 1999*. Ottawa: Health Canada.

FitzGerald, J., Wang, L. and Elwood, R. (2000). "Tuberculosis: Control of the disease among aboriginal people in Canada," *Canadian Medical Association journal* 162 (3), 351–5.

Food Security Bureau. (2001). Canada's action plan for food security (2001). Ottawa: Agriculture Canada. Online at www.agr.gc.ca/misb/fsb/fsap/fsape.html.

Government of Canada. (1995). "Indian Act: An Act respecting Indians." Online at www.solon.org/Statutes/Canada/English/I/I–5.html.

Government of Canada. (2002). Aboriginal Canada Portal. See www.aboriginalcanada.gc.ca.

Hanselmann, C. (2001). *Urban aboriginal people in Western Canada: Realities and policies.* Calgary: Canada West Foundation.

Kirby, M. and LeBreton, M. (2002). *The health of Canadians: The federal role. Vol 2: Recommendations for reform.* Chapter Five. Ottawa: The Standing Senate Committee on Social Affairs, Science and Technology.

Luepker, R. (1998). "Heart disease," in Wallace, R. (Ed.), *Public health and preventive medicine 14th edition.* Stamford: Appleton & Lange.

MacMillan, H., MacMillan, A., Offord, D. et al. (1996). "Aboriginal health," *Canadian Medical Association journal* 155 (11), 1569–78.

Manitoba Centre for Health Policy. (2002). *The health and health care use of registered First Nations people living in Manitoba: A population-based study.* Winnipeg: Manitoba Centre for Health Policy.

Myers, T., Bullock, S., Calzavara, L., Cockerill, R., Marshall, V. and Mandoka, G. (1999). "Culture and sexual practices in response to HIV among Aboriginal people living on-reseve in Ontario," *Culture, health & sexuality,* 1 (1), 19–37.

Myers, T., Calzavara, L. M., Cockerill, R., Marshall, V. W. and Bullock, S. L. (1993). *Ontario First Nations, AIDS and healthy lifestyle survey.* Toronto: LB Publishing Services.

Richards, J. (2001). *Neighbors matter: Poor neighborhoods and urban aboriginal policy.* Toronto: C. D. Howe Institute.

Royal Commission on Aboriginal Peoples. (1996). *Report of the Royal Commission on Aboriginal Peoples: Gathering strength: Vol 3.* Ottawa: Canada Communication Group.

Royal Commission on Aboriginal Peoples. (1997). *Report of the Royal Commission on Aboriginal Peoples: Gathering strength: Canada's Aboriginal Action Plan.* Ottawa: Canada Communication Group.

Shah, C. P. and Dubeski, G. (1993). "First Nations peoples in urban settings: Health issues," in Masi, R., Mensah, L., McLeod, K. A. and Oakville, K. (Eds.), *Health and cultures: Exploring the relationships.* Oakville: Mosaic Press.

Siggner, A. J. (1986). "The socio-demographic conditions of registered Indians," *Statistics Canada: Canadian social trends* 1 (1), 1–9.

SOGC. (2000). "Guide for health professionals working with Aboriginal peoples: The sociocultural context of aboriginal peoples in Canada," *Journal of Society for Obstetricians and Gynecologists of Canada* 22 (12), 1070–81.

Statistics Canada. (2003). *Aboriginal peoples of Canada: A demographic profile* (Vol. 9, January 2003). Ottawa: Statistics Canada. Online at www12.statcan.ca/english/census01/products/analytic/companion/abor/pdf/96F0030XIE2001007.pdf.

Task Force on Suicide in Canada. (1994). *Suicide in Canada.* Ottawa: Minister of National Health and Welfare.

Tjepkema, M. (2002). *The health of the off-reserve Aboriginal population.* Online at www.statcan.ca/english/freepub/82–003–SIE/82–003–SIE2002003.pdf.

Waldram, J. B., Herring, D. A. and Young, T. K. (1995). *Aboriginal health in Canada: Historical, cultural and epidemiological perspectives.* Toronto: University of Toronto Press.

Young, T., Reading, J., Elias, B. and O'Neill, J. (2000). "Type 2 diabetes mellitus in Canada's First Nations: Status of epidemic in progress," *Canadian Medical Association journal* 163 (5), 561–566.

# Chapter 19

Adams, M. (2003). Fire and ice: The United States, Canada and the myth of converging values. Toronto: Penguin.

Albo, G., Langille, D. and Panitch, L. (1993). A different kind of state: Popular power and democratic administration. Toronto: Oxford University Press.

Broadbent, E. (Ed.). (2001). Democratic equality: What went wrong? Toronto: University of Toronto Press.

Brodie, J. and Jenson, J. (1988). Crisis, challenge and change: Party and class in Canada revisited. Ottawa: Carleton University Press.

Canadian Council of Chief Executives (2004). CFO Website. Online at www.ceocouncil.ca.

Centre for Social Justice. (2003). "Prime Minister and CEO of Canada: Martin's ties to 'big business' too close for comfort." Press release. Toronto: Centre for Social Justice.

Centre for the Study of Living Standards. (2004). Online at csls.ca/data/ipt8.pdf (based on Statistics Canada data).

Clarkson, S. (2002). Uncle Sam and us: Globalization, neoconservatism, and the Canadian state. Toronto: University of Toronto Press.

Coburn, D. (2000), "Income inequality, social cohesion and the health status of populations: The role of neo-liberalism," Social science and medicine 51/1, 135-146.

Court, Jamie. (2003). Corporateering: How corporate power steals your personal freedom … and what you can do about it. New York: Tarcher/Putnam.

Crozier, M. J., Huntington, S. P. and Watanuki, J. (1975). The crisis of democracy: Report on the governability of democracies to the Trilateral Commission. New York: New York University Press.

D'Aquino, T. P. and Stewart-Patterson, D. (2001). Northern edge: How Canadians can triumph in the global economy. Toronto: Stoddart.

Department of Finance, Canada. (2003). Fiscal reference tables, October 2003. Online at www.fin.gc.ca/frt/2003/frt03_e.pdf.

Dobbin, M. (2003). Paul Martin: CEO for Canada? Toronto: Lorimer.

Dobbin, M. (2003 b). "Paul Martin's mea culpa," Winnipeg Free Press, November 9, 2003 (online edition).

Dunbar, A.C. and Derry, D.L. (Eds.)(1984). The Empire Club of Canada Speeches 1982-1983. Toronto, Canada: The Empire Club Foundation.

Frank, T. (2000). One market under God: Extreme capitalism, market populism, and the end of economic democracy. New York: Doubleday.

Glasbeek, H. (2002). Wealth by stealth: Corporate crime, corporate law, and perversion of democracy. Toronto: Between the Lines.

Grinspun, R. (2003). "Placing democracy and sovereignty at the top of the policy agenda in Canada," Canadian dimension 37/5, 35-36.

Hofrichter, Richard (Ed.). (2003). Health and social justice: Politics, ideology, and inequity in the distribution of disease. San Francisco: Jossey-Bass.

Hurtig, M. (2003). The vanishing country: Is it too late to save Canada? Toronto: McClelland and Stewart.

Langille, D. (1987). "The Business Council on national issues and the Canadian State," Studies in political economy (Autumn) 24, 41–85.

Laxer, J. (1998). The Undeclared War: Class conflict in the age of cyber capitalism. Toronto: Viking.

Marchak, P. (1991). The integrated circus: The new right and the restructuring of global markets. Montreal and Kingston: McGill-Queen's University Press.

McBride, S. (2001). Paradigm shift: Globalization and the Canadian state. Halifax: Fernwood.

McBride, S. and Shields, J. (1997). Dismantling a nation: The transition to corporate rule in Canada. Halifax: Fernwood.

McCann, T. C. (1986). Taking reform seriously: Perspectives on public interest liberalism. Ithaca: Cornell University Press.

McQuaig, L. (2002). All you can eat: Greed, lust and the new capitalism. Toronto: Penguin Viking.

Model, D. (2003). Corporate rule: Understanding and challenging the New World Order. Montreal: Black Rose.

Montbiot, G. (2000). Captive state: The corporate takeover of Britain. London: Macmillan.

Moscovitch, A. and Albert, J. (Eds.). (1987). *The benevolent state: The growth of welfare in Canada.* Toronto: Garamond.

Navarro, V. and Shi, L. (2003). "The political context of social inequalities and health," in Hofrichter, R. (Ed.) (2003). *Health and social justice: Politics, ideology, and inequity in the distribution of disease.* San Francisco: Jossey-Bass.

Navarro, V. and Shi, L. (2001). "The political context of social inequalities and health," *Social science and medicine* 52, 481-491.

Panitch, L. and Leys, C. (2003). *The new imperial challenge.* Halifax: Fernwood.

Phillips, K. (2002). *Wealth and democracy: A political history of the American rich.* New York: Broadway.

Stanford, J. (1999). *Paper boom: Why real prosperity requires a new approach to Canada's economy.* Toronto: Canadian Centre for Policy Alternatives, and James Lorimer.

Stanford, J. (2003). "NAFTA @ 10: Hold the propaganda please," *Globe and Mail.* December 21.

Teeple, G. (2000). *Globalization and the decline of social reform: Into the twenty-first century.* Aurora: Garamond.

# Chapter 20

Anis, A. H, Lynd, L. D., Wang, X., et al. (2001). "Double trouble: Impact of inappropriate use of asthma medication on the use of health care resources," *Canadian Medical Association journal* 164, 625–631.

Barratt, A., Irwig, L., Glasziou, et al. (1999). "A paper prepared for a workshop on intersectoral action and health sponsored by Health Promotion and Programs Branch Alberta/NWT/Nunavut Region, Health Canada," March 1999. See "Users guides to the medical literature XVII: How to use guidelines and recommendations about screening," *Journal of the American Medical Association* 281, 2029–2034.

Beaglehole, R. and Bonita, R. (1998). "Public health at the crossroads: Which way forward?" *Lancet* 351, 590–592.

Gibbs V. (2000). "Diabetes in the Capital Health Region. Update 1998/99. Capital Health Region." Victoria: Capital Health Region.. Online at www.viha.ca/mho/chronic/pdf/MSPUpdate.pdf.

Bragaglia, P., Apostolon, C., Wetzl, T. and Lee, H. (2001). *The health promotion initiative in diabetes (HPID) outcomes management program at the group health centre.* Presentation to the Canadian Diabetes Association Annual Meeting.

Citrin, T. (1998). "Topics for our times: Public health: community or commodity? Reflections on healthy communities," *American journal of public health* 88, 351–352.

Daniel, M., Green, L. W., Marion, S. A., et al. (1999). "Effectiveness of community-directed diabetes prevention and control in a rural Aboriginal population in British Columbia, Canada," *Social science and medicine* 48, 815–832.

Douglas, T. (1982). *The future of Medicare.* Archived Speech online at www.healthcoalition.ca/tommy.html.

Fabre, C., Chamari, K., Mucci, P., et al. (2002). "Improvement of cognitive function by mental and/or individualized aerobic training in healthy elderly subjects," *International journal of sports medicine* 23, 415–21.

Fortin, J.-P., Groleau, G., Lemieux, V., O'Neill, M. and Lamarche, P. (1994). *Intersectoral action for health.* Laval: Laval University, mimeo.

Fortmann, S. P.and Varady, A. N. (2000). "Effects of a community-wide health education program on cardiovascular disease morbidity and mortality: The Stanford five-city project," *American journal of epidemiology* 152, 316–323.

French, S. A., Jeffrey R. W. and Story, M. (2001). "Pricing and promotion effects on low-fat vending snack purchases: The CHIPS study," *American journal of public health* 91, 112–117.

Gowans, S. E., DeHueck, A. and Abbey, S. E. (2002). "Measuring exercise-induced mood changes in fibromyalgia: A comparison of several measures," *Arthritis & rheumatism* 47, 603–9.

Hall, N., De Beck, P., Johnson, D., Mackinnon, K., Gutman, G. and Glick, N. (1992). "Randomized trial of a health promotion program for frail elders," *Canadian journal on aging* 11, 72–91.

Hancock, T. (1992). "Public policies for healthy cities: Involving the policy makers," in Flynn, B.C. (Ed.),

*Proceedings of the Inaugural Conference of the World Health Organization Collaborating Center on Healthy Cities.* Indianapolis: Institute of Action Research for Community Health, Indiana School of Nursing.

Heart and Stroke Foundation of Canada. (2000). *The changing face of heart disease and stroke in Canada.* Online at www.hc–sc.gc.ca/pphb–dgspsp/ccdpc–cpcmc/cvd–mcv/publications/pdf/card2ke.pdf 030327.

Hertzman, C. (1996). Presentation to annual meeting of the Canadian Public Health Association, July 4, 1996.

Hoffman, C., Rice, D. and Sung, H. Y. (1996). "Persons with chronic conditions: Their prevalence and costs," *Journal of the American Medical Association* 276, 1473–9.

Hutchison, B., Woodward, C., Norman, G., et al. (1998). "Provision of preventive care to unannounced standardized patients," *Canadian Medical Association journal* 158, 185–193.

Institute for Clinical Evaluative Sciences. (2002). *Diabetes in Ontario: An ICES practice atlas.* Online at www.ices.on.ca 030108.

Joffres, M. R., Ghadian, P., Fodor J.G., et al. (1997). "Awareness, treatment, and control of hypertension in Canada," *American journal of hypertension* 10, 1097–1102.

King, M. (1992). "Comprehensive care management: A closer look," *New York doctor.*

Kokkinos, P. F., Narayan, P., Colleran, J. A., et al. (1995). "Effects of regular exercise on blood pressure and left ventricular hypertrophy in African-American men with sever hypertension," *New England journal of medicine* 333, 1462–1467.

Laville, J.L. and Nyssens, M. (2001). The social enterprise: Toward a theoretical approach," in Borzaga, C. and Defourny, J. (Eds.), *The emergence of social enterprise.* London: Routledge.

Lee, H., Garniss, D., Oliver, R., et al. (2001). "A community hospital-based heart failure program decreases readmission rates." Abstract for Society of General Internal Medicine meeting in San Diego May 2001.

Macaulay, A. C., Paraids, G., Potvin, L., et al. (1997). "The Kahnawake schools diabetes prevention project: Intervention, evaluation, and baseline results of a diabetes primary prevention program with a native community in Canada," *Preventive medicine* 26, 779–790.

Markel, H. (2002). "Diagnosis supersize," *New York Times* March 24, 2002, A4.

Marmot, M. (1998). "Improvement of social environment to improve health," *Lancet* 351, 57–60.

McKeown, T. (1979). *The role of medicine: Dream, mirage or memesis.* Oxford: Blackwell.

Mellor, C. (2000). "Uncontrolled asthma worse in Nova Scotia," *Halifax Mail Herald*, May 10, 2000, A4.

Nygard, J. F., Skare, G. B. and Thoresen, S. (2002). "The cervical cancer screening programme in Norway, 1992–2000: Changes in Pap Smear coverage and incidence of cervical cancer," *Journal of medical screening* 9, 86–91.

Ornish, D., Brown, S. E., Scherwitz, L. W., et al. (1990). "Can lifestyle changes reverse coronary heart disease?" *Lancet* 336, 129–133.

Ornish D., Scherwitz, L. W., Billings, J. H., et al. (1998). "Intensive lifestyle changes for reversal of coronary heart disease," *JAMA* 280, 2001–7.

Ortega, F., Toral, J., Cejudo, P., et al. (2002). "Comparison of effects of strength and endurance training in patients with chronic obstructive pulmonary disease," *American journal of respiratory & critical care medicine* 166, 669–74.

Pearce, N.(1997). "Pearce responds," *American journal of public health* 87, 2051.

Puska, P., Vartiainen, E., Tuomilehto, J., et al. (1998). "Changes in premature deaths in Finland: Successful long-term prevention of cardiovascular diseases," *Bulletin of the World Health Organization* 76, 419–425.

Putnam, R. D., Leonardi, R., and Nanetti, R. Y. (1993). *Making democracy work: Civic traditions in modern Italy.* Princeton: Princeton University Press.

Rachlis, M.M. (1999). A paper prepared for a workshop on intersectoral action and health sponsored by Health Promotion and Programs Branch Alberta/NWT/Nunavut Region, Health Canada. Available from the author at michaelrachlis@rogers.com.

Ransohoff, D.F. and Sandler, R.S. (2002). "Screening for colorectal cancer," *New England journal of medicine* 346, 40–44.

Social Determinants of Health

Raphael, D. and Farrell, E.S. (2002). "Beyond medicine and lifestyle: Addressing the societal determinants of cardiovascular disease in North America," *Leadership in health services* 15, 1–5.

Richmond Health Board. (2001). *Evaluation of clinical paths for congestive heart failure patients: Spanning the continuum of care.* Vancouver: Richmond Health Board.

Rochon, P.A., Anderson, G.M., Tu, J.V., et al. (1999). "Use of beta-blocker therapy in older patients after acute myocardial infarction in Ontario," *Canadian Medical Association journal* 161 (11), 1403–8.

Rose, G. (1981). "Strategy of prevention: Lessons from cardiovascular diseases," *British medical journal* 282, 1847–1851.

Rose, G. (1985). "Sick individuals and sick populations," *International journal of epidemiology* 14, 32–38.

Rosen, G.A. (1958). *History of public health.* New York: MD Publications.

Ross, L.H. (1989). "Lost and found: The drunk-driving problem in Finland," in Best, J. (Ed.), *Images of issues: Typifying contemporary social problems.* New York: De Gruyter.

Rowley, K.G., Daniel, M., Skinner, K., at al. (2000). "Effectiveness of a community-directed 'healthy lifestyle' program in a remote Australian aboriginal community," *Australian and New Zealand journal of public health* 24, 136–144.

Schuler, G., Hambrecht, R., Schlierf, G., et al. (1992). "Regular physical exercise and low-fat diet: Effects on progression of coronary artery disease," *Circulation* 86, 1–11.

Sox, H.C. (1998). "Benefit and harm associated with screening for breast cancer," *New England journal of medicine* 338, 1145–1146.

Stampfer, M.J., Hu, F.B., Manson, J.E., et al. (2000). "Primary prevention of coronary heart disease in women through diet and lifestyle," *New England journal of medicine* 343, 16–22.

Taylor, R. and Rieger, A. (1985). "Medicine as social science: Rudolf Virchow on the typhus epidemic in upper Silesia," *International journal of health services* 15, 547–559.

UK Prospective Diabetes Study Group. (1998). "Intensive blood glucose control with sulphonylureas or insulin compared with conventional treatment and risk of complications in type 2 diabetes: UKPDS 33," *The Lancet* 352, 837–853.

Wagner, E. H., Sandhu, N., Newton, K. M., et al. (2001). "Effect of improved glycemic control on health care costs and utilization," *Journal of the American Medical Association* 285, 182–189.

Wagner, E. H. (1997). "Preventing decline in function: Evidence from randomized trials around the world," *Western journal of medicine* 167, 295–8.

Walker, A. G. (2002). "Mohawks take charge to prevent type 2 diabetes," *Medical Post* January 15, 5.

Wolf, H. K., Andreou, P., Bata, I. R., et al. (1999). "Trends in the prevalence and treatment of hypertension in Halifax County from 1985 to 1995," *Canadian Medical Association journal* 161, 699–704.

Young, T. K., Reading, J., Elias, B. and O'Neil, J. D. (2000). "Type 2 diabetes mellitus in Canada's first nations: Status of an epidemic in progress," *Canadian Medical Association journal* 163, 561–566.

# Chapter 21

Arpin, R. (1999). *La complémentarité du secteur privé dans la poursuite des objectifs fondamentaux du système public de santé au Québec.* Quebec: Rapport Arpin.

Aubry, F. (2001). *Trente ans déjà: Le mouvement syndical et le développement des services de garde au Québec.* Montreal: Confédération des syndicats nationaux et table ronde pour le développement des ressources humaines du secteur des services de garde.

Axworthy, L. (1994). *Improving social security in Canada: A discussion paper.* Ottawa: Government of Canada.

Battle, K., Torjman, S. and Mendelson, M. (2002). "Foundations and future of social policy in Canada: Three short speeches from the Caledon Institute's 10th anniversary celebration, November 6, 2002," Ottawa: Caledon Institute of Social Policy. Online at www.caledoninst.org.

Battle, K. and Torjman, S. (2002). *Architecture for national child care.* Ottawa: Caledon Institute of Social Policy.

Beresford, P. and Holden, C. (2002). "We have choices: Globalization and welfare user movements," *Disability and society* 19, 7, 973–989.

Canadian Center for Philanthropy and Associates (CCP). (2003). *The capacity to serve.* Toronto: CCP.

Chantier de l'économie sociale. (1996). *Osons la solidarité, rapport du groupe de travail sur l'économie sociale.* Québec: Sommet sur l'économie et l'emploi.

Chantier de l'économie sociale. (2001). *De nouveau nous osons, document de positionnement stratégique.* Montréal: Chantier de l'économie sociale.

Chantier de l'économie sociale. (2003). *L'Économie sociale en mouvement, Actualités* novembre 2003, 6.

Charbonneau, C. (2002). "Développer l'intégration au travail en santé mentale, une longue marche à travers des obstacles sociopolitiques," *Santé mentale au Québec* 27, 1.

Charbonneau, C. (2004). *Travail et santé mentale: Les défis à relever.* Montréal Cahiers du LAREPPS and Fondation Travail, santé mentale, UQAM, no 04–01.

Comité de la santé mentale du Québec (CSMQ). (1997). *Bilan d'implantation de la politique de santé mentale.* Québec: Ministère de la Santé et des Services sociaux.

Clair, M. (2000). *Les solutions émergentes: Rapport et recommandations.* Rapport Clair Québec.

Conseil de la santé et du bien-être (CSBE). (2002). *Avis pour une stratégie du Québec en santé: Décider et agir.* Québec: Conseil de la santé et du bien-être.

D'Amours, M. (2002). "Économie sociale au Québec: Vers un clivage entre entreprise collective et action communautaire," *RECMA: Revue internationale de l'économie sociale* 284, 31–44.

Donnelly-Cox, G., Donoghue, F. and Taylor, R. (Eds.). (2001). "The third sector in Ireland, North and South," *Voluntas* 12, 3.

Ducharme, M.-N. and Vaillancourt, Y. (Forthcoming). "À l'orée d'une gouvernance associative? L'expérience du Fonds québécois d'habitation communautaire," *Économie et solidarité.*

Dumais, L. (2001). Accès-Cible (SMT): *Monographie d'un organisme d'aide à l'insertion pour les personnes ayant des problèmes de santé mentale.* Montréal: UQAM, Cahiers du LAREPPS 01–06.

Esping-Andersen, G. (1999). *Les trois mondes de l'État-providence: Essai sur le capitalisme moderne.* Paris: PUF, coll. Le Lien social.

Esping-Andersen, G. (2000). "Prologo," in Montagu, T. (2000). *Politica social. Una introduccion.* Barcelona: Ariel Sociologia.

Federal/Provincial/Territorial Ministers Responsible for Social Services. (1998). *In unison: A Canadian approach to disability issues. A vision paper.* Ottawa: Human Resources Development Canada.

Fonds québécois d'habitation communautaire. (1999). *Rapport annuel 1998–99.* Québec.

Fortin, S., Noël, A. and St-Hilaire, F. (Eds.). (2003). *Forging the Canadian social union: SUFA and beyond.* Montréal: Institute for Research on Public Policy.

Forum national sur la santé. (1997a). *La santé au Canada: Un héritage à faire fructifier. Rapport final.* Ottawa: Forum national sur la santé.

Forum national sur la santé. (1997b). *La santé au Canada: Un héritage à faire fructifier. Rapports de synthèse et documents de référence.* Ottawa: Forum national sur la santé.

Fuchs, D. (1987). "Breaking down barriers: Independent living resource centres for empowering the physically disabled," in Ismael, J. S. and Thomlison, R. J. (Eds.), *Perspectives on social services and social issues.* Ottawa: Canadian Council of Social Development.

Jerôme-Forget, M. (1998). "Canada's social union: Staking out the future of federalism," *Policy options* November 1998, 3–5.

Jetté, C., Lévesque, B., Mager, L. and Vaillancourt, Y. (2000). *Économie sociale et transformation de l'État–providence dans le domaine de la santé et du bien-être. Une recension des écrits (1990–2000).* Montréal: Presses de l'Université du Québec.

Jetté, C., Lévesque, B. and Vaillancourt, Y. (2001). *The social economy and the future of health and welfare in Québec and Canada.* Montréal: UQAM, Cahier du LAREPPS 01–04.

Jetté, C., Thériault, L., Mathieu, R. and Vaillancourt, Y. (1998). *Évaluation du logement social avec support communautaire à la Fédération des OSBL d'habitation de Montréal (FOHM).* Montréal: UQAM, LAREPPS.

Lauzon, G. and Charbonneau, C. (with the collaboration of G. Provost). (2001). *Favoriser l'intégration au travail: l'urgence d'agir.* Québec: Association québécoise pour la réadaptation psychosociale.

Larose, G., Vaillancourt, Y., Shields, G. and Kearney, M. (2003). "Contributions of the social economy to the renewal of policies and practices in the area of welfare to work in Québec during the years 1983–2003," paper presented at the National Forum Welfare to Work, St-John's, Newfoundland, November 16–18 2003.

Laville, J.-L. (Ed.). (2000). *L'économie solidaire: Une perspective internationale, 2nd edition*. Paris: Desclée de Brouwer.

Laville, J.-L. and Nyssens, M. (Eds.). (2001). *Les services sociaux entre associations, État et marché. L'aide aux personnes âgées*. Paris: La Découverte/Mauss/Crida.

Lévesque, B. and Ninacs, W. A. (1997). "The social economy in Canada: The Québec Experience" (issues paper for the conference "Local Strategies for Employment and the Social Economy"), Montreal, June 18–19 1997. Montréal: Les Publications de l'IFDEC.

Lévesque, B., Girard and Malo, M.-C. (1999). "L'ancienne et la nouvelle économie sociale. Deux dynamiques, un mouvement : le cas du Québec," in Defourny, J., Develtere, P. and Fonteneau, B (Eds.), *L'Économie sociale au Nord et au Sud*. Brussels: De Boeck Université.

Mendelson, M. and Battle, K. (2003). *Why Canada needs a federal–provincial social security review now*. Ottawa: Caledon Institute of Social Policy.

Mercier, C., Provost, G., Denis G. and Vincelette, F. (1999). *Le développement de l'employabilité et l'intégration au travail pour les personnes ayant des problèmes de santé mentale*. Montréal: Centre de recherche de l'hôpital Douglas.

Ministère de l'Industrie et du Commerce. (2002). *Portrait des entreprises en aide domestique*. Québec: Gouvernement du Québec.

Ministère de la Santé et des Services sociaux (MSSS). (1992). *La politique de la santé et du bien-être*. Québec: Gouvernement du Québec.

Noël, A. (2003). "Power and purpose in intergovernmental relations," in Fortin, S., Noël, A. and St-Hilaire, F. (Eds.), *Forging the Canadian social union: SUFA and beyond*. Montreal: Institute for Research on Public Policy.

Office des personnes handicapées du Québec (OPHQ). (1984). *À part ... égale. L'intégration sociale des personnes handicapées : un défi pour tous*. Drummondville: Gouvernement du Québec.

Polanyi, K. (2001). *The great transformation*. Boston: Beacon.

Pomeroy, S. (1996). "Final comments," *The role of housing in social policy*. Ottawa: Caledon Institute of Social Policy.

Puttee, A. (Ed.). (2002). *Federalism, democracy and disability policy in Canada*. Montreal and Kingston: McGill-Queen's University Press.

Quarter, J., Mook, L. and Richmond, B. J. (2003). *What counts: Social accounting for nonprofits and cooperatives*. Upper Saddle River, NJ: Prentice Hall.

Quarter, J. (1992). *Canada's social economy: Cooperatives, non-profits, and other community enterprises*. Toronto: Lorimer.

Ramon, S. (Ed.). (1991). *Beyond community care: Normalisation and integration work*. London: Macmillan.

Roeher Institute. (1993). *Social well-being: A paradigm for reform*. North York: Roeher Institute.

Salamon, L., Anheier, H. K., List, R., Toepler, S., Sokolowski, S. and Associates (Eds.). (1999). *Global civil society: Dimensions of the nonprofit sector*. The John Hopkins Comparative Nonprofit Sector Project. Baltimore: The John Hopkins Center for Civil Society Studies.

Shragge, E. and Fontan, J. M. (2000). *Social economy: International debates and perspectives*. Montreal: Black Rose.

Taylor, M. (1995). "Voluntary action and the state," in Gladstone, D. (Ed.), *British social welfare: Past, present and future*. London: UCL Press.

Thériault, L., Jetté, C., Mathieu, R. and Vaillancourt, Y. (2001). *Social housing with community support: A study of the FOHM experience*. Ottawa: Caledon Institute of Social Policy. Online at www.caledoninst.org.

Vaillancourt, Y. (1996). "Remaking Canadian social policy: A Québec viewpoint," in Pulkingham, J.and Ternowetsky, G. (Eds.). (1996). *Remaking Canadian social policy: Staking claims and forging change*. Halifax: Fernwood.

References

Vaillancourt, Y. (1999). "Tiers secteur et reconfiguration des politiques sociales," *Nouvelles pratiques sociales* 11, 2 and 12, 1, 21–39.

Vaillancourt, Y. (2003a). *Jalons théoriques pour l'examen des politiques sociales touchant les personnes handicapées*. Montréal, UQAM: Cahiers du CRISES, no 0304.

Vaillancourt, Y. (2003b). "The Quebec model in social policy and its interface with Canada's social union," in Fortin S., Noël, A .and St-Hilaire, F. (Eds.), *Forging the Canadian social union: SUFA and beyond*. Montreal: Institute for Research on Public Policy.

Vaillancourt, Y. and Ducharme, M.-N. (with the collaboration of Cohen, R., Roy, C. and Jetté, C.). (2001). *Social housing: A key component of social policies in transformation: The Québec experience*. Ottawa: Caledon Institute of Social Policy. Online at www.caledoninst.org.

Vaillancourt, Y. and Favreau, L. (2001). "Le modèle québécois d'économie sociale et solidaire," *Revue internationale de l'économie sociale: RECMA* 281, 69–83.

Vaillancourt, Y. and Jetté, C. (1997). *Vers un nouveau partage de responsabilité dans les services sociaux et de santé: rôles de l'État, du marché, de l'économie sociale et du secteur informel*. Montréal, UQAM: Cahiers du LAREPPs.

Vaillancourt, Y. and Laville, J. L. (1998). "Les rapports entre les associations et l'État: un enjeu politique," *La revue du MAUSS semestrielle* 11, 119–135.

Vaillancourt, Y. and Tremblay, L. (Eds.) (2002). *Social economy: Health and welfare in four Canadian provinces*. Montreal/Halifax: LAREPPS/Fernwood.

Vaillancourt, Y., Aubry, F., Jetté, C. and Tremblay, L. (2002). "Regulation based on solidarity: A fragile emergence in Québec," in Vaillancourt, Y. and Tremblay, L. (Eds). *Social economy: Health and welfare in four Canadian provinces*. Montreal/Halifax: LAREPPS/Fernwood.

Vaillancourt, Y. Aubry, F., D'Amours, M., Jetté, C. Thériault, L. and Tremblay, L. (2000). "Social economy, health and welfare: The specificity of the Quebec model with the Canadian context," *Canadian review of social policy* 45/46, 55–88.

Vaillancourt, Y., Caillouette, J. and Dumais. L. (Eds.). (2002). *Les politiques sociales s'adressant aux personnes ayant des incapacités au Québec*. Montréal: LAREPPS/ARUC–Economie Sociale/UQAM

Vaillancourt, Y., Aubry, F., Tremblay, L., Kearney, M. and Thériault, L. (2003). *Social policy as a determinant of health and well-being: Lessons from Québec on the contribution of the social economy* (SPR Occasional Paper). Regina: Social Policy Research Unit, University of Regina, ,

Vaillancourt, Y., Aubry, F. and Jetté, C. (Eds.). (2003). *L'économie sociale dans les services à domicile*. Quebec: Presses de l'Université du Québec.

World Health Organization (WHO). (1998). *Social determinants of health: The solid facts*. Copenhagen: World Health Organization Regional Office for Europe.

# Chapter 22

Armstrong, P. and Armstrong, H. (2002). "Women, privatization and health care reform: The Ontario case," in Armstrong, P. et al.(Eds.), *Exposing privatization: Women and health care reform in Canada*. Aurora: Garamond.

Armstrong, P. and Cornish, M. (1997). "Restructuring pay equity for a restructured workforce: Canadian perspectives," *Gender, work and organization* 4: 2 (April 1997), 67–86.

Benoit, C., Carroll, D. and Millar, A. (2002). "But is it good for non-urban women's health? Regionalizing maternity care services in British Columbia," *Canadian review of sociology and anthropology* 39, 4 November 2002, 373–396.

Bernier, J. and Dallaire, M. (2002). "What price have women paid for health care reform? The situation in Quebec," in Armstrong, P., et al.(Eds.), *Exposing privatization: Women and health care reform in Canada*. Aurora: Garamond.

Boivin, L. and Fournier, M. (1998). *L'Économie sociale: l'Avenir d'une illusion*. Montreal: Fides.

Cohen, M. G. (2001). "Do comparisons between hospital support workers and hospitality workers make sense?" Report Prepared for the Hospital Employees Union, Vancouver B.C.

Commission on the Future of Health Care. (2002). *Building on values. The future of health care in Canada*.

Ottawa: Commission on the Future of Health Care in Canada.

Dion Stout, M., Kipling, G. D. and Stout, R. (2001). Aboriginal women's health research synthesis project. Online at www.cwhn.ca

Doré, G. (1991). "Les relations réseau–communautaire: Vers la coopèration conflictuelle," *Circuit socio-communitaire* 3 (1).

Horne, T., Donner, L. and Thurston, W. E. (1999). *Invisible women: Gender and health planning in Manitoba and Saskatchewan and models for progress*. Winnipeg: Prairie Women's Health Centre of Excellence.

Jackson, A. and Sanger, M. (2003). *When worlds collide: Implications of international trade and investment agreements for non-profit social services*. Ottawa: Canadian Centre for Policy Alternatives.

Knapp, M., Hardy, B. and Forder, J. (2001). "Commissioning for quality: Ten years of social care markets in England," *Journal of social policy* 30 (2), 283–306.

Morris, M(2001). *Gender-sensitive home and community care and caregiving research: A synthesis paper*. Ottawa: Health Canada.

National Forum on Health. (1997). Synthesis report and issues papers. Ottawa: National Forum on Health.

Rekart, J. (1993). *Public funds, private provision*. Vancouver: University of British Columbia Press.

Renaud, M. (1987). "Reform or illusion? An analysis of the Quebec state intervention in health," in Coburn, D., et al. (Eds.), *Health and Canadian society, 2nd edition*. Markham: Fitzhenry and Whiteside.

Statistics Canada. (2000). *Women in Canada*. Ottawa: Industry Canada.

Tremblay, L., Aubrey, F., Jetté, C. and Vaillancourt, Y. (2002). "Introduction," in Vaillancourt, Y., et al. (Eds.), *Social economy, health and welfare in four Canadian provinces*. Halifax: Fernwood.

# Chapter 23

Agren, G. and Hedin, A. (2002). *The new Swedish public health policy*. National Institute of Public Health. Online at www.fhi.se/pdf/roll_eng.pdf.

Ashton, J. (1992). *Healthy cities*. London: Routledge.

Atlantic Centre of Excellence for Women's Health. (2000). *Social and economic inclusion in Atlantic Canada*. Atlantic Centre of Excellence for Women's Health. Online at www.medicine.dal.ca/acewh/inclusion–preface.htm.

Burstrom, B., Diderichsen, F., Ostlin, P. and Ostergren, P. O. (2002). "Sweden," in Bakker, M. (Ed.), *Reducing inequalities in health: A European perspective*. London: Routledge.

Canadian Labour Congress. (2003). *Economy: Economic review and outlook* 14, 2. Ottawa: Canadian Labour Congress.

Curry-Stevens, A. (2003). *An educator's guide for changing the world: Methods, models and materials for anti-oppression and social justice workshops*. Toronto: Centre for Social Justice.

Curry-Stevens, A. (2004). "Arrogant capitalism: Changing futures, changing lives," *Canadian review of social policy* 52 (forthcoming).

Coburn, D. (2000). "Income inequality, social cohesion and the health status of populations: The role of neo-liberalism," *Social science and medicine* 51, 1, 135–146.

Davies, J. K. and Kelly, M. P. (Eds.). (1993). *Healthy cities: Research and practice*. New York: Routledge.

Ehrenreich, B. (2001). *Nickel and dimed: On (not) getting by in America*. New York: Holt.

Fischer, F. (2000). *Citizens, experts, and the environment: The politics of local knowledge*. Durham: Duke University Press.

Hatfield, J. (2002). *Fortunate son: George W. Bush and the making of an American president*. New York: Soft Skull Press.

Hobgood, M. (2000). *Dismantling privilege: An ethics of accountability*. Cleveland: Pilgrim.

Hulchanski, D. (2002). *Can Canada afford to help cities, provide social housing, and end homelessness? Why are provincial governments doing so little?* Toronto: Centre for Urban and Community Studies, University of Toronto. Online at www.tdrc.net/2rept29.htm.

Jackson, A. (2002). *Canada beats USA – but loses gold to* Sweden. Canadian Council on Social Development (CCSD). Online at www.ccsd.ca/pubs/2002/olympic/indicators.htm.

Lahelma, E., Keskimaki, I. and Rahkonen, O. (2002). "Income maintenance policies: The example of Finland," in Bakker, M. (Ed.), *Reducing inequalities in health: A European perspective*. London: Routledge.

Mackenbach, J. and Bakker, M. (Eds.). (2002). *Reducing inequalities in health: A European perspective*. London: Routledge.

McLaren, P. (2003). "Critical pedagogy: A look at the major concepts," in Darder, A. (Ed.), *The critical pedagogy reader*. New York: Routledge Falmer.

Ministry of Social Affairs and Health. (2001). *Government resolution on the Health 2015 public health program*. Helsinki: Ministry of Social Affairs and Health.

Moore, M. (2003). *Dude, where's my country?* New York: Warner.

Navarro, V. (Ed.). (2002). *The political economy of social inequalities: Consequences for health and quality of* life. Amityville: Baywood Press.

Navarro, V. and Shi, L. (2001). "The political context of social inequalities and health," *Social science and medicine* 52, 481–491.

Nettleton, S. (1997). "Surveillance, health promotion and the formation of a risk identity," in Peberdy, A. (Ed.), *Debates and dilemmas in promoting health*. London: Open University.

Phillips, K. (2002). *Wealth and democracy*. New York: Broadway.

Popay, J. and Williams, G. H. (Eds.). (1994). *Researching the people's health*. London: Routledge.

Raphael, D. (2001). "From increasing poverty to societal disintegration: how economic inequality affects the health of individuals and communities," in Armstrong, P., Armstrong, H. and Coburn, D. (Eds.), *Unhealthy times: The political economy of health and care in Canada*. Toronto: Oxford University Press.

Raphael, D. (2002a). "Addressing health inequalities in Canada," *Leadership in health services* 15, 3, 1–8.

Raphael, D. (2002b). *Poverty, income inequality and health in Canada*. Centre for Social Justice Foundation for Research and Education (CSJ). Online at www.socialjustice.org/pubs/income&Health.pdf.

Raphael, D. (2002c). *Social justice is good for our hearts: Why societal factors—not lifestyles—are major causes of heart disease in Canada and elsewhere*. Centre for Social Justice Foundation for Research and Education (CSJ). Online at www.socialjustice.org/pubs/justiceHearts.pdf.

Raphael, D. (2003a). "Towards the future: Policy and community actions to promote population health," in Hofrichter, R. (Ed.), *Health and social justice: A reader on politics, ideology, and inequity in the distribution of disease*. San Francisco: Jossey-Bass/Wiley

Raphael, D. (2003b). "A society in decline: the social, economic, and political determinants of health inequalities in the USA," in Hofrichter, R. (Ed.), *Health and social justice: A reader on politics, ideology, and inequity in the distribution of disease*. San Francisco: Jossey-Bass/Wiley.

Raphael, D. (2003c). "Barriers to addressing the determinants of health: Public health units and poverty in Ontario, Canada," *Health promotion international* 18, 415–423.

Raphael, D. (2003d). "Bridging the gap between knowledge and action on the societal determinants of cardiovascular disease: How one Canadian community effort hit—and hurdled—the lifestyle wall," *Health education* 103, 177–189.

Raphael, D. (2003e). "Addressing the social determinants of health in Canada: Bridging the gap between research findings and public policy," *Policy options* 24, 3, 35–40.

Raphael, D., Anstice, S., Raine, K., et al. (2003). "The social determinants of the incidence and management of Type 2 Diabetes Mellitus: Are we prepared to rethink our questions and redirect our research activities?" *Leadership in health services* 16, 10–20.

Raphael, D. and Bryant, T. (2004). "The welfare state as a determinant of women's health: Support for women's quality of life in Canada and four comparison nations," *Health policy* 68, 63–79.

Raphael, D., Renwick, R., Brown, I., Phillips, S., Sehdev, H. and Steinmetz, B. (2001a). "Community quality of life in low income urban neighbourhoods: Findings from two contrasting communities in Toronto, Canada," *Journal of the community development society* 32, 2, 310–333.

Raphael, D., Renwick, R., Brown, I., Steinmetz, B., Sehdev, H. and Phillips, S. (2001b). "Making the links between community structure and individual well-being. Community quality of life in Riverdale,

Social Determinants of Health

Toronto, Canada," *Health and place* 7/3, 17–34.

Romanow, R. J. (2002). *Building on values: The future of health care in Canada.* Saskatoon: Commission on the Future of Health Care in Canada.

Sauve, Roger. (2002). *The dreams and the reality: Assets, debts and net worth of Canadian households.* Ottawa: Vanier Institute on the Family.

Statistics Canada. (2001). *The assets and debts of Canadians: An overview of the results of the survey of financial security.* Ottawa: Statistics Canada.

Shaw, M., Dorling, D. and Davey Smith, G. (1999). "Poverty, social exclusion, and minorities," in Marmot, M. and Wilkinson, R. G. (Ed.), *Social determinants of health.* Oxford: Oxford University Press.

Teeple, G. (2000). *Globalization and the decline of social reform.* Aurora: Garamond.

Tesh, S. (1990). *Hidden arguments: Political ideology and disease prevention policy.* New Brunswick: Rutgers University Press.

Williams, G. and Popay, J. (1997). "Social science and the future of population health," in Sidell, M. (Ed.), *The challenge of promoting health.* London: Open University.

World Health Organization. (1986). *Ottawa charter for health promotion.* World Health Organization, Europe Office. Online at www.who.dk/policy/ottawa.htm.

World Health Organization. (1997). *Twenty steps for developing a Healthy Cities project.* Copenhagen: World Health Organization Regional Office for Europe.

World Health Organization Regional Office for Europe. (2003). *Healthy cities: Books and published technical documents.* Online at http://www.who.dk/healthy-cities/Documentation/20010914_2.

Zweig, M. (2000), *The working class majority: America's best kept secret.* Ithaca: Cornell University Press.

# CONTRIBUTORS' BIOGRAPHIES

**Pat Armstrong** is co-author or editor of such books on health care as *Exposing privatization: Women and health reform in Canada; Unhealthy times, heal thyself: Managing health care reform; Wasting away: The undermining of Canadian health care; Universal health care: What the United States can learn from Canada; Medical alert: New work organizations in health care; Vital signs: Nursing in transition;* and *Take care: Warning signals for Canada's health system*. She has also published on a wide variety of issues related to women's work and social policy. She has served as Chair of the Department of Sociology at York University and Director of the School of Canadian Studies at Carleton University. Currently, she is a partner in the National Network on Environments and Women's Health and chairs a working group on health reform that crosses the Centres of Excellence for Women's Health. She holds a CHSRF/CHIR Chair in Health Services.

**François Aubry** is an economist and has been a member of LAREPPS since 1999. For several years, his work at the research unit of the CSN (Confederation of National Trade Unions) focused on the social and economic situation, the reduction and the adjustment of working time, tax issues, social security, and social economy.

**Nathalie Auger** has a Master's degree in Epidemiology and Biostatistics from McGill University and is presently in her last year of residency in Community Medicine at the Montreal Public Health Unit.

**Gina B. Browne** is founder and director of the System-Linked Research Unit (SLRU) on Health and Social Service Utilization based at McMaster University, Hamilton, Ontario. She is a Professor, Nursing and Clinical Epidemiology and Biostatistics, at McMaster University, Faculty of Health Sciences.

Dr. Browne has also functioned as a Halton Health Service Organization part-time family therapist since 1978 and has a long track record of conducting research in chronic illness and service utilization, in developing others in the conduct of research, linking and coordinating a variety of clinical and research initiatives. She is particularly interested in clientele shared by health and social sectors, the combination of problems that guides simultaneous use of services, factors which explain the variability of client outcomes and the cost of a "life without purpose" to society. It has been said that, "Gina often thinks the unthinkable, says the unsayable and does the undoable!"

**Toba Bryant** is a post-doctoral fellow at the Centre for Health Studies at York University. Her doctoral thesis examined how housing and health activists used different forms of knowledge to influence policy development during the "Common Sense Revolution" in Ontario. She is currently investigating how the ideological stances of government policy-makers shape state receptivity to the theoretical concepts and demonstrated importance of the social determinants of health. Dr. Bryant's recent publications have been concerned with the policy-change process, hospital restructuring in Ontario, housing policy, and Toronto seniors' quality of life as revealed through a participatory policy process.

**Tracey Burns** is a Research Analyst with the Organization for Economic Cooperation and Development in Paris evaluating programs for youth at risk. She holds a PhD (Northeastern University) in Psychology with a specialty in early language acquisition.

**Robert Choinière** is in charge of population health surveillance at the Montreal Public Health Unit and clinical adjunct professor in the Department of Social and Preventive Medicine at the University of Montreal.

**Ann Curry-Stevens** has been both overseeing research on the growing income gap and conducting original research for the last five years. Ann is based in Toronto where she has been active with social movements for the last 12 years. She was the lead researcher and author of the Centre for Social Justice's third annual update on inequality in Canada, "When markets fail people." She is formerly Co-Director of Management and Research at the Centre for Social Justice and today continues her association with the organization as a Research and Education Associate. Ann is currently completing her PhD at the University of Toronto's Ontario Institute for Studies in Education. Ann lives in Toronto with her partner, Timothy, and their 6-year old daughter, Michele.

**Janice Foley** completed her PhD in Organizational Behaviour from the University of British Columbia in 1995. She assumed her first academic position at the University of Winnipeg in 1998, and moved to the University of Regina in 2000. Current research interests include organized labour's response to globalization and changing workplace practices and their impact on employee health and worklife quality.

**Martha Friendly** is a Senior Research Associate at the University of Toronto and Co-ordinator of the Childcare Resource and Research Unit at the University of Toronto. CRRU is a policy research facility that specializes in early childhood education and care (ECEC). Born in New York City and educated in the U.S., she immigrated to Canada in 1971. She has two grown children. She has been actively involved in advocating for progressive social

Social Determinants of Health

policy for many years and works closely with a variety of community and advocacy groups as well as with government policy-makers, supporting the formation of a universal system of early childhood education and care for all children.

Martha's recent publications include *Early childhood education and care in Canada 2001* (2002), and *Social inclusion through early childhood education and care* (2002). She co-authored Canada's background paper on ECEC for the international Organisation for Economic Co-operation and Development (2004).

*Grace-Edward Galabuzi* is a research associate at the Centre for Social Justice in Toronto and a professor at Ryerson in the department of political science. He earned his PhD from York. He has worked in the Ontario government as a senior policy analyst on justice issues, and he is a former provincial co-ordinator of the Alliance for Employment Equity. Dr. Galabuzi has been involved in many community campaigns around social justice issues such as anti-racism, anti-poverty, community development, human rights, education reform, anti-poverty, and police reform.

*Andrew Jackson* has been Senior Economist with the Canadian Labour Congress since 1989 and is a Research Associate with the Canadian Centre for Policy Alternatives. His areas of interest include the labour market and the quality of jobs, income distribution and poverty, macro-economic policy, tax policy and the impacts of globalization on workers and on social democratic economic policy. He has written numerous articles for popular and academic publications, and has co-authored three books, including *Falling behind: The state of working Canada 2000*.

Mr. Jackson returned to the CLC in June, 2002 after a two year leave of absence to serve as Director of Research with the Canadian Council on Social Development. He was educated at the London School of Economics (BSc (Econ); MSc (Econ) and at the University of British Columbia.

*Muriel Kearney* graduated from McGill University with an MBA in 1989. She worked in the private sector from 1990 to 2001. She is currently a Masters degree candidate at UQAM in Social Work (Social Economy stream), and she has been a member of the LAREPPS research team since 2002. Her research projects relate to the evolution of co-operative and solidarity-based initiatives and professional integration of welfare recipients through local community development.

*Ronald Labonte* is Director, Saskatchewan Population Health Evaluation and Research Unit (SPHERU), and Professor, Community Health and Epidemiology, University of Saskatchewan, and Kinesiology and Health Studies, University of Regina. For the first twenty-five years of his career, his work focused on the practice and policy implications of community empowerment approaches to health promotion and population health, a field to which he contributed extensively. Over the past five years his research has examined the health impacts of economic globalization and trade/investment liberalization, development of community level population health indicators, and the effects of health system reform Canada on health promotion, community development, and health determinants practice. He currently holds a

Canadian Institutes of Health Research RPP Investigator Award in Globalization and Health, and has worked with the World Health Organization and the Pan-American Health Organization on health and globalization issues, and represented health NGOs in several multilateral meetings on health and globalism. His most recent book, *Fatal indifference: The G8, Africa and global health*, has just been published by University of Cape Town Press.

**David Langille** is currently at the Centre for Social Justice, where he is the Public Affairs Director. The Centre for Social Justice is an advocacy organization that seeks to strengthen the struggle for social justice. It is committed to working for change in partnership with various social movements and recognize that effective change requires the active participation of all sectors of our community. With Gregory Albo and Leo Panitch, he is co-author of *A different kind of state?: Popular power and democratic administration*.

**Richard Lessard** is Director of the Montreal Public Health Unit and clinical associate professor in the Department of Social and Preventive Medicine at the University of Montreal.

**Lynn McIntyre** is a Professor in the Faculty of Health Professions at Dalhousie University where she has served as Dean since January 1, 1992. Dr. McIntyre holds both a medical degree and master's degree in Community Health and Epidemiology from the University of Toronto. She is also a Fellow of the Royal College of Physicians of Canada in Community Medicine, the specialty that deals with public health.

In addition to her administrative duties, Dr. McIntyre continues to be an active food security researcher. She has investigated children's feeding programs, and child hunger in Canada. She recently turned her attention to maternal hunger and food insecurity with the completion of a large study of low-income lone mothers in Atlantic Canada, and is now investigating feast and famine cycling among food insecure women.

Dr. McIntyre has been a member of several expert groups supporting poverty issues including the National Longitudinal Survey of Children and Youth, the Canadian Institute of Child Health's Child Health Profile Project, and the Canadian Council on Social Development's Progress of Canada's Children reports. She is a member of the Board of Trustees of the National Institute of Nutrition and a member of the Advisory Board for the Canadian Institutes of Health Research Aboriginal Peoples' Health Institute.

**Michael Polanyi** has worked professionally in community development and health promotion. He has a PhD in Environmental Studies from York University. He is a Faculty Researcher with the Saskatchewan Population Health Research and Evaluation Unit (SPHERU), and an Assistant Professor in the Faculty of Kinesiology and Health Studies, University of Regina. Polanyi's research interests include the impacts of changing labour markets and organizational practices on the health of workers, and collaborative and community-based interventions to improve workplace and community health.

**Michael Rachlis** earned his MD from the University of Manitoba and his MSc from McMaster University. He is a specialist in community medicine and a part-time Associate Professor in the Department of Health Policy, Management and Evaluation, Faculty of Medicine, University of Toronto. He practices as a private consultant in policy analysis. His most recent publication is *Prescription for excellence: How innovation is saving Canada's health care system*, published by HarperCollins Canada in 2004.

***Dennis Raphael***, PhD, is an Associate Professor at the School of Health Policy and Management and a member of the Atkinson Faculty of Liberal and Professional Studies at York University in Toronto. A native of New York City, he has lived in Canada since 1973. Dr. Raphael was trained in human development and education, and has applied his skills in the areas of educational evaluation, developmental disabilities, community health, and health promotion. The most recent of his over 100 scientific publications have focused on the health effects of income inequality and poverty, the quality of life of communities and individuals, the impact of governmental decisions on North Americans' health and well-being, and international comparisons of policy environments and how these influence the health of citizens.

***Marie-France Raynault*** is Director of the Observatoire montréalais des inegalitées sociales et de la santé and chair of the Department of Social and Preventive Medicine at the University of Montreal.

***Barbara Ronson***, a former high school teacher and graduate of the doctoral program at OISE/UT, is currently a consultant at the University of Toronto's Centre for Health Promotion, Department of Public Health Sciences. As a member of the core team, she handles special programs in literacy and health, child and youth health, and school and workplace health. She has initiated, co-ordinated, and participated in health and literacy related workshops and surveys across Canada. Barbara is also the co-chair of the Ontario Health Schools Coalition, an active work group of the Ontario Public Health Association and the Centre for Health Promotion. Founded in 2000 with the amalgamation of three Ontario school health groups, the coalition now has over 200 members and has been playing an important role in education reform across the province.

***Irving Rootman*** is a Michael Smith Foundation for Health Research Distinguished Scholar and Professor in the Faculty of Human and Social Development at the University of Victoria. He was the first Director of the Centre for Health Promotion at the University of Toronto, a World Health Organization Collaborating Centre, from 1990–2001 and a Professor in the Department of Public Health Sciences. Currently, he is a member of the Health Promotion and Disease Prevention Advisory Board and the Health Literacy Committee of the U.S. Institute of Medicine. He has published widely in the health promotion and drug abuse fields. His most recent book is *Health Promotion Evaluation* published by the European Office of the World Health Organization. He received the R.F. Defries Award, the highest award of the Canadian Public Health Association, in October 2001. His main area of research interest is Literacy and Health. He received his PhD in sociology from Yale University in 1970.

***Chandrakant Shah***, Professor Emeritus at the University of Toronto, is a practising physician, a public health practitioner, and an advocate for improving the health and well-being of marginalized groups in Canadian society. He was a Professor in the Department of Public Health Sciences, University of Toronto from 1972 –2001. He held cross appointments in the Departments of Health Policy, Management and Evaluation, Paediatrics, Family and Community Medicine in the Faculty of Medicine and also in the Faculties of Social Work and Nursing at the University of Toronto. Dr. Shah was instrumental in developing the Endowed Chair in Aboriginal Health and Wellbeing at the University, the first of its kind in Canada.

In 1999, Dr. Shah received the highest award of the Canadian Public Health Association, the R.D. Defries Award and Honorary Life Membership for his contribution to furthering medical education in public health as well as his advocacy for the disadvantaged populations such as homeless, unemployed and poor. He is the recipient of the highest award "Eagle Feather" from the First Nations House at the University of Toronto for his lifetime work with the aboriginal community and particularly for developing annual program of Visiting Lectureship on Native Health series. He received an Honorary Life Membership from the Ontario Medical Association in 2002 and designation of Senior Member from the Canadian Medical Association in 2003 for his lifetime devotion for improving the health of Canadians and particularly the marginalized population.

*Michael Shapcott* has been a housing and homeless advocate for 20 years. He is Co-ordinator of the Community/University Research Partnerships Unit at the University of Toronto's Centre for Urban and Community Studies. He is Co-Chair of the National Housing and Homelessness Network and is a founding member of a number of groups, including the Housing and Homelessness Network in Ontario, the Toronto Disaster Relief Committee, the Ontario Smart Growth Network, and the Bread Not Circuses Coalition.

*Valerie Tarasuk* is an associate professor in the Department of Nutritional Sciences at the University of Toronto. Her primary research interest is in the study of social and economic determinants of nutritional health and well-being. Much of her work focuses on problems of domestic food insecurity, considering their origins and nutrition implications and examining current policy and program responses. This work includes a recent ethnographic study of front-line work in food banks, a study of nutritional vulnerability, and food insecurity among women in families using food banks in Toronto, and an examination of social assistance benefit levels in relation to costs of basic needs. Current research initiatives include a study of food access, nutritional vulnerability and social exclusion among homeless youth in Toronto and an analysis of Statistics Canada food expenditure data to elucidate the impact of changing social and economic conditions on food consumption patterns within specific population subgroups.

*Luc Theriault* holds a PhD in sociology from the University of Toronto and is currently an Associate Professor in the Faculty of Social Work at the University of Regina. Specializing in social policy and third sector studies, he is a regular collaborator on research projects based at LAREPPS where he once was a post-doctoral fellow.

*Emile Tompa* holds a PhD in Economics from McMaster University. He is a labour and health economist with a background in aging and retirement issues. Dr. Tompa is a Scientist at the Institute for Work and Health in Toronto, and an Adjunct Assistant Professor in the Department of Economics at McMaster University in Hamilton. His current research agenda is centered on the health impacts of labour-market policies and programs, labour-market experiences and their health and human development consequences, and workplace interventions directed at improving the health of workers.

*Diane-Gabrielle Tremblay* is the Canada Research Chair of Socio-Organizational Challenges of the Knowledge Economy. She is professor and director of research at the Télé-université of the Université du Québec. She is a member of the Committee on Sociology of Work of the International Sociological Association, the Executive Council of the Society for the Advancement of Socio-Economics. She is also president of the Political Economy Association of Quebec and editor of the electronic journal *Interventions économiques.* Also co-chair of the Bell Canada Research Chair on Technology and Work Organization, she has published many articles and books on employment and types of employment, job training, innovation in the workplace and work organization, as well as work–life balance. See www.teluq.uquebec.ca/chaireecosavoir/cvdgt.

*Louise Tremblay* has a doctorate in linguistics. She is a research associate at LAREPPS where she has contributed to many studies and publications related to the social economy. She also participates in the work of other research units dealing with communication issues and the sociology of language.

*Charles Ungerleider*, Professor of the Sociology of Education at the University of British Columbia, was Deputy Minister of Education for British Columbia from 1998 to 2001. His most recent book, *Failing our kids: How we are ruining our public schools*, was published by McClelland and Stewart in 2003.

*Yves Vaillancourt* holds a PhD in political science from the Université de Montréal. He is a Professor at the School of Social Work, Université du Québec à Montréal, where he leads a research unit (LAREPPS) studying social policy and social practices. Dr. Vaillancourt has written extensively in the area of social policy.

# COPYRIGHT ACKNOWLEDGEMENTS

# Statistics Canada tables

Figure 1.1, Figure 1.2, Table 1.1, Table 6, Table 4.1, Table 4.2, Table 6.1, Table 6.2, Box 10.1, Box 10.2, Table 13.1, Table 16.1, Table 16.2, Table 16.3, Figure 22.1, Figure 22.2: *Statistics Canada information is used with the permission of the Minister of Industry, as Minister responsible for Statistics Canada. Information on the availability of the wide range of data from Statistics Canada can be obtained from Statistics Canada's Regional Offices, its World Wide Web site at www.statcan.ca, and its toll-free access number 1-800-263-1136.*

# INDEX

*Achieving Health for All: A Framework for Health Promotion* (Epp), 4

Action Plan for Food Security, 176

*Action Statement for Health Promotion in Canada* (CPHA), 4

active labour force, concept of, 55

adequate income from work, 102

adolescents
post-secondary education, and family income, 141
self-perceived health, 142–143

adult-onset diabetes. *See* diabetes

Affordable Housing Framework Agreement, 212

age-appropriate arts and recreation services, 131–132

aggressive behaviour, 143

Agreement on Government Procurement, 260

Agreement on Trade-Related Investment measures, 260

alcohol abuse, and Aboriginal health, 270–271

anomie, 259

appreciative work, 103–104

appropriate work arrangements, 102

Armstrong, Pat, 282, 331

Atlantic Canada study of hunger and food insecurity, 177–178, 180–181, 181*f*, 182*f*

Aubry, François, 282, 311

Auger, Nathalie, 19–20, 39

available work, 100–102

average income, 21–22

average wealth measure, 31

# B

Bank of Canada, 291

basic income policy, 101

BC Homelessness and Health Research Network, 232

behavioural risk factors, as weak predictor, 10

Bell Canada Chair on Technology and Work Organization, 66

Benedict, Phyllis, 168

*A Better You: The Benefits of a Healthy Lifestyle,* 165

*Black Report* (Townsend, Davidson and Whitehead), 3, 11–12

body mass index, 181, 191–193, 271

Books for Babies, 163

boom and bust cycles, 24–26

boundaryless careers, 54–55

British research, 3–4

Browne, Gina M., 107–108, 125

Bryant, Toba, 172, 217

Burns, Tracey, 108, 139

Business Council on National Issues (BCNI), 287–289, 290, 293

# C

Caledon Institute of Social Policy, 228, 309, 311

Campaign 2000 and the Child Poverty Working Groups, 38, 123

Canada
budgetary expenditures as percentage of GDP, 350*f*
early childhood education and care (ECE), 110
federal budgetary expenses and GDP, 1961–2002, 284*f*
fiscal policy needs, 294
food insecurity. *See* food insecurity
health care administrative costs, 307
hunger. *See* hunger
individualism, increasing, 146
long-term unemployment, 82
monetary policy needs, 294
owner households in, 203
political divisions, 146
politics, *vs.* U.S. politics, 286
post-secondary education in, 147
precarious work, 82–83
provincial/territorial jurisdiction and social policy, 121
public education. *See* public education
renter households in, 203
self-centredness, increasing, 146
social exclusion, in, 238–239
sweatshops, 244
transformation, 139
United States, integration with, 292
work-related mortality rate, 71
workplace change, 81
workplace injuries, 71

Canada Mortgage and Housing Corporation (CMHC), 201, 210, 219, 222, 325

Canada Research Chair on the Knowledge Economy, 66

Canada Trust Survey, 356

Canadian Alliance for Trade and Job Opportunities, 290

Canadian Association of Food Banks, 177, 185, 200

Canadian Auto Workers (CAW), 89

Canadian Centre for Policy Alternatives (CCPA), 18, 38, 153, 295, 310

Canadian Chamber of Commerce, 293

Canadian Council of Chief Executive (CCCE), 288–289, 290, 292, 293, 295

Canadian Council on Social Development (CCSD), 18

Canadian ECEC programs. *See* early childhood education and care (ECEC)

Canadian families
income distribution trends, 26–28
market income distribution, 1980-2000, 27*f*
poorest Canadians, 31–32

Canadian Health Coalition, 359

Canadian Housing Renewal Association, 213

Canadian income-health studies
described, 41–43
Montreal health study (1998), 43
Montreal health study (2002), 43–49

# D

Dahrendorf, Ralf, 255
D'Aquino, Tom, 290
Dartmouth Literacy Network, 165
daycare. *See* early childhood education and care
  (ECEC)
death, causes of, 274
debt, 354
debt and deficit mania, 290–291
deciles, 23, 23*t*
deinstitutionalization, 144
demographics
  changes, and public education, 144
  measures, as predictor of health status, 10
determinants of health
  Aboriginal peoples, 269–272
  conditions of living, 12–15
  hierarchy, 15
  political determinants of health. *See* political
    determinants of health
  social determinants of health. *See* social
    determinants of health
  social distance, 15
  social infrastructure, 14–15
  various, outline of, 5–6
developed countries
  hunger in. *See* food insecurity
  trade unions, decrease in, 68
developing countries
  and hunger, 174
  women and social inclusion/exclusion concept,
    261
diabetes
  and Aboriginal peoples, 301–303
  and childhood circumstances, 10
  Chronic Care Model, 301
  complications of, 300
  food insecurity, 190
  life-course perspective, 16
dietary compromise, implications of, 188–189
disability-free life expectancy, 11*f*
disabled persons, 144, 316–317
disadvantaged workers, 69
discrimination, and mental health, 236
disease
  chronic disease management, 190–191,
    299–300
  chronic diseases, 299
  early detection, 298–299
  income differences, and adult incidence and
    death, 10
  income-related premature years of life lost, 10*f*
  screening, 298–299
diversity
  Canadian students, 144
  linguistic diversity in schools, 144
Dobbin, Murray, 291
Donner Task Force, 93
Douglas, Tommy, 308

drinking and driving, 305
drop-out rates, 148–150
Durkheim, Emile, 259

# E

Early Childhood Development Initiative, 121
early childhood education and care (ECEC)
  agencies, 127
  in Canada, 110, 113–121
  child development, enhancement of, 111–112
  concerns about Canada's approach, 121–122
  directorate for, 121–122
  equity, 113
  fiscal issues, 122
  and health. *See* integrated health promotion
    programs
  high quality in, 111–112
  integrated programs. *See* integrated health
    promotion programs
  integration of services, 125, 128–130
  international use of term, 109–110
  literacy and, 163
  national childcare program, 109–110, 121
  OECD policy study, 114–121
    *see also* OECD ECEC policy study
  parental support, 112
  percentage of children in regulated childcare,
    116*f*
  policy goals, 110–113
  public spending per child capita by province,
    118*f*
  in Quebec, 314, 323–324
  regulated child-care spaces, 115*f*
  social cohesion, fostering, 112–113
  as social determinant of health, 110–113
  unregulated child-care, 119
  wages, 120*f*
  *You Bet I Care!* (YBIC!) study, 118–119
early detection, 298–299
early learning and care. *See* early childhood
  education and care (ECEC)
Economic and Employment Summit, 314–315
economic exclusion in labour market, 243–245
economic inequality. *See* income inequality
education
  early childhood education and care. *See* early
    childhood education and care (ECEC)
  and healthy work, 73–74
  public education. *See* public education
effort-reward imbalance model (ERI), 96
EKOS/CPRN survey, 80, 356
emergency shelter standards, 207
empirical evidence, 7–8
Emploi-Quebec, 322
Employability Assistance for People with
  Disabilities (EAPD), 321
employee benefits coverage, 83–84, 83*t*
employee commitment, 68

employee ill-health
  and employer flexibility, 71–73
  growing employer-employee power imbalance,
    76
  and income security, 73
  and intensification of work, 71–72
  job insecurity, 72–73
  and longer working hours, 72
  non-standard work hours, 72
  precarious work arrangements, 72
employer-provided training, 88
employers
  flexibility, and employee ill-health, 71–73, 98
  growing power imbalance, 76
  high quality employment practices, 97–98
  social accountability, 75
employment
  Aboriginal peoples, 269
  contingent employment, 68
  flexibility, age of, 55
  "good job," 80–81
  healthy work. *See* healthy work
  and ill-health. *See* employee ill-health
  new types of, 54
  non-standard forms, 69*f*, 75
  occupational integration, 322–323
  opportunities, and employee ill-health, 73
  part-time employment, 58*f*, 82
  positive employment measures, 83
  poverty-reducing jobs, 260
  precarious employment, 59, 70, 72, 82–84,
    244
  quality of, 80–81
  self-development opportunities, 88
  self-employment, 82
  strain, 74*t*
  unemployment rate, 55
  unequal access to full employment, 242*t*
  unregulated piecemeal homework, 244
  variable intensity of, 55
  workers' empowerment, and social economy,
    317–318
employment conditions. *See* working conditions
Employment Insurance, 83
employment policies, 59–60
employment standards, 89
Engels, Friedrich, 2–3
Enquête sociale et de santé, 42–43
environmental contaminants, 270
environmental determinants of health, 5
epidemiological model of housing effects, 224
equality in outcome, 261
equity
  early childhood education and care (ECE), 113
  growing employer-employee power imbalance,
    76
equivalence scales, 41
European Foundation for the Improvement of
  Work and Living, 77, 86, 94

European Office of the World Health Organization,
  6
European Union
  and downward convergence and
    homogenization, 61
  early childhood programs, 114
  long-term unemployment, 82
  paid vacation leave entitlement, 90
  precarious employment, and legislation, 83
  program to combat social exclusion, 266
  working hours, 90
"Evidence That Informs Practice and Policy"
  (Browne), 130–131

# F

fair share approach, 25–26
fair trade framework, 75
"false" self-employment, 54
familiarization of human services, 327
family literacy classes, 163
federal budget surplus, 209–210, 291–292, 320
Fédération des Organisations d'habitation sans but
  lucratif (OSBL) de Montréal, 326
Federation of Canadian Municipalities, 209, 213,
  227
feminist perspective on minimum integration
  income, 63
fetal alcohol effects (FAE), 270
fetal alcohol syndrome (FAS), 270
financial autonomy, 64
financial strain, 73
First Nations and Inuit Health Branch (FNIHB), 272
First Nations peoples. *See* Aboriginal peoples
flexible organizational strategies. *See* flexible
  production strategies
flexible production strategies
  described, 67–69
  and the experience of work, 69–71
  functional flexibility, 68
  health impact. *See* employee ill-health
  numerical flexibility, 68
  potential benefits, 98
  staffing flexibility, 68
  task flexibility, 68
"flexicurity" framework, 98–99
Foley, Janice, 20, 67
Fontana, Joe, 210
food bank recipients, 194–195
food banks, 179–180, 197
food insecurity
  *see also* hunger
  Atlantic Canada study, 177–178, 180–181,
    181*f*, 182*f*
  best estimate of, 178
  and body mass index, 181, 191–193
  and child development, 193–196
  chronic, 181
  chronic disease management, 190–191
  community-based responses, 176

coping strategies, 179–180
current status in Canada, 177–183
definition of, 173–174
dietary compromise, implications of, 188–189
dynamics of hungry households, 182–183
and emotional and mental health problems, 193
health implications, 193–197, 196*f*
and health inequalities, 179
"healthy eating" barriers to, 190
history of, in Canada, 175–176
and income insecurity, 198
increasing, 171
individual food security, and societal issues, 175
measurement of, 175
nutritional implications, 180–181, 188–193
nutritional status, 189–190
obesity, 192*f*
and obesity, 181, 191–193
policy implications, 197–198
prevalence in Canada, 177–178
risk factors, 178–179
second cheque of the month effect, 180
self-appraisals of, 188
statistics, 178*t*
studies of, 177–178
T3 effect, 180
understanding, 173–175
Food Security Core Module, 175, 178
for-profit sector, and social economy approach, 338–339
Foucault, Michel, 256
fragmentation in communities, 167–168
France, view of unemployed persons, 61, 258–259
Francophones, and literacy rates, 161
Fraser Institute, 293
free trade fight, 290
Friendly, Martha, 107, 109
Fuchs, Don, 317
functional flexibility, 68

**G**

Galabuzi, Grace-Edward, 233
*gemeinshaft,* 254
gender
    and drop-out rates, 148
    and educational achievement, 150
    and life expectancy, in Montreal study, 46
    and literacy, 162
    as social determinant of health, 7, 331
    wage gap, 338*f*
gender trap, 62
gendered analysis of social economy approach, 332–338
General Agreement on Trade in Services, 260
General social survey, 87, 91
*gesellschaft,* 254
global perspective
    net social expenditure, percentage of GDP, 350*f*

social economy approach, 342
and social inclusion/exclusion concept, 261–262
Global School Health Initiative, 158
globalization
    and job insecurity, 56–57
    as political process, 285
    reforms, impact on, 16–17
"good job," 80–81
government spending, 118*f*, 211*t*, 214*t*, 284, 357
government transfers, 29–30, 45
graduation rates, 145, 148–150
Grass Roots Press, 166
Group Health, 300, 301
guaranteed income, 62–63, 101
*The Guide for Health Professionals Working with Aboriginal Peoples* (SOGC Policy Statement), 277

**H**

Habitat Agenda, 201
Harvard School of Public Health, Health Literacy Studies, 168
health. *See* social determinants of health
*Health and Social Organization: Towards a Health Policy for the 21st Century* (Blane, Brunner and Wilkinson), 5
Health Canada, 5, 166, 280, 331
Health Canada's Policy Research Program, 2
health care
    administrative costs, 307
    chronic care model, 300–301, 301*f*, 302
    chronic disease management, 299–300
    chronic diseases, 299
    medical model, and social economy approach, 339–340
    origins of public health, 308
    primary prevention, 301–308
    re-engineered health care, 297–298
    secondary prevention, 298–301
    and teamwork, 306–307
    tertiary prevention, 297–298
    universal access to, 246
health differences, and socio-economic status, 3
*Health Divide* (Townsend, Davidson and Whitehead), 3, 11–12
Health for Two, 163
health inequalities
    British research on, 3–4
    exclusion from mainstream society, 4
    food insecurity and, 179
    housing and, 223
    and income, 4
    materialist approach, 12–14
    neo-materialist approach, 14–15
    and policy agenda, 353–354
    and poverty, 4
    social comparison approach, 15
    social determinants of, 8–11
    sources of, 14

Health Promoting Schools, 158
health promotion programs for children. *See*
    integrated health promotion programs
health services, as social determinants of health, 6
health tips, 13
health-work relationship policy, 99–104
Healthy Babies, Healthy Children, 134
Healthy Cities Movement, 351
"healthy eating" barriers to, 190
healthy work
    culture change, 75
    education, need for, 73–74
    framework for promoting, 96f
    institutional change, 75
    legislative changes, 76
    policy, 75–76
    research, need for, 73–74
    work-health linkage. *See* work-health
        relationship
heart disease
    and childhood circumstances, 10
    congestive heart failure, 300
    death rates, 297
    health promotion programs, 303
    income-health association, 43
    and job strain, 96
    life-course perspective, 16
    rehabilitation approach, 297–298
Heart Health Nova Scotia, 165
hierarchy, 15
high quality employment practices, 97–98
high stress jobs, 87
historical perspective, 2–5
homecare services, 324–325
homelessness
    Aboriginal peoples, 269
    in Canada, 205–207
    First Nations people, 207–208
    growth in, 201, 205–207
    and health, 220–221
    national homelessness strategy, 212
    overview of, 205
    premature death, risk of, 220–221
    and racialized groups, 246
    and recent immigrants, 246
    shelter conditions, 207
    shelter use, 219
    as social exclusion, 246
    solutions, 206
    statistics, 205, 217
    in Toronto, 205
    in United Kingdom, 220
housing
    Aboriginal peoples, 207–208, 270
    affordable housing, 202–203
    Affordable Housing Framework Agreement,
        212
    children, 208
    core need situations, 219

federal government, role of, 209–210, 211–
    212
"filtering," 208–209
government spending on, 211t, 214t
and health. *See* housing and health issues
homelessness, growth in, 205–207
housing crisis, 202, 203–205, 218–219
insecurity, increasing, 171
international commitments, violation of, 211
national social housing program, 209
One Percent Solution, 212–214, 227
poor living conditions, 219, 221–222
and private sector, 208–209
provincial and territorial government, role of,
    210–211, 212
real estate investment trusts, 202
secondary rental market, 204
as social determinant of health, 6, 226
social housing, 325–326
"tale of two Canadas," 203
TD study, 204–205
weakening of other social determinants of
    health, 219
women, 208, 218
housing advocacy groups, 227
Housing Again, 215
housing and health issues
    childhood housing conditions, impact of, 222
    complexities of, 226–227
    dose-response relationship, 222
    excessive spending on housing, impact of,
        222–223, 223f
    expanded model, 225–226, 225f
    narrow focus of research, 224–225
    neglect of research, 224–225
    poor housing conditions, 221–222
    research, 219–220, 224–225
    traditional epidemiological model, 224
Housing and Health Website, 232
housing policy
    legal approach, 229
    National Affordable Housing Strategy, 227
    One Percent Solution, 227
    personal stories approach, 229
    policy change process, 228–230, 229f
    policy framework, 228–230
    and political ideologies, 230
    political-strategic approach, 229
    and public perceptions, 230
    public relations, 229
    recent developments, 228
Housing Supply Working Group, 208
Hulchanski, David, 203–204, 212
Human Resources Development Canada (HRDC),
    66, 167, 319
hunger
    *see also* food insecurity
    and absolute *vs.* relative poverty, 175
    Atlantic Canada study, 177–178, 180–181,
        181f, 182f

Canadian debate, 175
child hunger, 178
coping strategies, 179–180
current status in Canada, 177–183
definition of, 175
developing *vs.* developed countries, 174
dynamics of hungry households, 182–183
elements of, 175
and health inequalities, 179
logistical regression models, 179
maternal hunger, 178, 180–181, 189
nutritional implications, 180–181
predictors of, 179
prevalence in Canada, 177–178
risk factors, 178–179, 183*t*
second cheque of the month effect, 180
studies of, 177–178
T3 effect, 180
understanding, 173–175
HUNGERCOUNT 2003, 185

# I

immigrants and immigration
*see also* racialized groups; social exclusion
economic performance of, 32–33
employment rates, 242*t*
high-poverty neighbourhoods, 245
and homelessness, 246
"immigration factor," 241
labour market integration difficulties, 241
literacy, 161
literacy programs, 166
marginalization, 239
mental health issues, 248–249
in Montreal, 44
poverty, incidence of, 242
and public education, 144, 150–151
and racism, 248
recent immigrants, 241
skill deployment, barriers to, 249
and social exclusion, 239
statistics, 239
under-utilization of immigrant skills, 242–243
unequal access to full employment, 242*t*
youth, and integration stresses, 249
improvements in health, 7–8
Improving Chronic Illness Care (ICIC), 300
*In Unison,* 321, 322
income
adequate income from work, 102
annual disposable income, 41
average income, 21–22
citizen's income, 62–63, 101
as determinant, 8
family disposable income, 71
guaranteed income, 62–63, 101
and health inequalities, 4
income-related premature mortality, 8–11
by level of prose literacy and sex, 159*f*

and literacy, 159–161
low income incidence, reduction of, 349
material advantage, indicators of, 13
median income, 22–23
minimum integration income, 62–63, 101
misleading measures of, 21–22
and owner households, 203
polarization of income, 70–71
and policy agenda, 353–354
and post-secondary education, 141
post-transfer and post-tax income, changes in,
    29*f*
premature years of life lost, 8–11
reported gains, 22
stagnation, 70–71
and sub-optimal nutrient intake, 180
volatility, 41
and work conditions, 79
income and health issues. *See* income-health studies
income distribution measures
boom and bust cycles, 24–26
changing population income distribution,
    1973–1996, 27*f*
horizontal measures, 24–26
market incomes, 22–26
misleading "average" income reports, 21–22
population measures of inequality, 26–28
wealth measures, 30–31
income gap. *See* income inequality
income-health studies
absolute deprivation hypothesis, 49
absolute income hypothesis, 49
Canadian children, 42
Canadian studies, 41–43
cardiovascular diseases, 43
characteristics of, 40–41
confounders, 41
ecologic study, 42
health status, and gross annual income, 43
indicators, drawbacks of, 41
individual level data, 42–43
methodological constraints, 41
Montreal health study, 43–49
Montreal health study (1998), 43
poverty, definition of, 40
poverty measures, 40–41
trends over time, 42
underlying concepts, 40–41
income-health theories, 49–50
income inequality
and family disposable income, 71
government tolerance of, 29–30
government transfers, 29–30
growth of government-driven inequality, 29*f*
hardest hit populations, 31–34
health, effect on, 49–50
market incomes. *See* market incomes
measures of. *See* income distribution measures
national differences, 14–15
people of colour, 32–34

policy solutions, 35
poorest Canadians, 31–32
redistributive factors, 29–30
summary of findings, 34–35
taxes, 29–30
vision-based solutions, 36
income insecurity
and employee ill-health, 73
and food insecurity, 198
income security
benefits of, 101
promotion of, 76
welfare state, association with, 56
Independent Living Movement, 316–317
Independent Living Resource Centres, 317
Industry Canada, 167
inequalities in opportunity, 261
infant mortality, 274–275
infectious diseases, 275
Innovation Agenda, 167
Institut de la statistique du Québec, 42–43
Institute for Research on Public Policy, 153, 296
Institute for Work and Health, 94, 105
institutional change, 75
institutional racism, 34
integrated health promotion programs
age-appropriate arts and recreation services,
131–132
development impediments, 132–133
effective strategies, 127–128
implementation challenges, 128
implementation model, 133–136
integration, effectiveness and efficiency of,
130–133
integration of services, 128–130
intersectoral integration, 128
investments in, 132
measures of system integration, 134t
mental health services, 129, 130
Ontario programs, examples of, 135f
risk factors and, 128–129
school-based delivery model, 135
three-dimensional model of integration, 133f
integration of services, 125, 128–130
intensification of work, 69–70, 71–72
interest groups, 103, 286–287
internal markets model, 54
International Adult Literacy Survey (IALS), 159,
161
international context. See global perspective
international division of labour, 56
international financial institutions, 254
International Labour Organization, 77, 94
International Monetary Fund, 254
International Year of Shelter for the Homeless, 205
intersectoral action, 305–308
intervention youth services. See integrated health
promotion programs
Interventions Économiques, 66

the Inuit. See Aboriginal peoples
Ipsos-Reid, 356

**J**

Jackson, Andrew, 20, 79
Jérôme-Forget, Monique, 320
job control, 87–88, 96
job insecurity
see also job security
and health, 72–73, 97
increased, 70
meaning of, 56–59
perceived, 57
in precarious labour market, 83
reduction of, 57
risk perception, 57
job market
employment policies, effect of, 59–60
regulation of, 56
Job Quality, 94
job quality
"good job," 80–81
job control, 87–88
job security, 81–84
participation, 92–93
physical conditions of work, 84–88
self-development opportunities, 88
social relations, 92–93
stress, sources of, 87–88
work hours, 88–91
work-life balance issues, 91–92
work pace, 87–88
job security
see also job insecurity
assuring, 63–64
concept of, 55
employment policies, effect of, 59–60
enhancement of, 76
and globalization, 56–57
importance of, 62–63
Japanese companies, 56
and job flexibility, 62
and job quality, 81–84
measurement, 57
objective measures, 57
social policy, effects of, 60–62
social security, 63–64
standard-bearer for, 55
subjective measures, 57
job strain, 96

**K**

Kahnawake Schools, 301, 303
Kearney, Muriel, 282, 311
Keynesian tools, 287, 290
knowledge economy, 53–54
Kyoto Accord, 290

# L

Labonte, Ronald, 233–234, 253
Laboratoire de recherche sur les pratiques et les
  politiques sociales, 311, 329
labour force participation rates
  described, 57–59, 58*f*
  immigrants and immigration, 242
  men, 57
  mothers, 109, 112
  women, 57, 63
labour market
  boundaryless careers, 54–55
  economic exclusion, 243–245
  and economic insecurity, 57–59
  internal markets model, 54
  and knowledge economy, 53–54
  mobility within, 54
  neo-liberal restructuring, effect of, 243
  norms, changing, 68
  opportunities, and employee ill-health, 73
  precarious employment, 59
  racially stratified, 243–244
  segregation, 243–244
  structures, changing, 68
  transformation of, 53–54
  unemployment, 57–59
labour market flexibility
  and disadvantaged workers, 69
  increase in, 69
  and increased job insecurity, 70
  intensification of work, 69–70
  polarization of income, 70–71
  stagnation of income, 70–71
Laidlaw Foundation, 251, 264–265
laissez-faire approach, 61
Lalonde report. *See A New Perspective on the
  Health of Canadians* (Lalonde)
Langille, David, 281, 283
layoffs, 68
Layton, Jack, 217
lean production, 68
LEAP (Learning, Earning, and Parenting), 135–136
legislation
  and healthy work, 6
  precarious employment in European Union, 6
Lessard, Richard, 19–20, 39
liberal model, 61
Liberal Party, 290
life-course perspective, 15–16
life expectancy
  and gender, in Montreal study, 46
  homelessness, 220–221
  Montreal health study data, 46*f*
  variation, proportion of, 11*f*
"life-style" approaches, 12
literacy
  adult literacy resources, 166
  Canadian literacy and health milestones, 157*f*
  Canadian literacy specialists, 165

community development approaches, 166
comparative distribution of literacy levels,
  160*f*
and culture, 161–162
direct effects on health, 156–158
early childhood and, 162–163
empirical evidence, 156–158
evolution of definition, 155
family literacy classes, 163
and gender, 162
health status, prediction of, 155
importance of, as health determinant,
  156–158
and income, 159–161
indirect effects on health, 158
life-long learning strategy, 167
and living conditions, 161
mechanisms and pathways of influence,
  158–164
other factors, 163–164
parental attitudes and, 162–163
participatory approaches, 165
policy, role of, 164–168
  *see also* literacy policy recommendations
policy solutions, 161
and quality of education system, 161
school libraries, threats to, 164
and socio-economic status, 159–161
testing, 166
and working conditions, 161
*Literacy and Health Promotion: Four Case Studies,*
  165–166
literacy education, 167
literacy policy recommendations
  goals and accountabilities, new definitions of,
    166–167
  interministerial collaborations, new
    mechanisms for, 167–168
  research needs, 165–166
living conditions, and literacy, 161
living wage, 102
Lloyd Axworthy Green Paper, 319
local community access centres, 339
long-term care facilities, 339
longer work hours. *See* work hours
longitudinal studies, 16
low employment-level groups, 3
low-paying work systems, 75–76

# M

MacDermid, Robert, 290–291, 292
market incomes
  average income, 21–22
  boom and bust cycles, 24–26
  bottom 30% of Canadian families, 26
  deciles, 23, 23*t*
  distribution, 1980 to 2000, 27*f*
  horizontal measures, 24–26
  inequality, creation of, 29

median income, 22–23
middle class trends, 26–28
population distribution, 28*f*
population measures of inequality, 26–28
quintiles, 22–23, 23*t*
ratios, 23
during recessions, 25*t*
during recoveries, 25*t*
Martin, Paul, 209–210, 290, 291–292, 319
material conditions of life, 12–14
material deprivation, effects of, 226
materialism, 258
materialist approach, 12–14
materialistic/structuralist approach, 12
maternal hunger, 178, 180–181, 189
McColl Institute for Healthcare Innovation, 300
McIntyre, Lynn, 171, 173
McMahon, 146
median income, 22–23
median net worth comparison, 30*f*
medical model, and social economy approach,
    339–340
men
    *see also* gender
    average household work hours, 339*f*
    labour participation rate, 57
    parenting and family responsibilities,
        participation in, 63
    unpaid care or assistance to seniors, 334*f*
mental health
    discrimination and, 236
    and food insecurity, 193
    immigrants, 248–249
    and racism, 236, 248–249
    and social exclusion, 248–249
    stigma of mental illness, 248–249
mental health services, 129, 130
the Métis. *See* Aboriginal peoples
middle class trends, 26–28
minimum integration income, 62–63, 101
minimum wages, 102
minority groups. *See* social exclusion
Montreal health study (1998), 43
Montreal health study (2002)
    behavioural risk factors, 46
    census tract, 44
    CLSC district, 44
    comparisons, 44
    findings, 44–49
    gender, and life expectancy, 46
    geographic sub-regions, 46–47, 48*t*
    government transfers, 45
    health status, variations in, 45
    income quintiles, relationship across, 45–46
    infant mortality rate, by income status, 45–46,
        45*f*
    life expectancy data, 46*f*
    methodology, 43–44
    mortality rate for leading causes of death, 47*f*

pregnancy rate among adolescents, 49*f*
    suicide rates, 48–49
Montreal Municipal Housing, 326
Montreal Public Health Unit, 52
Moore, Michael, 356–357
morbidity, and Aboriginal peoples, 275–276
mortality rates
    Aboriginal peoples, 274–275
    demographic measures, 10
    homelessness, 220–221
    income-related premature mortality, 8–11
    socio-economic measures, 10
mothers, labour force participation rate of, 109,
    112
multi-employer bargaining systems, 103
Multilateral Framework on Early Learning and Care,
    121–122
municipal policies, 351

## N

National Adult Literacy Database, 169
National Advisory Council on Aging, 276
National Affordable Housing Strategy, 227
National Child Benefit, 321
national childcare program, 109–110, 121
National Children's Agenda, 121
National Citizens' Coalition, 293
National Council of Welfare (NCW), 18, 199
National Crime Prevention Council of Canada, 143
national differences
    income gaps and, 14–15
    in overall population health, 5, 11, 12*t*
National Forum on Health, 333, 337
National Health and Nutrition Examination Survey
    III, 189–190, 190, 193–194
National Housing and Homelessness Network
    (HNHN), 205, 212–213, 228
National Institute for Occupational Safety and
    Health, 105
National Institute of Public Health, 359
National Literacy Action Agenda, 167
National Literacy and Health Research Program,
    163
National Longitudinal Study of Children and Youth
    (NLSCY), 129, 150, 161, 177, 179
National Population Health Survey (NPHS), 88, 93,
    177, 179, 181, 188, 190, 191–193, 198
*National Post,* 173
national social housing program, 209
National Swedish Health Policy, 348
National Workshop on Literacy and Health
    Research, 167
neighbourhood selection, racialized, 245–246
neo-conservatism, 284–285
neo-liberalism
    approaches, 16–17
    Canadian institutions of, 288
    effect of, 311
    impact of, 284–285

and racially stratified labour market, 243
and social exclusion, 237
and social inclusion/exclusion concept,
254–255
neo-materialist approach, 14–15
New Democratic Party, 290
*A New Perspective on the Health of Canadians*
(Lalonde), 4, 5
new social economy, 314
New Zealand, 260–261
Nixon, Gordon, 292
Non-Insured Health Benefits Program (NIHB), 272
non-profit sector. *See* social economy
non-standard forms of employment, 69*f*, 75
*see also* precarious employment
non-standard work hours, 72
non-Status Indians. *See* Aboriginal peoples
North America
palliative and passive employment policy
measures, 60
working hours, 90
numerical flexibility, 68
nutritional status, 189–190

# O

obesity, 181, 191–193, 192*f*
Observatoire montréalais des inegalitées sociales et
de la santé (OMISS), 52
occupational diseases, 84–86
occupational exposures, 86
occupational integration, 322–323
OECD ECEC policy study
data collection, systematic, 120
education system, partnership with, 115–116
high-quality ECEC programs, 116
monitoring, systematic, 120
policy lessons of, 114–121
regulation and monitoring of program,
118–119
substantial public investment, need for,
117–118
sustained research investment, 120–121
systemic and integrated policy approach, need
for, 114–115
training and working conditions, 119–120
universal approach to access, 116–117
oecd.org/linklist, 123
On Lok Senior Health Services, 298
One Percent Solution, 212–214, 227
Ontario Community Care Access Centres, 338–339
Ontario Ministry of Education, 167
Ontario Public Health Association report, 167
Ontario Teachers' Federation, 168
Organization for Economic Cooperation and
Development (OECD), 57, 62, 71, 82
Ornstein report, 242
Ottawa Charter for Health Promotion, 5, 217,
347–348, 351–352

# P

paid work, 100–101
parental support, 112
part-time employment, 58*f*, 59, 82
peace movement, 290
Pearce, Neil, 305
people of colour
*see also* racialized groups; social exclusion
Aboriginal peoples, marginalization of, 33–34
*see also* Aboriginal peoples
immigrants, economic performance of, 32–33
and income inequality, 32–34
racism, 33, 34
*see also* racism
Peterborough (Ontario) Social Planning Council,
205–206
phased-in retirement process, 90
PISA. *See* Programme for International Student
Assessment (PISA)
Polanyi, Michael, 20, 67
polarization of income, 70–71
policy agenda and low priorities
biomedical focus, 352
blaming other marginalized groups, 354
cost assumptions, 357
debt of Canadians, 354
general public, 353
health workers' priorities, 353
hidden failings, 354
income issues, 353–354
individual responsibility focus, 352
inequality issues, 353–354
low priority of social determinants of health,
352–356
politicians, distrust of, 355–356
promise of riches, 356–357
real human dilemmas, 355
self-blame, 354–355
policy change process, 228–230, 229*f*
policy environments, 16–17
policy recommendations
*see also* social policy reforms
food insecurity and hunger, 183–184
literacy. *See* literacy policy recommendations
strengthening social determinants of health,
348–352
Policy Research Initiative of Canada, 265–266
political determinants of health
*see also* social policy
balance of forces, 289–290
chief executives, power of, 293
continental integration, push for, 292
corporate power, 292–294
corporate rule, new era of, 287–289
debt and deficit mania, 290–291
democracy and, 287
democratic resistance, 292–294
health as politics, 304
historical perspective, 285–287

homecare services, 324–325
housing issues, 228
occupational integration, 322–323
population health objectives, 39
poverty, programs to diminish, 43
poverty effects on health, 39
regulated child-care spaces, growth of, 116
social economy, use of, 314–315
social housing, 325–326
social policy reforms, 321–326
Quebec Family Policy, 324
Quebec Women's Federation, 335
quintiles, 22–23, 23*t*

# R

Rabble.ca, 359
Rachlis, Michael, 282, 297
racialization
    *see also* racialized groups
    and health, 246–247
    and health status, 247–248
    international research, 247–248
    of poverty, 235, 239–243
    and social exclusion, 246–247
racialized groups
    *see also* immigrants and immigration; people
        of colour; racism; social exclusion
    growth rate of, 239
    and homelessness, 246
    impact of racialization, 240
    and low income cut off, 241
    marginalization experiences, 248
    and racialization of poverty, 240–243
    and social exclusion, 239, 258
racialized neighbourhood selection, 245–246
racialized spatial concentration of poverty, 245
racism
    *see also* racialized groups
    and differential earnings level, 33
    gendered racism, 244
    and health status, 247–248
    hypertension, source of, 247
    and immigrants, 248
    institutionalized racism in health care, 248
    and mental health, 236, 248–249
    in public education, 145
    stress, source of, 247
    systemic racism, 34
Raphael, Dennis, 1, 282, 345
Raynault, Marie-France, 19–20, 39
re-engineering, 68, 297–298, 318–321
real estate investment trusts, 202
"Realizing the Promise of Public Education" Forum,
    168
recessions, 24, 25*t*, 26
recovery periods, 24–25, 25*t*, 26
redistribution patterns, 29–30
reduced work time, 89
repetitive work, 86

Report of the Collective Reflection on the
    Changing Workplace, 93
*Report on the Health of Canadians,* 109
resistance, 256
retirement age, 90
Rhymes that Bind, 163
Robert Wood Johnson Foundation, 300
Roeher Institute, 317
Romanow Commission on the Future of Health
    Care, 333, 339, 343, 352
Romanow Royal Commission on Health Services
    Reports, 308
Ronson, Barbara, 108, 155
Rootman, Irving, 108, 155
Royal Commission on Aboriginal Peoples, 277
Royal Commission on the Status of Women,
    109–110, 121
Rozanski, Mordechai, 168

# S

Salamon, Lester, 315
Santé Quebec, 322
Santé Québec survey, 42–43
Scandinavian nations
    commitment to progressive public policy,
        348–349
    job entry policies, 59–60
    national differences in population health, 5
    National Swedish Health Policy, 348
    unemployed persons, view of, 60–61
School Achievement Indicators program (SAIP),
    148
school-based delivery model, 135
school libraries, threats to, 164
schooling. *See* public education
screening, 298–299
second cheque of the month effect, 180
secondary prevention
    chronic care model, 300–301, 301*f,* 302
    chronic disease management, 299–300
    and chronic diseases, 299
    early detection, 298–299
    screening, 298–299
sector-based representation systems, 103
security
    *see also* job security
    definitions of, 55, 56
    individual security, 56
    need for security, 56
self-development opportunities at work, 88
self-employment, 54, 55, 82
Sen, Amartya, 255
seniority standard, 56
Shah, Chandrakant P., 234, 267
Shapcott, Michael, 172, 201
shared resources, advantages of, 41
shelter. *See* housing
Silesia, typhus in, 303–304

cancer incidence and mortality, 47–48
in childhood, and later health risks, 236
explanation of recent trends, 283–285
and literacy, 159–161
material advantage, indicators of, 13
and PISA literacy tests, 148
as predictor of health status, 10, 12
and school achievement, 139–140
Special Committee on Child Care, 121–122
special education, 144
staffing flexibility, 68
stagnation of income, 70–71
Stanford, Jim, 291–292
Stanford Five Cities study, 303
*The State of Food Insecurity in the World* (FAO),
174
*State of the Crisis, 2001* (NHHS), 205
Statistics Canada, 66, 152, 354
Status Indians, 267
*see also* Aboriginal peoples
Stewart, Jane, 121
strengthening social determinants of health
actions to, 346–352
back to basics, 347–348
community action, 351–352
low income incidence, reduction of, 349
municipal policies, 351
national policy options, 348–349
Ottawa Charter for Health Promotion,
347–348, 351–352
political economy perspective, 347
privatization, resistance to, 347
social exclusion, reduction of, 349
social infrastructure policies, 349–351
targets for action, 347
stress
high stress jobs, 87
immigrant youth integration stress, 249
psychosocial stress, 14
racism as source of, 247
and social exclusion, 248–249
sources of, and job quality, 87–88
time stress, 91–92
work stress, 79, 87–88, 91–92
stroke, 10, 16
"subsidized" daycare, 323
substance abuse, and Aboriginal health, 270–271
Supporting Community Partnerships Initiative
(SCPI), 212
suppression, 255
Survey of literacy skills used in daily living
(LSUDA), 159, 165
sweatshops, 244
System-Linked Research Unit on Health and Social
Service Utilization, 137

# T

T3 effect, 180
*Taking Action on Population Health* (Health
Canada), 4

Tarasuk, Valerie, 172, 187
task flexibility, 68
Task Force on Defence and International Security
(BCNI), 290
Task Force on the Environment (BCNI), 290
taxes, 29–30
TD Economics, 204–205
tertiary prevention, 297–298
Thériault, Luc, 282, 311
third sector initiatives. *See* social economy
*The Three L's Literacy and Life-Long Learning*
(Calamai), 167
time stress, 91–92
Tommy Douglas Research Institute, 309
Tompa, Emile, 20, 67
Toronto Charter on the Social Determinants of
Health, 358, 361–365
Toronto Disaster Relief Committee, 207, 212–214,
215, 227, 232
Townsend Centre for International Poverty
Research, 251
trade unions
benefits coverage, 83*t*
decrease, in developed countries, 68
development of, 56
paid vacation, 90
reduced work time, 89
transnational corporations, 345–346
Tremblay, Dianne-Gabrielle, 20, 53
Tremblay, Louise, 282, 311
Tremblay, Richard, 143
Trilateral Commission, 287
type 2 diabetes. *See* diabetes
typhus, 303–304

# U

U.N. Committee on Economic, Social and Cultural
Rights, 211
U.N Human Rights Committee, 211
unemployment
long-term unemployment, 82
and precarious work, 57–59
rate, 55, 70, 81–82, 269
Ungerleider, Charles, 108, 139
unhealthy work. *See* working conditions
unionization. *See* trade unions
United Kingdom
homelessness in, 220
poor living conditions, 221–222
social inclusion and labour market attachment,
259–260
United Nations Food and Agriculture Organization,
174, 185
United Nations' Human Development Index, 176
United States
anti-combines legislation, 286
child hunger rates, 177
health care administrative costs, 307
integration with, 292

international health differences, 5
politics, *vs.* Canadian politics, 286
population surveys, and food intake, 188
unemployed persons, view of, 60
United States Current Population Study, 177
universal programs, 261
University of Montreal, 52
unpaid work, 100–101
unregulated piecemeal homework, 244
Unsworth, Barry, 257
U.S. Department of Health and Human Services, Indian Health Service, 280

# V

Vaillancourt, Yves, 282, 311
Vanier Institute for the Family, 153, 354
violence
    family violence in Aboriginal communities, 269
    learning capacity, threat to, 161
Virchow, Rudolf, 3, 303–304
vision-based solutions, 36
Vocational Rehabilitation of Disabled Persons, 321
volatility of income, 41
voluntary sector. *See* social economy
Voluntary Sector Initiative (VSI), 327

# W

wage gap, 338*f*
wage levels, 102
Wagner, Ed, 300
wealth measures, 30–31
weekend working, 90
welfare state
    and Canadian ECEC programs, 113–114
    citizen's income, 62–63
    corporate offensive against, 285–287, 287
    development of, in Canada, 16
    future of, 345–346
    health of, 345–346
    and income security, 56
    origins of, 346
    slow emergence of, 285–286
    "subsidized" daycare, 323
    typology, 60
    welfare state typology, for analysis, 60
*What the Health! A Literacy and Health Resource for Youth,* 166
"When Markets Fail People" (Curry-Stevens), 24–26
"When the Bough Breaks" study, 130
Winning Workplaces, 77
women
    *see also* gender
    autonomous rights, ensuring, 64
    average household work hours, 339*f*
    conscription into care work, 333, 337
    in developing countries, 261

    and educational attainment, 147
    gender trap, 62
    housing, 208, 218
    labour participation rate, 57, 63
    literacy levels, 162
    maternal hunger, 178, 180–181, 189
    mothers, labour force participation rate of, 109, 112
    "natural" caregivers, 337
    and part-time work, 59, 82
    and poverty, 334
    and precarious work, 70
    racialized women, and unregulated piecemeal homework, 244
    social policy, effects of, 61
    social risks, major, 61–62
    and social safety net gaps, 334–335
    time stress, 91–92
    unpaid care or assistance to seniors, 334*f*
    work intensity, increase in, 69
    work-life balance issues, 87, 91–92
    work stress, 87, 91–92
Women's March on Poverty, 335
work, restructuring of, 81
work conditions. *See* working conditions
work environment. *See* working conditions
work-health relationship
    adequate income from work, 102
    advocating for action, 104–105
    analysis, 97–99
    appreciative work, 103–104
    appropriate work arrangements, 102
    available work, 100–102
    effort-reward imbalance model (ERI), 96
    employer flexibility, 98
    evidence, 95–97
    fairness of rewards, 96
    "flexicurity" framework, 98–99
    high quality employment practices, 97–98
    job insecurity, impact of, 97
    and job strain, 96
    pillars of workplace health, 100*f*
    shared vision, possibility of, 100
    wage levels, 102
    work–life balance, 96
work hours
    changing trends, 89
    and health, 72
    high demand jobs, 90
    increase in, 70
    and job quality, 88–91
    and negative health symptoms, 96
    overtime, 89
    prevalence of, 89
    reduced work time, 89
    weekend working, 90
    worker control, increasing, 102
work intensification, 69–70, 71–72
work–life balance, 87, 91–92, 96
work pace, 87–88